Pathophysiology of Blood Disorders

a LANGE medical book

Pathophysiology of Blood Disorders

H. Franklin Bunn, MD
Professor of Medicine
Harvard Medical School
Hematology Division
Brigham and Women's Hospital
Boston, Massachusetts

Jon C. Aster, MD, PhD
Professor, Department of Pathology
Harvard Medical School
Staff Pathologist,
Department of Pathology
Brigham and Women's Hospital
Boston, Massachusetts

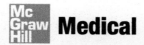

New York Chicago San Francisco Lisbon London Madrid Mexico City
Milan New Delhi San Juan Seoul Singapore Sydney Toronto

Pathophysiology of Blood Disorders

1 2 3 4 5 6 7 8 9 0   CTP/CTP   14 13 12 11 10

ISBN 978-0-07-171378-8
MHID 0-07-171378-6

This book was set in minion pro by Glyph International.
The editors were Jim Shanahan and Karen G. Edmonson.
The production supervisor was Catherine Saggese.
The illustration manager was Armen Ovsepyan.
Project management was provided by Ranjit Kaur, Glyph International..
China Translation & Printing Services Ltd. was printer and binder.

This book is printed on acid-free paper

Library of Congress Cataloging-in-Publication Data

Bunn, H. Franklin (Howard Franklin), 1935-Pathophysiology of blood disorders / H. Franklin Bunn, Jon Aster.
   p. ; cm.
"A Lange medical book."
Includes bibliographical references.
ISBN-13: 978-0-07-171378-8 (alk. paper)
ISBN-10: 0-07-171378-6 (alk. paper)
1. Blood—Pathophysiology.   2. Blood—Diseases—Pathophysiology.   I. Aster, Jon. II. Title.
[DNLM: 1. Hematologic Diseases—physiopathology.   2. Blood Physiological
Phenomena.   WH 120]
RB145.B78 2011
616.1′5—dc22

                                                               2010037908

Contents

PART **IV**

TRANSFUSION MEDICINE 301

Contributors

Joseph H. Antin, M.D.
  Professor of Medicine
  Dana Farber Cancer Institute
  Boston, Massachusetts

Kenneth A. Bauer, M.D.
  Professor of Medicine
  Beth Israel Deaconess Medical Center
  Boston, Massachusetts

Nancy Berliner, M.D.
  Professor of Medicine
  Director of Hematology
  Brigham and Women's Hospital
  Boston, Massachusetts

Daniel J. DeAngelo, M.D., Ph.D.
  Associate Professor of Medicine
  Dana Farber Cancer Institute
  Boston, Massachusetts

Mark D. Fleming, M.D., Ph.D.
  Professor of Pathology
  Children's Hospital Boston
  Boston, Massachusetts

Arnold S. Freedman, M.D.
  Associate Professor of Medicine
  Department of Medical Oncology
  Division of Hematologic Malignancies
  Dana-Farber Cancer Institute
  Boston, Massachusetts

Bruce Furie, M.D.
  Professor of Medicine
  Beth Israel Deaconess Medical Center
  Boston, Massachusetts

Richard M. Kaufman, M.D.
  Assistant Professor of Pathology
  Medical Director,
  Adult Transfusion Service
  Brigham & Women's Hospital
  Boston, Massachusetts

Matthew M Heeney, M.D.
  Assistant Professor of Pediatrics
  Hematology/Oncology Fegan 704
  Children's Hospital Boston
  Boston, Massachusetts

Samuel E. Lux IV, M.D.
  Professor of Pediatrics
  Division of Hematology/Oncology
  Children's Hospital Boston
  Boston, Massachusetts

David G. Nathan, M.D.
  Professor of Pediatrics
  Dana Farber Cancer Institute
  Boston, Massachusetts

David T. Scadden, M.D.
  Professor of Medicine
  Massachusetts General Hospital
  Harvard Stem Cell Institute
  Boston, Massachusetts

Preface

The study of blood and hematologic disorders has special appeal for medical students as well as physicians at all stages of their training. Few specialties have such a broad impact on other medical disciplines. A competent hematologist must be well-grounded in pathology, internal medicine, pediatrics, and surgery. Conversely, both generalists and other specialists regularly encounter patients with anemia, hemorrhage, thrombosis, and hematologic malignancies. For many students, the close kinship of hematology with laboratory medicine is an added virtue. Few medical disciplines enjoy such a rich array of reliable and informative diagnostic tests, and none has stronger underpinnings in contemporary molecular and cell biology and molecular pathology.

Our book is designed to introduce medical students to the physiological principles underlying the regulation and function of blood cells and hemostasis as well as the pathophysiologic mechanisms responsible for the development of blood disorders. We have placed more emphasis on principles than on practice. Accordingly, we have avoided technical details pertaining to diagnostic tests and procedures as well as the compilation of specific drugs and dosages. Instead, issues pertaining to diagnosis and management are covered primarily within a framework of pathogenesis.

The organization and contents of the book are based on a 3-week hematology course given to students in their second year at Harvard Medical School. All of the authors of individual chapters are lecturers in this course, and many of the figures have been taken directly or adapted from their lectures. We wrote the first drafts of all the co-authored chapters and revised them following in-depth input from our colleagues. Moreover, each of us provided thorough reviews of the others' chapters. All figures in this book were redrawn by a single artist and vetted by both of us. We hope that these measures have enabled our book to achieve uniformity of style and clarity along with a high level of scientific rigor and clinical relevance.

We are indebted to a number of individuals who helped bring our book to fruition. James Shanahan, Karen Edmonson, and Armen Ovsepyan at McGraw-Hill provided critical editorial advice including guidance on how to make the book useful and interesting to students. Jessica Hughes and Muriel Goutas provided invaluable secretarial help. Dr. Jeff Kutok (Brigham and Women's Hospital) and Carola von Kapff contributed images of some of the peripheral smears used in the book. About 10 months prior to publication, a draft of this book was provided to 180 Harvard medical students, class of 2012. Many were remarkably conscientious and astute in picking up technical as well as conceptual errors. We are grateful for their input, which improved the final version of the book substantially. Finally, we thank our wives, Erin Malone and Betsy Bunn for their love and support.

H. Franklin Bunn
Jon C. Aster
August 2010

Introduction to Blood and Hematopoietic Tissues

Jon C. Aster

1

LEARNING OBJECTIVES

After studying this chapter you should know:
- The components of the blood.
- The methods used to assess these components.
- The identity and function of the major hematopoietic and lymphoid tissues: the bone marrow, spleen, thymus, and lymph nodes.

Regardless of what kind of doctor a student decides to become, a well-grounded understanding of disorders of the blood and the hematopoietic tissues is essential. Primary hematologic disorders are commonly encountered in community and hospital-based clinical practices, and a wide variety of other diseases come to attention by producing secondary abnormalities of the blood. Beyond their everyday clinical importance, studies of hematologic diseases have yielded seminal insights into the molecular pathogenesis of cancer and basic aspects of stem cell biology. These lessons have had far-reaching influences on biomedical research and are beginning to shape the practice of molecular medicine.

The goal of this book is to provide students with a foundation in the area of blood disorders that they can build on as they train to become physicians and/or research scientists. In this chapter, we will commence with a description of the cast of characters—the blood, the primary blood-forming (hematopoietic) tissues, and the secondary hematopoietic tissues that support the maturation and function of some of the elements of the blood—accompanied by a brief description of commonly used laboratory tests. In Chapter 2, the origins of blood cells and the regulation of blood cell production will be discussed in detail. The remainder of the text will then be devoted to specific hematologic disorders.

BLOOD

Normal adult men have about five liters of blood, whereas women average closer to four. The blood has two main components—the *blood cells* (or *formed elements*)—and the *plasma*, the fluid phase of the blood. These two components can be separated from one another by centrifugation at low speed. Red cells are dense and

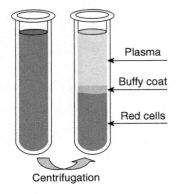

Centrifugation

collect in the bottom of the tube, whereas white cells and platelets are of intermediate density and tend to collect at the interface between the red cells and the plasma in a thin gray-white layer referred to as *the buffy coat*.

THE FORMED ELEMENTS

Most formed elements can be recognized by their morphologic appearance in smears of whole blood, which can be prepared, stained, and visualized under the light microscope in just a few minutes' time. In days past, clinicians skilled in the art of morphology could sometimes confirm a suspected diagnosis based on a patient's history and physical findings through the inspection of blood smears prepared at the bedside. In the modern era, the evaluation of blood is usually left to laboratory technicians and pathologists, but to fully understand blood disorders, students must have a working knowledge of the morphology of the formed elements and their precursors.

The formed elements of the blood are of three major types—red cells (erythrocytes), white cells (leukocytes), and platelets (thrombocytes). The normal values for these cells are listed in Table 1-1.

- *Red cells* are the most numerous of the formed elements. In humans they lack nuclei, appearing in smears prepared from peripheral blood as biconcave disks filled with cytoplasm rich in the oxygen-carrying protein hemoglobin (Fig. 1-1). Although simple in appearance and structure, red cells are elegantly designed to fulfill their major functions—the delivery of oxygen from the lungs to the peripheral tissues and the transport of carbon dioxide from peripheral tissues to the lungs for elimination via respiration. Normal red cells have a life span of about 120 days.

- *White cells* are of several different types (Fig. 1-2). *Granulocytes* are short-lived, marrow-derived cells that can be distinguished by their appearance in peripheral smears. The most numerous kind is the *neutrophil* (or polymorphonuclear leukocyte), which has three to five nuclear lobes and moderately abundant cytoplasm containing pale, lilac-colored granules. Neutrophils are phagocytes that provide protection against certain types of acute infections, particularly those caused by bacteria and fungi. They are very short-lived, persisting in the circulation for only a few hours. *Eosinophils* are cells with two nuclear lobes and abundant red cytoplasmic granules (as befits cells named for Eos, the goddess of dawn). They have an important role in certain chronic immune responses, particularly those associated with helminthic worm infections, asthma, and certain types of allergic reactions. *Basophils*, the least common granulocyte, have abundant dark blue cytoplasmic granules that obscure their nuclei. Basophils may be slightly increased in number in many of the same conditions that are associated with

TABLE 1-1 Normal Blood Cell Counts*

Cell Type	No. of Cells (per μL)
Red cells	4.5-6.4 × 10⁶
White cells	4-10 × 10³
Neutrophils	1.9-7.6 × 10³ (48%-76%)†
Eosinophils	0.0-0.5 × 10³ (<5%)†
Basophils	0.0-0.2 × 10³ (<1.5%)†
Monocytes	0.1-0.8 × 10³ (2.5%-8.5%)†
Lymphocytes	0.8-4.1 × 10³ (18%-41%)†
Platelets	150-450 × 10³

*Adult patients, Brigham and Women's Hospital.
†% of total white blood cell count.

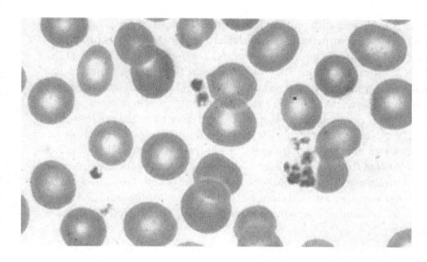

FIGURE 1-1 **Red cells and platelets, peripheral smear.**

elevated eosinophil counts. The other types of white cells are so-called mononuclear cells lacking the nuclear segmentation that is characteristic of granulocytes. *Monocytes* are the largest white blood cell, being 12 to 20 μm in diameter. They are characterized by folded or kidney-shaped nuclei and abundant light blue cytoplasm containing a few small granules. Like neutrophils, monocytes are highly phagocytic, but these cells differ from neutrophils in other important ways. Most notably, upon emigration into

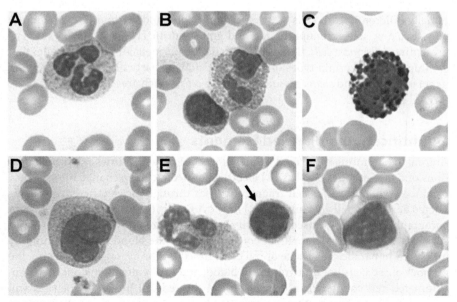

FIGURE 1-2 **White cells, peripheral smear.** A) Neutrophil, B) eosinophil, C) basophil, D) monocyte, E) resting small lymphocyte, F) activated "atypical" lymphocyte.

tissues, monocytes differentiate into relatively long-lived macrophages, which serve as sentinels capable of detecting "danger" signals produced by infection or tissue injury. *Lymphocytes* are the key components of the adaptive immune system. They vary widely in size; resting lymphocytes are about the size of normal red blood cells (7-9 μm in diameter) and have round, condensed nuclei and scant cytoplasm, whereas activated lymphocytes can be up to 20 μm in size and have enlarged nuclei and abundant cytoplasm, which may contain a few granules. Circulating lymphocytes may be B cells, T cells, or natural killer cells, which can be distinguished from one another reliably only by testing for the presence of certain lineage-specific markers. Some B and T cells (so-called memory cells) may live for years; this longevity is the basis for the immune system's ability to "remember" exposures to pathogens that occurred many years in the past.

- *Platelets (thrombocytes)* are small, anucleate cell fragments replete with purplish granules that are shed from megakaryocytes in the bone marrow (Fig. 1-1). Together with clotting factors present in the plasma, platelets play a critical role in the regulation of hemostasis. Platelets have a life span of 7 to 10 days. The structure and function of normal platelets are covered in Chapter 14.

As will be discussed in Chapter 2, red cells, platelets, granulocytes, and monocytes originate from a common precursor in the marrow and are referred to as *myeloid cells*, whereas various kinds of lymphocytes arise from a different common precursor and are referred to as *lymphoid* cells.

In addition to macrophages, there are a number of other types of bone marrow–derived white cells that exist mainly in tissues. These include *osteoclasts*, monocyte-derived multinucleated cells that line and resorb bone; *plasma cells*, terminally differentiated B cells that secrete antibodies and are found mainly in the bone marrow, spleen, lymph nodes, and gut; *dendritic cells*, specialized antigen-presenting cells; *mast cells*, tissue cells with dark blue, metachromatic granules that are important in certain types of immune responses, particularly those involving hypersensitivity; and *stem cells* and *progenitor cells*, which are the precursors of the formed elements.

Quantification of Formed Elements

Automated counting of formed elements in clinical laboratories relies on variations of two methods (Fig. 1-3): 1) electrical impedance, the change in resistance produced when a cell or cell fragment passes through an electric current conducted across a small aperture; and 2) flow cytometry (described in the following paragraph). Both can be used to identify, count, and size individual types of blood cells in a sample. The hemoglobin concentration of the blood is most commonly measured in parallel in a lysate of red cells. Based on the average red cell size, the number of red cells per unit volume of blood, and the hemoglobin concentration, automated cell counters can calculate all of the red cell indices, which (as will be explained in Chapter 3) are very useful in the classification and diagnosis of anemias. These indices include the mean red cell volume (MCV), the mean cell

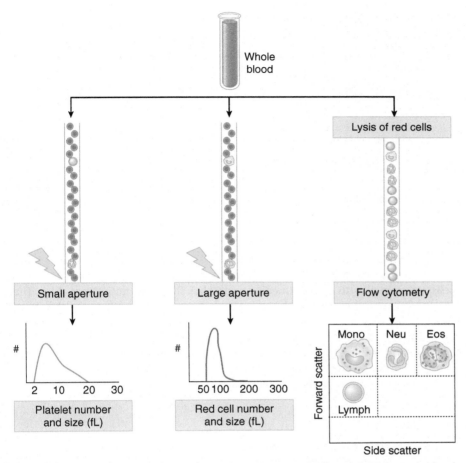

FIGURE 1-3 **Automated counting of formed elements.** Red cells and platelets are sized and counted by electrical impedance, whereas white cells are enumerated by flow cytometry. See text for details. fL, femtoliter; eos, eosinophil; mono, monocyte; neu, neutrophil; lymph, lymphocyte.

hemoglobin concentration (MCHC), the mean cell hemoglobin (MCH), and the hematocrit; normal red cell indices for adult males and females are given in Table 1-2. The sizing of platelets by automated cell analyzers also provides useful information, because an increase in the mean platelet size usually signifies a population of young platelets with a shortened life span.

Specific types of white cells are quantified by flow cytometry, in which a stream of droplets containing individual cells is passed through a laser. Cells deflect light forward based on their size and to the side based on their cytoplasmic granularity. Light sensors located forward and to the side of the incident beam of light allow each cell's light scattering properties to be measured and plotted on a graph. Different kinds of white cells (lymphocytes, monocytes, neutrophils, etc.) fall within particular regions of the light scatter plot (Fig. 1-3), allowing them to be quantified in both absolute and relative terms.

TABLE 1-2 Normal Red Cell Indices∗

Measurement	Male	Female
Hemoglobin (g/dL)	14.5-18.0	13.5-16.5
Hematocrit (% red cells)	44-54	40-50
Mean cell volume (fL)	80-95	
Mean cell hemoglobin (pg)	27-32	
Mean cell hemoglobin concentration (pg/fL)	32-36	

∗Adult patients, Brigham and Women's Hospital.

A limitation of forward and side scatter is that they do not discriminate among morphologically similar cells, such as B and T lymphocytes. To accomplish this, cells are stained with lineage-specific antibodies linked to fluorescent dyes. The stained cells are then passed through the flow cytometer equipped with a laser tuned to the excitation wavelength of the dyes and a system of mirrors and filters that allows the detection of light corresponding to each dye's emission wavelength. This method is used to quantify T helper (CD4-positive) cells in the peripheral blood of patients who are infected with human immunodeficiency virus as well as in the diagnosis of hematologic malignancies (Chapters 19-24).

PLASMA

Plasma, the fluid phase of the blood, consists of water and solutes such as proteins, lipids, and electrolytes. The homeostatic mechanisms that regulate plasma volume, electrolytes, and lipids are beyond our scope. Here, our chief focus will be on the plasma proteins that are involved in the formation and dissolution of blood clots. The most important of these are the proteins of the coagulation cascade, certain coagulation cascade regulatory factors, von Willebrand factor, and proteins that promote the lysis of clots, such as plasmin. The laboratory tests that are used to assess these factors as well as the function of platelets, which have an essential role in hemostasis, are described in Chapters 14 and 15.

BONE MARROW

Under normal circumstances, the bone marrow is the only site of blood cell production (hematopoiesis) following birth. Early in life, most bones contain hematopoietically active marrow, but by adulthood hematopoiesis is normally confined to the axial skeleton, the proximal long bones, and the skull. The marrow is supplied by nutrient arteries, which divide and eventually give rise to venous sinusoids that are lined by endothelial cells and adventitial cells. The frond-like tissue between the sinusoids contains a mixture of fibroblasts, fat cells, mononuclear cells (including lymphocytes and macrophages), and hematopoietic cells at

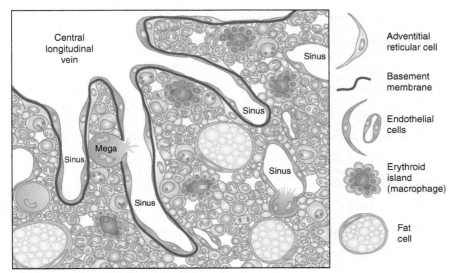

Central
longitudinal
vein

Sinus

Sinus

Mega

Sinus

Sinus

Sinus

Sinus

Adventitial
reticular cell

Basement
membrane

Endothelial
cells

Erythroid
island
(macrophage)

Fat
cell

FIGURE 1-4   **Organization of normal bone marrow.**

various stages of maturation (Fig. 1-4). Although it is difficult to appreciate in microscopic sections, hematopoietic cells in the marrow are spatially organized in ways that are crucial for their normal development and function. For example, megakaryocytes are positioned next to sinusoids, allowing them to shed platelets directly into the blood; red cell precursors are often clustered around centrally placed macrophages; plasma cells are found along capillaries, an arrangement that presumably aids the secretion of antibodies into the blood; and (as will be discussed in Chapter 2) stem cells are nurtured within a special niche that lies close to blood vessels and osteoblasts lining the bone. It has been appreciated recently that fat cells appear to negatively regulate hematopoiesis, an interrelationship that may shape both the amount and distribution of hematopoietic tissue in the marrow.

EXAMINATION OF THE BONE MARROW

Indications for performing a bone marrow examination include an unexplained decrease or increase in blood cell counts beyond the normal range and the presence of abnormal cells in the blood (such as immature marrow precursors). Because myeloid elements (red cells, neutrophils, and platelets) have short life spans relative to lymphocytes, a decrease in marrow function, whatever the cause, affects these formed elements first. A decrease in all of the myeloid elements is called *pancytopenia* and usually indicates the existence of a disorder that causes a decrease in marrow output. An increase in all of the myeloid elements is an unusual circumstance referred to as *pancytosis*. Other terms used to describe increases or decreases in various blood counts are listed in Table 1-3.

When the marrow is examined, in most instances both an aspirate and a biopsy are taken, usually from the posterior iliac crest. The aspirated marrow and admixed blood are spread out on a slide and stained for microscopic examination. Normal

TABLE 1-3 Nomenclature of Abnormal Blood Cell Counts

Alteration in Counts	Descriptor(s)
Decrease in all myeloid elements	Pancytopenia
Increase in all myeloid elements	Pancytosis
Decrease in red cell count	Anemia
Increase in red cell count	Erythrocytosis, polycythemia
Decrease in white cell count	Leukopenia
Increase in white cell count	Leukocytosis
Decrease in neutrophil count	Neutropenia
Increase in neutrophil count	Neutrophilia
Increase in eosinophil count*	Eosinophilia
Increase in basophil count*	Basophilia
Decrease in monocyte count	Monocytopenia
Increase in monocyte count	Monocytosis
Decrease in lymphocyte count	Lymphopenia
Increase in lymphocyte count	Lymphocytosis
Decrease in platelet count	Thrombocytopenia
Increase in platelet count	Thrombocytosis

*Normal counts close to zero; eosinopenia and basopenia not recognized.

aspirates contain spicules of marrow made up of a heterogeneous mixture of cells of various lineages at all stages of differentiation (Fig. 1-5), with myeloid cells predominating over lymphoid cells. The excellent cytologic detail that is achieved in aspirates makes it possible to identify most myeloid precursors and formed elements by morphology alone (Fig. 1-6). Other cell types, such as immature tumor cells or lymphocytes, can be characterized further by other tests such as flow cytometry.

The limitation of marrow aspiration is that many pathologic processes induce fibrosis that renders the marrow inaspirable, a phenomenon referred to as a "dry tap." Such disorders often are recognized only in bone marrow biopsies (Fig. 1-7). In this procedure, a cutting needle is used to remove a slender core of bone of a centimeter or so in length, which is decalcified and used to prepare tissue sections. Biopsies lack the cytologic detail of aspirates but are excellent for judging overall marrow cellularity and diagnosing marrow involvement by disorders that produce fibrosis, such as granulomatous disease (e.g., tuberculosis), metastatic cancer, and some hematologic malignancies.

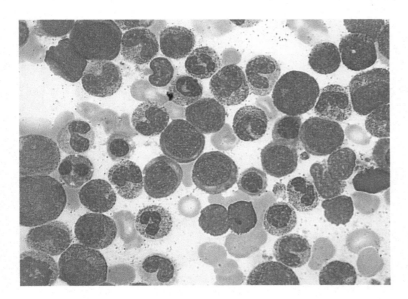

FIGURE 1-5 Normal bone marrow aspirate. A heterogeneous mixture of maturing erythroid and granulocytic precursors is present.

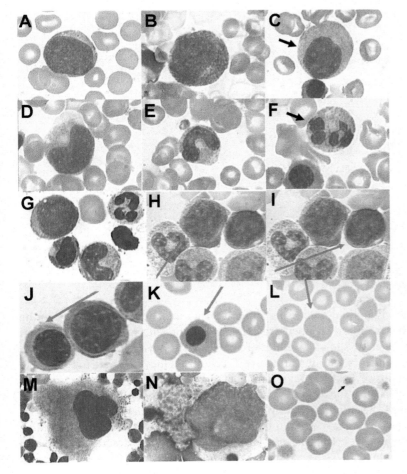

FIGURE 1-6 Myeloid elements and precursors, bone marrow aspirate. A-F, Sequential stages of neutrophil differentiation. A) Myeloblast, B) Promyelocyte, C) Myelocyte, D) Metamyelocyte, E) Band form, F) Neutrophil. G-L, sequential stages of red cell differentiation. G) Erythroblast, H-I) basophilic normoblasts, J) Polychromatophilic normoblast, K) Orthochromic normoblast, L) Reticulocyte. M-O, sequential stages of platelet development. M) Megakaryocyte, N) Megakaryocyte with fragmented cytoplasm shedding platelets, O) Peripheral blood platelets. Other bone marrow cells present in small numbers in normal aspirates include lymphocytes, plasma cells, mast cells, and macrophages (not shown).

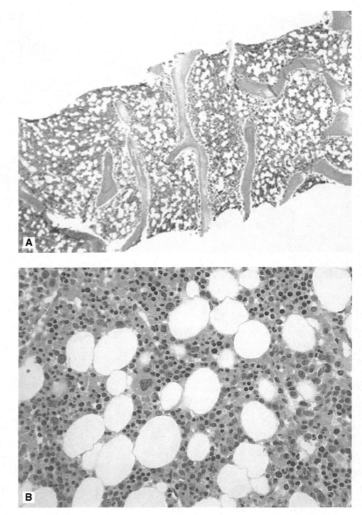

FIGURE 1-7 Bone marrow biopsy. A) Low-power view showing trabecular bone and intramedullary marrow, B) higher-power view showing an even mixture of fat and hematopoietic elements, which include red cell and granulocytic precursors and scattered megakaryocytes.

THYMUS

Certain early lymphoid precursors emigrate from the bone marrow through the blood to the thymus, a bi-lobed organ located in the anterior mediastinum that serves as the major site of T-cell differentiation. The thymus is subdivided into the cortex, which is rich in immature T cells (thymocytes), and the medulla, which contains fewer thymocytes and scattered Hassall corpuscles, clusters of epithelial cells that have undergone squamous differentiation (Fig. 1-8). The entire organ is heavily invested by a meshwork of epithelial cells and dendritic cells, both of which play a part in the presentation of peptide antigens to differentiating thymocytes. This process, termed *thymopoiesis*, is described in greater detail in Chapter 2.

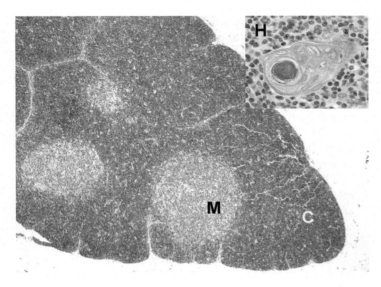

FIGURE 1-8 **Thymus.** Low-power view showing the thymocyte-rich cortex (C) and pale, centrally placed medulla (M). Inset shows a medullary Hassall corpuscle (H).

SECONDARY LYMPHOID TISSUES

Once released from the marrow, terminally differentiated myeloid elements (red cells, granulocytes, monocytes, and platelets) have defined fates and life spans. The story is quite different for T and B lymphocytes. After their release from the marrow or the thymus, these cells circulate through the blood and home to the secondary lymphoid tissues—the spleen, the lymph nodes, and the mucosa-associated lymphoid tissues (the most important of which are the Peyer patches of the small intestine and tonsillar tissues of the oropharynx). The anatomy of these tissues serves to optimize the probability that cells of the adaptive and innate immune systems will encounter pathogens and foreign antigens. If activated by antigen at these sites, T and B cells begin to proliferate and may undergo further differentiation to a variety of fates, which are dictated by factors produced locally at the site of the immune reaction. T cells can differentiate into effector T cells (helper and cytotoxic T cells), regulatory T cells, or memory T cells, whereas B cells can become memory B cells or plasma cells secreting one of a number of possible types of immunoglobulin.

The spleen has two chief functions: 1) it serves as a filter for particulate matter in the blood, and 2) it is a site of adaptive immune responses. Blood enters the splenic hilum through the splenic artery, which divides within the substance of the spleen to give rise to small arteries (Fig. 1-9). During their course, these small arteries give rise to branches that are surrounded by lymphoid follicles, organized collections of T cells and B cells that are poised to respond to immunologic stimuli; these constitute the splenic *white pulp*. The arteries eventually give rise to small, arborizing arterioles, which empty into the splenic *red pulp*, an interstitial space separated from the venous sinuses of the spleen by a basement membrane with slit-like openings. Red cells that have

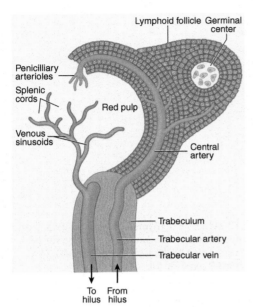

Penicilliary arterioles

Splenic cords

Red pulp

Venous sinusoids

Lymphoid follicle **Germinal center**

Central artery

Trabeculum

Trabecular artery

Trabecular vein

To hilus   From hilus

FIGURE 1-9   Spleen. Illustration showing the relationship of the splenic blood supply to the white pulp and the red pulp. (From Robbins Pathologic Basis of Disease, 8th edition, Kumar V, Abbas A, Fausto N, Aster J, eds. Elsevier, Philadelphia, 2010, p. 633.)

normal deformability are able to push through the slits and return to the circulation, but cells that are rigid are retained and removed by resident macrophages. The same phagocytes also remove particulate matter, including bacteria, making the spleen an important first line of defense against sepsis. Antigens derived from blood borne pathogens are readily presented to T and B lymphocytes in the white pulp, which can differentiate into effector T cells or plasma cells, respectively. The splenic red pulp contains many plasma cells and is an important site of antibody production.

Primary disorders of the spleen are rare. In contrast, the spleen is secondarily involved by many different disorders, which often cause splenic enlargement (splenomegaly) (Table 1-4). The spleen normally weighs about 150 g, but can increase in weight 10-fold or more in some pathologic conditions.

Just as the spleen serves to filter the blood, *lymph nodes* act as a filter for the lymphatic fluid. With the exception of the central nervous system, all tissues contain lymphatic vessels that collect interstitial fluid (lymph). This low-pressure system delivers lymph to lymph nodes positioned along the lymphatic drainage system. Resting lymph nodes are small (<1.5 cm), encapsulated structures that contain highly organized collections of B lymphocytes, T lymphocytes, antigen-presenting

TABLE 1-4   Causes of Splenomegaly

I. Infection
   Bacterial: endocarditis, sepsis, tuberculosis
   Viral: infectious mononucleosis
   Fungal: histoplasmosis
   Protozoal: malaria, babesiosis

II. Congestion
   Portal hypertension due to cirrhosis, portal vein or splenic vein thrombosis, cardiac failure

III. Hematologic malignancies
   Lymphoid malignancies: non-Hodgkin lymphoma, lymphocytic leukemia, Hodgkin lymphoma
   Myeloproliferative disorders

IV. "Work" hyperplasia
   Hemolytic anemias

V. Noninfectious immune reactions
   Sarcoidosis
   Connective tissue disorders (e.g., rheumatoid arthritis)

VI. Miscellaneous
   Amyloidosis
   Storage disorders (e.g., Gaucher disease)
   Metastatic tumors
   Primary splenic cysts and neoplasms (very rare)

dendritic cells, phagocytic macrophages, and antibody-producing plasma cells (Fig. 1-10). Lymph suffuses slowly through the lymph nodes, enabling its contents to be examined thoroughly by resident immune cells. As anyone who has had a sore throat and tender lymph nodes realizes, lymphadenopathy is common in many different types of acute and chronic immune reactions. Much less often lymphadenopathy is a presenting symptom of lymphoma, a malignancy of lymph node–homing B or T cells.

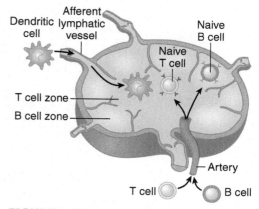

FIGURE 1-10 Lymph node. Illustration showing the organization of B and T cells into specific zones. (From Robbins Pathologic Basis of Disease, 8th edition, Kumar V, Abbas A, Fausto N, Aster J, eds. Elsevier, Philadelphia, 2010, p. 189.)

SELF-ASSESSMENT STUDY QUESTIONS

1. Which of the following is not true of the spleen?
   A. It serves as a filter for the blood.
   B. It is an important source of immunoglobulins.
   C. It is enlarged in many conditions associated with acute or chronic activation of the immune system.
   D. It is an important source of formed blood elements.
   E. It is a rare site of primary tumor development.

2. Which of the following is not true of lymph nodes?
   A. They filter the lymph.
   B. They contain mainly B cells and few T cells.
   C. They may become painfully enlarged in acute immune reactions.
   D. They are a major source of immunoglobulins.
   E. They contain numerous antigen-presenting cells.

3. Which of the following is not true of the bone marrow?
   A. It serves as the major source of formed blood elements after birth.
   B. In patients who are suspected of having metastatic carcinoma, biopsy of the marrow is the best way to establish a tissue diagnosis.
   C. It is often examined to determine the cause of pancytopenia.
   D. It is the primary site of hematopoiesis during embryonic development.
   E. It contains fat cells that may negatively regulate hematopoiesis.
   F. It contains a niche that nurtures stem cells.

2

Hematopoiesis

Jon C. Aster and David Scadden

LEARNING OBJECTIVES

After studying this chapter you should know:

- The developmental origins of the blood-forming tissues.
- The properties and functions that define hematopoietic stem cells.
- The role of growth factors and transcription factors in the regulation of hematopoiesis.
- The therapeutic roles of growth factors and hematopoietic stem cell transplantation.

In Chapter 1, we introduced the morphologically recognizable marrow progenitors and their progeny, the red cells, white cells, and platelets that make up the formed elements of the blood. Here we turn to the topic of hematopoiesis (from the Greek "to make blood"), the process by which these elements are created. As we will discuss, hematopoiesis depends on rare, morphologically inconspicuous progenitor cells that have remarkable functional properties. Unraveling how hematopoiesis is maintained and regulated has provided a paradigm for understanding the biology of tissue stem cells and has resulted in the development of effective therapies for certain cancers and genetic disorders as well as a variety of conditions in which bone marrow output is inadequate to maintain normal blood cell counts.

DEVELOPMENT OF BLOOD-FORMING TISSUES

The developmental origins of hematopoietic cells are complex and incompletely understood. Cells with the properties of hematopoietic stem cells (HSCs; described in the following section) arise several times in different tissues during prenatal development, producing successive waves of hematopoiesis (Fig. 2-1). Hematopoiesis first appears around day 16 of gestation in the embryonic yolk sac; at this site, it is limited to the production of red cells, which are needed for oxygen transport in the newly developed circulatory system. Hematopoietic cells arise anew around 3 to 4 weeks of gestation in a portion of the ventral mesoderm referred to as the aorta-gonad-mesonephros region. HSCs derived from this region (and possibly the yolk sac as well) are believed to migrate through the blood and take up residence in the liver, which becomes a hematopoietic organ at around 6 weeks of

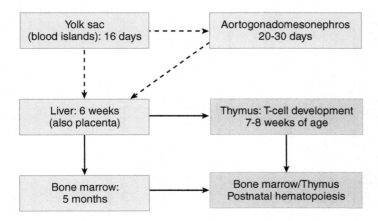

FIGURE 2-1 **Ontogeny of human hematopoiesis.** Dotted lines indicate migrations of hematopoietic stem cells or early progenitors that are suspected but not proven.

gestation and serves as the major source of hematopoietic cells throughout much of fetal development. HSCs and some hematopoietic progenitors also appear by around 6 weeks of gestation in the placenta and umbilical cord blood and persist in these sites until birth. By 7 to 8 weeks of gestation, lymphoid progenitors derived from the liver begin to seed the newly developed thymus, which is the major site of T-lymphocyte development. Around 5 months of age, HSCs derived from the liver (and possibly other sites) home to the bone marrow, which becomes the dominant source of hematopoietic elements by birth, around the time that hepatic hematopoiesis ceases.

Under normal circumstances, hematopoiesis is confined to the marrow throughout postnatal life, but under stress (e.g., severe inherited anemias) it can persist or reappear in the liver and spread to other extramedullary sites, such as the spleen and the lymph nodes. Hematopoietic neoplasms such as chronic myelogenous leukemia also tend to involve the same organs, sometimes producing massive hepatosplenomegaly and more modest lymphadenopathy.

HEMATOPOIETIC STEM CELLS AND PROGENITORS

Hematopoiesis is a remarkably dynamic process. The marrow normally produces approximately 200 billion red cells, 100 billion platelets, and 60 billion neutrophils each day, numbers that are just sufficient to match the rate of peripheral destruction of these formed elements. Hematopoiesis must persist throughout life and be finely tuned and highly responsive to changes in peripheral blood counts, because both cytopenias (too few formed elements) and cytoses (too many formed elements) can have serious or fatal consequences.

The ability of the hematopoietic system to meet these homeostatic challenges involves a hierarchy of progenitor cells with distinct roles (Fig. 2-2). At the top of this hierarchy lies the HSC. HSCs are essential for the maintenance of hematopoiesis and are by definition multipotent, meaning they can give rise to all other hematopoietic cells. When HSCs divide, under homeostatic conditions, it is thought that at least one of the two daughter cells remains an HSC, a critical property

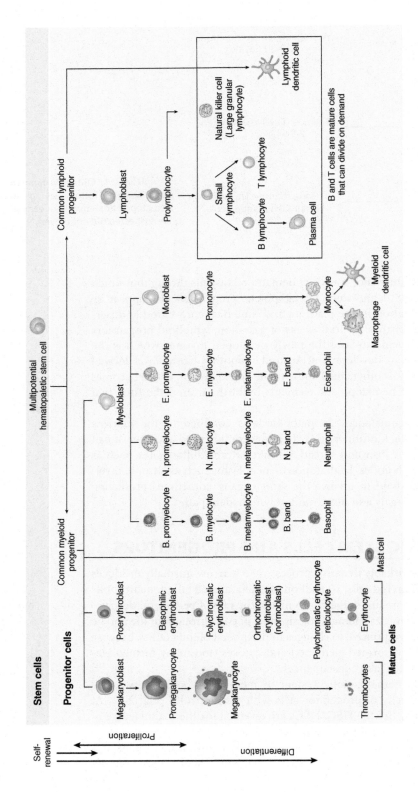

FIGURE 2-2 The hierarchy of hematopoietic cells. Self-renewal is confined to true multipotent hematopoietic stem cells, which lie at the top of the hierarchy, giving rise to all of the cells of the myeloid and erythroid lineage. Immature myeloid cells and both immature and mature lymphoid cells are capable of cell division.

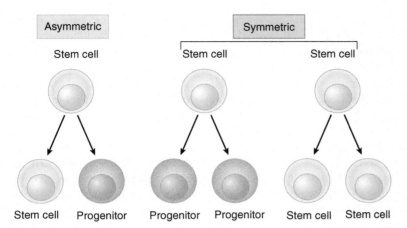

FIGURE 2-3 **Symmetric and asymmetric divisions of hematopoietic stem cells.**

referred to as *self-renewal* that maintains HSC numbers. Some HSC divisions may be symmetric, such that both daughter cells either become HSCs or begin to differentiate into progenitors (Fig. 2-3). Symmetric divisions that give rise to two HSCs may occur in the fetal liver, a stage of development during which HSC numbers increase. Symmetric divisions in which both daughter cells begin to differentiate into an early hematopoietic progenitor, a process termed *commitment*, may occur following periods of hematopoietic stress. Other HSC divisions are asymmetric, such that one cell remains an HSC, and the second commits to differentiation. Asymmetric cell divisions are dominant in the bone marrow, in which the number of HSCs remains fairly constant. Details still remain to be worked out, but it appears that the potential of very early committed progenitors is first restricted to myeloid (red cell, granulocyte, and megakaryocyte) or lymphoid (B cell, T cell, and natural killer cell) differentiation. With subsequent divisions, the differentiation potential of progenitors is further refined, so that it is ultimately restricted to a single cell type.

Bone marrow HSCs normally spend most of the time in a resting state referred to as *quiescence*, only "awakening" to divide, at most, every few months. Quiescence may help to maintain the multipotent state and protect HSCs against the acquisition of mutations that could lead to transformation and cancer development. Under conditions of increased hematopoietic demand, however, HSCs in the marrow divide more frequently and are more likely to divide symmetrically, expanding their numbers. In extreme circumstances, substantial numbers of HSCs and early progenitors may leave the marrow and migrate to the liver, spleen, and lymph nodes, where they can produce *extramedullary hematopoiesis*.

Given that HSCs have the ability to circulate in the blood, why is postnatal hematopoiesis normally confined to the marrow? One important contributing factor is active homing of HSCs. Circulating HSCs adhere to and migrate across bone marrow capillaries at sites where there are high levels of the chemokine CXCL12. Upon entering the interstitium, the HSCs nestle between blood vessels and osteoblasts (cells that line trabecular bone), which create a specialized microenvironment, or niche. These "niche" cells release factors (such as CXCL12) that regulate

HSC behavior in ways that are not yet completely understood. HSCs are resistant to stimulation by hematopoietic growth factors (described in the following section), possibly because niche factors actively promote quiescence. It may be that HSCs expand only when growth factors increase and quiescence factors decrease concomitantly. Another idea posits that HSC numbers are regulated by niche "vacancy," such that HSCs expand their numbers only when open niches are available. Under conditions of severe hematopoietic stress, it is possible that secondary niches appear in sites of extramedullary hematopoiesis, such as the liver.

Because HSCs are rare cells that are morphologically indistinguishable from lymphocytes, special means must be used to identify them. HSCs express particular surface markers such as CD34 and actively pump out certain dyes, properties that can be used to identify populations of cells that are enriched for HSCs. However, proof that viable HSCs are present in a sample requires functional testing. If a cell preparation can completely reconstitute long-term hematopoiesis when transfused into a host that has had its own marrow cells destroyed (e.g., by high doses of radiation), then it must contain HSCs, which can be quantified by serial dilution of the sample. Although this procedure, termed *stem cell transplantation*, was originally developed (and is still widely used) for experimental purposes, it was rapidly adopted as a means to treat a variety of diseases (described later in this chapter). It remains the only form of stem cell therapy that is widely used in clinical practice.

CONTROL OF MYELOPOIESIS BY GROWTH FACTORS

Myelopoiesis (the production of myeloid elements—red cells, granulocytes, and platelets) is regulated at the level of myeloid progenitors by hematopoietic growth factors. As differentiation proceeds, myeloid progenitors lose multipotency and the capacity for self-renewal, but in turn acquire two other key properties: 1) an increased capacity for cell division, and 2) surface expression of specific receptors for hematopoietic growth factors. By controlling the growth and survival of committed myeloid progenitors, growth factors regulate the production of red cells, granulocytes, and platelets from the marrow. Some growth factors, such as stem cell factor (also known as c-KIT ligand) and interleukin (IL)-3, have growth- and survival-promoting effects on multiple types of progenitors, whereas other factors, such as erythropoietin and thrombopoietin, have effects that are restricted to progenitors committed to a single line of differentiation (Fig. 2-4).

The marrow can increase its production of myeloid elements as much as 10-fold in response to growth factor stimulation. Three lineage-restricted growth factors are particularly important regulators of myeloid element production.

- *Erythropoietin* (Epo), a growth factor secreted by cells primarily located in the interstitium of the kidney, is a critical growth factor for early erythroid progenitors. Epo expression in the kidney is regulated by oxygen tension through the transcription factor hypoxia-inducible factor (HIF), described further in Chapter 3, such that when delivery of oxygen to tissues falls, HIF activity and Epo production rise (Fig. 2-5).

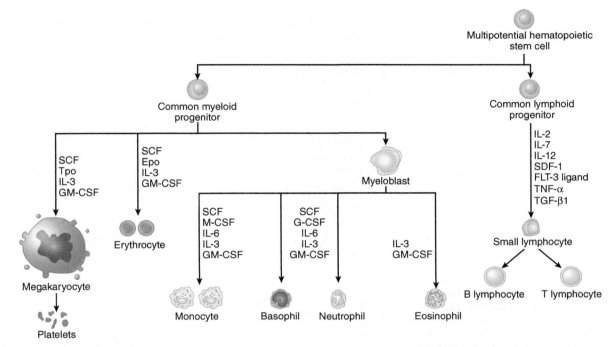

FIGURE 2-4 **Hematopoietic growth factors.** Factors that act on particular types of progenitors are listed. IL, interleukin; GM-CSF, granulocyte-macrophage colony stimulating factor; M-CSF, monocyte colony stimulating factor; Tpo, thrombopoietin; Epo, erythropoietin; SCF, stem cell factor (also known as c-KIT ligand); SDF-1, stromal cell-derived factor-1; FLT-3, Fms-like tyrosine kinase-3; TNF, tumor necrosis factor; TGF, transforming growth factor.

- *Thrombopoietin* (Tpo) is an important growth factor for megakaryocytes, the large polyploid marrow cells that shed platelets into the circulation. Tpo is secreted constitutively by hepatic parenchymal and endothelial cells as well as by bone marrow stromal cells. Unlike that of Epo, the activity of Tpo is not regulated by changes in its expression but rather through a competition between platelets and megakaryocyte progenitors for Tpo (Fig. 2-6). Platelets and marrow progenitors both express Tpo receptors, such that as platelet levels fall, the level of free Tpo available to stimulate megakaryocytic precursors in the marrow rises. Thus, platelet production is regulated by the total body platelet mass. This relationship explains why the sequestration of platelets in enlarged spleens fails to stimulate increased platelet production; these platelets still bind Tpo, keeping free Tpo levels relatively low even in the face of thrombocytopenia in the peripheral blood.

- *Granulocyte colony stimulating factor* (G-CSF) is an important growth factor for neutrophil progenitors. Like Tpo, G-CSF is secreted constitutively by several different cell types, including macrophages, endothelial cells, and fibroblasts. The production of G-CSF increases over basal levels in response to inflammatory cytokines such as IL-1 and tumor necrosis factor. By stimulating granulocytic progenitors in the marrow, G-CSF can markedly increase neutrophil production.

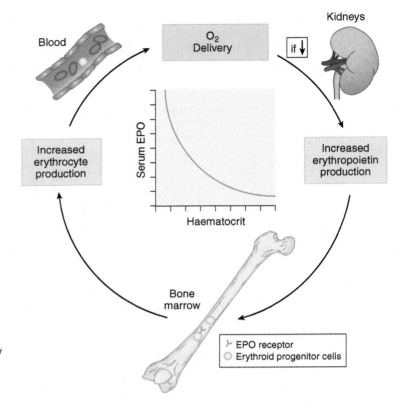

FIGURE 2-5 Regulation of red cell production by erythropoietin (Epo). Decreased oxygen delivery to specialized cells in the kidney results in increased expression and secretion of Epo, which stimulates marrow progenitors and increases red cell production. (Adapted from J. Spivak, Nature Reviews Cancer 5:543, 2005.)

Epo, Tpo, and G-CSF are glycoproteins that bind to specific members of the cytokine receptor family. When activated by growth factors, the Epo, Tpo, and G-CSF receptors all trigger signaling through several downstream pathways, including the JAK-STAT, Ras, and AKT pathways (Fig. 2-7). These pathways have effects on metabolism and gene expression that enhance the growth and survival of committed progenitor cells, the proliferating precursors that ultimately give rise to the formed myeloid elements. Following growth factor stimulation it generally

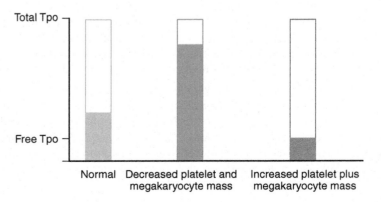

FIGURE 2-6 Regulation of platelet production by thrombopoietin (Tpo). Tpo is produced constitutively and binds to receptors on megakaryocytic progenitors, megakaryocytes, and platelets. When the megakaryocyte and platelet mass falls, the amount of free Tpo available to bind to Tpo receptors on marrow megakaryocyte progenitors rises; when the megakaryocyte and platelet mass rises, the converse is true.

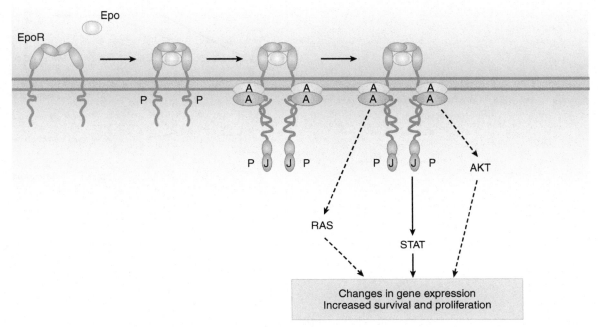

FIGURE 2-7 **Erythropoietin (Epo) signaling.** Binding of Epo causes the Epo receptor (EpoR) to undergo a conformational change and autophosphorylation, and recruit several adaptor proteins (A) and kinases of the JAK family (J). Through a series of additional phosphorylation events, these proteins transmit signals through the RAS, AKT, and JAK/STAT pathways, leading to increased expression of genes that augment the growth and survival of red cell progenitors. Certain other hematopoietic growth factors, such as Tpo, appear to activate the same set of signaling pathways in other kinds of hematopoietic progenitors.

takes about 10 days for the expanded pool of progenitors to mature, resulting in a lag between the elevation of growth factor levels and the appearance of increased numbers of newly formed elements in the peripheral blood.

LYMPHOPOIESIS

Regulation of lymphocyte production (lymphopoiesis) is more complicated than myelopoiesis, because it occurs at both the level of lymphocyte progenitors and mature lymphocytes. In the marrow, early progenitors with lymphoid potential expand under the influence of growth factors such as IL-7. These cells may differentiate into B cells, T cells, or natural killer cells, as follows:

- Some lymphoid progenitors remain in the marrow and differentiate into B cells (Fig. 2-8). This process involves sequential productive rearrangements of the immunoglobulin (Ig)H heavy chain gene followed by the kappa or lambda Ig light chain genes, which permits naïve B cells to express IgM and IgD on their cell surfaces. Upon emerging from the marrow, naïve mature B cells home to peripheral lymphoid tissues, where they can persist in a

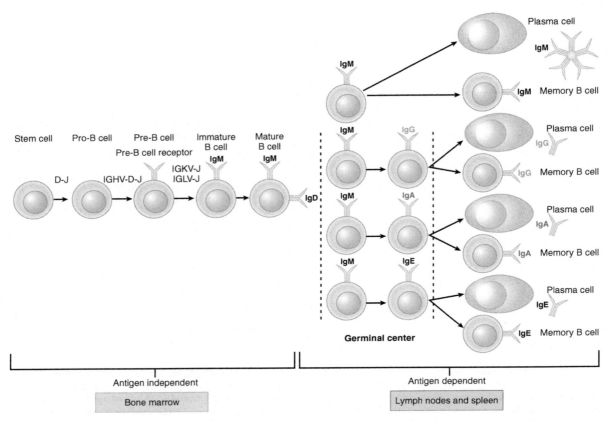

FIGURE 2-8 B-cell differentiation. D-J, IGHV-D-J, IGKV-J, and IGLV-J indicate segmental stages of IgH heavy chain and kappa and lambda light chain gene rearrangement. (Adapted from a figure prepared by Dr. M-P Lefranc and the International ImMunoGeneTics Information System.)

resting state for long periods. When stimulated by antigen, some of these cells proliferate and differentiate directly into IgM-secreting plasma cells or IgM-expressing memory B cells. However, most antigen-stimulated B cells migrate into germinal centers, a specialized niche found in peripheral lymphoid tissues such as lymph nodes. Many of these germinal center B cells die, but those that make high affinity antibodies survive and undergo class-switching, a process that allows B cells to express other types of immunoglobulin. These cells then leave the germinal center and become either long-lived memory cells or terminally differentiate into plasma cells.

- Other marrow-derived lymphoid progenitors migrate to the thymus. Here, these cells differentiate into T progenitors and rearrange their T-cell receptor genes (Fig. 2-9). The only cells expressing T-cell receptors that survive are those that bind antigen with low affinity in the context of major histocompatibility complex class I (also known as human leukocyte antigen [HLA] class I) or class II (HLA class II) antigens; this process is referred to as positive selection. Those that recognize self-antigens with high affinity die

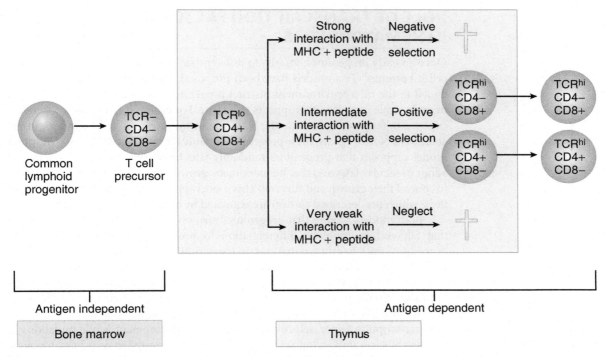

FIGURE 2-9 **T-cell differentiation (see text for details).** (Adapted from a figure prepared by Dr. Luc Van Kaer.)

by apoptosis (negative selection), which helps to prevent the development of autoimmunity, whereas cells that fail to rearrange their T-cell receptors productively or make receptors that fail to bind antigen die by neglect. Most cells emerging from the thymus express αβ T-cell receptors on their surfaces as well as the co-receptors CD4 or CD8. These cells circulate in the blood and home to lymphoid tissues throughout the body. When exposed to antigen in the proper cellular context, T cells become activated, enlarge, and begin to divide. Like B cells, activated T cells can either undergo terminal differentiation into antigen-specific effector cells (either CD4-positive Th1 or Th2 T-helper cells or CD8-positive cytotoxic T cells) or become long-lived memory T cells. A smaller number of progenitors in the thymus express a different type of T-cell receptor composed of γ and δ chains. These γδ T cells fail to express CD4 or CD8 and tend to home to the skin and the gut.

- The third type of lymphocyte is the natural killer cell. These cells also arise from lymphoid progenitors in the marrow, where their production is promoted by the cytokine IL-15, and subsequently migrate to peripheral lymphoid tissues. They do not express either antibodies or T-cell receptors on their surfaces but can be activated by certain cytokines or exposure to cells that have been infected by viruses or have abnormal patterns of surface antigen expression, such as cancer cells. Like CD8-positive cytotoxic T cells, natural killer cells have azurophilic granules containing enzymes that are capable of killing target cells.

ROLE OF TRANSCRIPTION FACTORS IN HEMATOPOIESIS

Once an early progenitor commits to differentiate, what determines which kind of cell it becomes? Two models have been proposed. One supposes that factors produced in the microenvironment instruct progenitors to differentiate along certain lines. In some instances, this appears to be true. For example, lymphoid progenitors exposed to factors that activate the Notch pathway become T cells, whereas, in the absence of Notch signals, these progenitors mainly become B cells instead. The other model supposes that progenitors randomly (stochastically) become competent to adopt particular fates and that hematopoietic growth factors act on this pool of cells to control their growth and survival. This model appears to hold for myeloid progenitors, which (as described earlier) are regulated by hematopoietic growth factors.

Both models require that progenitors turn on the expression of a set of genes that allows hematopoietic differentiation to proceed. Experimental work with "knockout" mice has shown that certain transcription factors, proteins that associate with DNA and control gene expression, are critically important in directing differentiation along particular lines (Fig. 2-10). For example, the loss of the transcription factor PAX5 specifically blocks B-cell development, while leaving other lineages intact. Similarly, loss of Notch1, a unique type of receptor that also acts directly as a transcription factor, selectively blocks T-cell development, while mutations in C/EBPα block granulocytopoiesis. Other factors are required in early hematopoietic progenitors, and, as a result, their loss causes a complete failure of hematopoiesis. MLL is an example of one such factor. On the other end of the developmental spectrum, some factors have no role in early progenitors or in lineage determination but are instead required for the further differentiation of mature cells. For example, loss of the transcription factor BCL6 prevents antigen-stimulated B lymphocytes from maturing into germinal center B cells. Thus, hematopoiesis is orchestrated by a complex interplay between extrinsic factors (hematopoietic growth factors and local factors produced in the microenvironment) and factors intrinsic to hematopoietic progenitors (growth factor receptors and hematopoietic transcription factors).

One important group of disorders in which these regulatory mechanisms go awry is the various kinds of hematologic malignancies, cancers of hematopoietic cells. These cancers are commonly associated with acquired mutations that alter the function of the same transcription factors that control differentiation. In fact, mutations in particular transcription factors tend to be found in tumors composed of cells that correspond to the stage in development at which the affected transcription factor normally acts. For example, PAX5 mutations are found in tumors composed of early B-cell progenitors, whereas BCL6 mutations are confined to tumors derived from germinal center B cells. In general, cancer-specific mutations in transcription factors interfere with differentiation, holding cells in an immature state. In addition to transcription factor mutations, mutations in one or another component of the signaling pathways that are normally activated by growth factors are often found in hematopoietic cancers. These mutations typically stimulate signaling even in the absence of growth factors, permitting tumors to proliferate in a growth factor–independent fashion. These themes are expanded upon in later chapters describing the hematopoietic neoplasms.

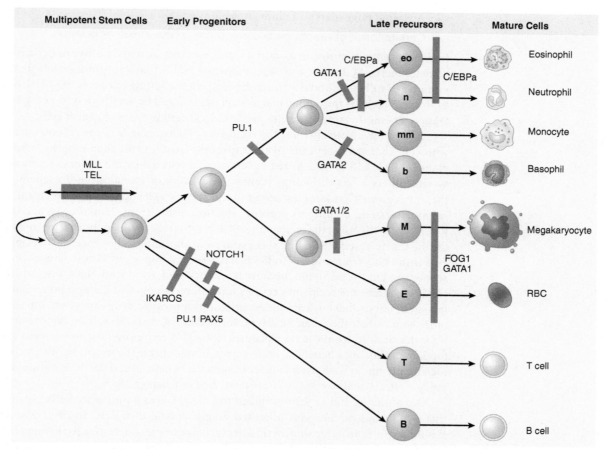

FIGURE 2-10 Hematopoietic transcription factors. Deficiencies of the indicated transcription factors block hematopoiesis at junctures indicated by the red lines in "knockout" mice.

STEM CELL TRANSPLANTATION

Stem cell transplantation (SCT) is described in detail in Chapter 26; we present only a brief overview here. The ability of HSCs to home to the bone marrow niche and completely reconstitute hematopoiesis makes it feasible to deliver these cells by simple transfusion into the peripheral blood. Tissue sources of HSCs used in SCT include bone marrow, the umbilical cord blood of newborns (a rich source of HSCs), and the peripheral blood. SCT may be *autologous* (in which case the HSCs are from the same patient) or *allogeneic* (in which case the HSCs are obtained from another individual). The source of the HSCs and the type of SCT that is performed vary according to the clinical indication.

A variety of disorders are treated with SCT, including:

- Inherited blood disorders that qualitatively or quantitatively impair the function of HSCs or their progeny.

- Acquired bone marrow failure (aplastic anemia).
- Certain forms of cancer, particularly those of hematopoietic origin.

In patients with inherited or acquired conditions that lead to defective or deficient hematopoiesis, SCT serves to supply normal HSCs that can produce adequate numbers of fully functional formed elements. In the setting of cancer, SCT is used to "rescue" patients from bone marrow aplasia induced by very high doses of radiation or chemotherapy, which are needed to kill certain types of cancer cells.

Except for identical twins, the recipients of allogeneic SCT are reconstituted with cells that are genetically distinct from the host. In this situation, the transplanted HSCs will be recognized as foreign and rejected by the patient's immune system unless a "conditioning" regimen consisting of radiation and/or chemotherapy is given. Conditioning serves two purposes: 1) it suppresses the recipient's immune system, helping to prevent rejection of the transplanted cells, and 2) it destroys or displaces the recipient's HSCs, creating vacancies in the marrow niche for the transplanted HSCs. The successful reconstitution of allogeneic SCT recipients with HSCs from another individual has several important immunologic consequences. On the one hand, because lymphocytes derived from the transplanted HSCs recognize the recipient's cells as foreign, recipients will develop potentially fatal graft-versus-host disease unless immunosuppressive drugs are given. On the other hand, when allogeneic SCT is performed in patients with cancer, donor lymphocytes derived from the transplanted HSCs also recognize host cancer cells as foreign, producing a beneficial graft-versus-tumor effect. The means by which clinicians attempt to walk the fine line between the beneficial and deleterious immunologic effects of allogeneic SCT are described in Chapter 26.

An attractive but as yet unfulfilled use of SCT is as a means to deliver "gene therapy" to individuals with inherited hematopoietic disorders. In principle, it should be possible to repair genetic defects (for example, a defective β-globin gene encoding sickle hemoglobin) in stem cells in the laboratory and then reconstitute the patient with "corrected" HSCs through autologous SCT. Recent advances in reprogramming of somatic cells into stem cells with the capacity for hematopoiesis provide a reason for optimism about the long-term prospects of this approach.

GROWTH FACTOR THERAPY

Growth factors are used clinically in a variety of settings to enhance the marrow output of formed myeloid elements.

- *Epo* is the most widely used growth factor. It is most effective when given to treat anemias associated with inappropriately low levels of Epo. These include the anemia of renal failure, in which the production of Epo is diminished by damage to the kidney parenchyma, and the anemia of chronic inflammation, in which inflammatory cytokines suppress the production of Epo. Anemia of inflammation is common in patients with certain inflammatory disorders and various forms of cancer (Chapter 7). Epo is also used with varied success in patients with hematopoietic neoplasms, such as myelodysplastic syndromes (Chapter 20), that are associated with ineffective hematopoiesis.

- *G-CSF* is primarily used in the treatment of drug induced neutropenia, particularly following high-dose chemotherapy, which causes a transient marrow aplasia that lasts roughly 21 days. G-CSF lessens the period of neutropenia, thereby decreasing the frequency of fevers related to infection. Granulocyte-macrophage colony stimulating factor, another growth factor that enhances the production of both granulocytes and macrophages, is also used in this setting and appears to have similar efficacy to that of G-CSF. G-CSF is also used in patients with congenital disorders associated with low neutrophil counts (neutropenia), as described in Chapter 18.

- *Tpo* and other factors that stimulate the production of megakaryocytes and shedding of platelets have proven to be beneficial in patients with immune thrombocytopenia (Chapter 14) but are not effective in patients with low platelet counts (thrombocytopenia) following chemotherapy or in those with primary disorders of the marrow that impede platelet production.

SELF-ASSESSMENT STUDY QUESTIONS

1. Which of the following is not true of hematopoietic growth factors?
   A. Thrombopoietin production increases in response to thrombocytopenia.
   B. Erythropoietin production increases in response to blood loss.
   C. Granulocyte colony stimulating factor is commonly given to patients with iatrogenic forms of neutropenia.
   D. Interleukin-7 is an important growth factor for lymphoid progenitors.
   E. Thrombopoietin therapy may benefit patients with immune-mediated thrombocytopenia.

2. Which of the following is not true of hematopoietic stem cells?
   A. They first appear during development in the yolk sac and the posterior aorta.
   B. They are rare cells that express particular surface markers and have a unique morphologic appearance.
   C. They are nurtured in a niche in the bone marrow that is close to blood vessels and stromal cells that express the chemokine CXCL12.
   D. They can be obtained for therapeutic purposes from the bone marrow, umbilical cord blood, or the peripheral blood.
   E. They are the only hematopoietic cells that possess the properties of self-renewal and multipotency.

3. Which of the following is not true of hematopoietic transcription factors?
   A. They include factors that are specifically required for the development of particular cell types.
   B. They include factors that control the development and maintenance of hematopoietic stem cells.
   C. They include factors that control the terminal differentiation of mature lymphocytes.
   D. They are directly controlled by hematopoietic growth factors.
   E. They collaborate with hematopoietic growth factors to orchestrate the production of hematopoietic cells.

PART I Anemia and Red Cell Disorders

In common parlance, the word *anemic* connotes weakness, apathy, lifelessness. In medicine, anemia refers specifically to a reduction in red cell mass. These two concepts merge with the realization that oxygen is essential for all forms of life and that red cells are responsible for the transport of oxygen. This painting shows a pale young woman clutching her chest, apparently complaining of palpitations. Her physician is feeling her pulse, documenting her rapid forceful heartbeat. These signs and symptoms, common in patients with very low hemoglobin levels, can be readily explained by the cardiovascular adjustments discussed in Chapter 3.

Physicians in the 17th century would readily conclude that this patient suffers from chlorosis, derived from the Greek word *chloris* (χλωριζ), meaning *greenish yellow*. This condition was also known as *morbus virgineus* (virgin's disease) or *mal d'amour* (love sickness) in recognition of its high prevalence in young women. We now realize that iron deficiency is by far the most prevalent cause of anemia worldwide.

During the last century, studies of hemoglobin, red cells, and disorders thereof have laid the cornerstones of contemporary molecular and cell biology and have greatly deepened our understanding of hematopoiesis, genetics, and oxygen homeostasis.

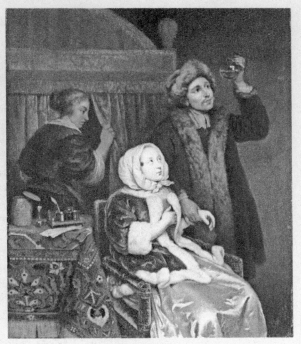

"The Sick Lady," a 17th century painting attributed to Caspar Netscher, from the Royal Collection, Buckingham Palace. The Royal Collection © 2010 Her Majesty Queen Elizabeth II.

3

Overview of the Anemias

H. Franklin Bunn

LEARNING OBJECTIVES

After studying this chapter you should:

- Understand how anemia impacts oxygen transport and the ways in which anemic patients compensate for decreased oxygen-carrying capacity.
- Develop a coherent approach to the clinical and laboratory evaluation of patients with anemia.
- Understand and use classification of anemia based on production versus destruction and on red cell size (mean cell volume).
- Be able to explain the phenomenon of ineffective erythropoiesis—its diagnosis and role in pathogenesis.
- Understand the process by which red cells are broken down, the catabolism of heme in macrophages, and the transport of bilirubin in the plasma and its conjugation in the liver.

DEFINITION OF ANEMIA

As stated in Chapter 1, the primary function of the red blood cell is to transport oxygen to respiring cells and tissues. Anemia is defined as a significant deficit in the mass of circulating red blood cells. As a result, the capacity of the blood to deliver oxygen is compromised. Clinicians document the presence of anemia by measurement of either the concentration of hemoglobin in the blood or the hematocrit, which is the ratio of the volume of red cells to the total volume of a blood sample. A patient is anemic if the hemoglobin or hematocrit value is more than two standard deviations below normal. As shown in Figure 3-1, the lower limits of normal vary with the age of the individual and, in adults, with gender. Occasionally, the documentation of anemia is confounded by a concurrent alteration in the plasma volume. For example, if a patient with a low mass of circulating red blood cells is also hypovolemic, owing to a concurrent loss of plasma volume from dehydration, the blood hemoglobin and hematocrit levels will be falsely elevated and may even be in the normal range. Another important example, discussed in more detail later in this chapter, is acute hemorrhage, in which there is concomitant loss of both red blood cells and plasma.

OXYGEN TRANSPORT IN ANEMIA

Oxygen transport to a given region in the body, as expressed in the Fick equation, is a product of three independent variables: blood flow, hemoglobin concentration, and the fraction of hemoglobin that has unloaded oxygen during transit

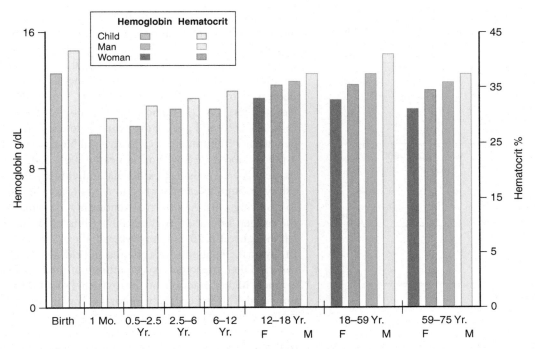

FIGURE 3-1 Lower limits of normal levels of hemoglobin and hematocrit at different ages. Mo, month; Yr, year; F, female; M, male.

from artery to vein. In anemic patients, the oxygen-carrying capacity of the blood is, by definition, low. As shown in Figure 3-2 and explained below, the two other components in the Fick equation undergo compensatory changes.

BLOOD FLOW

In all anemic individuals, there is enhanced shunting of blood to vital organs, including the heart, brain, liver, and kidneys, at the expense of non-vital organs. Anemic patients are pale because blood is shunted away from the skin to preserve oxygenation of these crucial organs. In patients with mild or moderate anemia, the cardiac output is normal at rest but, with exercise, increases more than that of a normal individual. In severe anemia, the resting cardiac output is increased, putting patients at risk of developing high-output cardiac failure, particularly those with coronary artery disease or other forms of preexistent cardiovascular disease.

OXYGEN UNLOADING

The variable (Asat-Vsat) in the Fick equation is the difference in percent oxygenation between the arterial (A) and venous (V) blood. This AV difference in oxygen saturation depends on the

Fick Equation – Adaptations in Severe Anemia

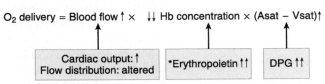

O_2 delivery = Blood flow ↑ × ↓↓ Hb concentration × (Asat − Vsat)↑

FIGURE 3-2 The Fick equation applied to anemia. Hb, hemoglobin; Asat, arterial O_2 saturation; Vsat, venous O_2 saturation; DPG, 2,3-diphosphoglycerate.
*Response to erythropoietin is blunted in underproduction anemias

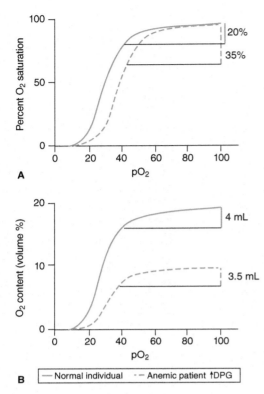

A

B   — Normal individual   - - Anemic patient ↑DPG

FIGURE 3-3 Oxygen-binding curves of a normal individual and a patient with anemia. Top: conventional plot of % O₂ saturation versus pO₂. Bottom: the Y-axis shows the volume of oxygen in mL per 100 mL of blood. DPG, 2,3-diphosphoglycerate.

oxygen-binding curve. Figure 3-3 compares curves from an anemic patient and a normal individual. As the top panel shows, the anemic curve is shifted to the right. At any given oxygen tension (pO₂), the oxygen saturation is lower in the anemic individual. Thus, red cells of anemic patients have decreased oxygen affinity. This change is due entirely to elevated levels of 2,3-diphosphoglycerate (2,3-DPG) in red cells. 2,3-DPG and pH are the primary determinants of oxygen affinity in human red cells. Arterial blood normally has a pO₂ of about 95 Torr and is nearly 100% saturated with oxygen. As red cells from a normal individual pass from an artery through its capillary bed to its vein, oxygen is released to respiring cells. At a normal venous pO₂ of about 40 Torr, the oxygen saturation is about 80%. Thus, as shown on the left in Figure 3-3, 20% of the oxygen in the blood is unloaded. In contrast, in patients with anemia and elevated levels of red cell 2,3-DPG, the lower oxygen affinity of the blood enables a much higher fraction of the oxygen (about 35%) to be unloaded. This is a critically important way in which anemic patients compensate for their major deficit in red cell mass.

This benefit is shown quantitatively in the bottom panel of Figure 3-3. Here, the oxygen-binding curves are depicted with the volume fraction of oxygen plotted on the Y-axis. One gram of hemoglobin binds up to 1.34 mL of oxygen under standard conditions of temperature and pressure. Thus, in a normal individual with a hemoglobin of 15 g/dL, the oxygen-carrying capacity of the blood will be 15×1.34 or 20 mL O₂/dL. In traversing the earlier-mentioned capillary bed, 20% of this oxygen will be unloaded, that is, 4 mL per 100 mL of blood. In contrast, an anemic patient with a hemoglobin of 7.5 g/dL has an oxygen-binding capacity that is half normal, that is, 10 mL O₂/dL. If this patient had red cells with normal oxygen affinity, 20% or only 2 mL of oxygen would be unloaded per 100 mL of blood. However, as shown on the right in Figure 3-3, because the patient's red cells have a lower affinity for oxygen, 3.5 mL is unloaded, nearly as much as normal.

STIMULATION OF ERYTHROPOIESIS BY ERYTHROPOIETIN

There are two ways in which anemia impacts the middle component of the Fick equation, depicted in Figure 3-2. As mentioned earlier, by definition, hemoglobin concentration is low in anemic patients. The reduction in the oxygen-carrying capacity of the blood results in cellular hypoxia. A molecular sensor in all cells of the body detects even mild degrees of hypoxia and induces a hypoxia-inducible transcription factor called *HIF*. In the kidney, and to a lesser extent in the liver, HIF up-regulates the expression of the hormone erythropoietin, which stimulates red blood cell production. The physiology and cell biology of erythropoietin is discussed in more detail in Chapter 2. The regulated production of erythropoietin enables normal individuals to maintain nearly constant levels of circulating red cells. In anemic patients, the hypoxic signal in the kidneys and liver results in a marked enhancement in erythropoietin production. As shown in Figure 3-4, plasma erythropoietin levels are inversely proportional to the hematocrit and, in severely anemic patients, can be 1000-fold higher than normal. The erythroid progenitors in patients with anemia due to impaired red cell production are unresponsive to such high levels of plasma erythropoietin. In contrast, in patients whose anemia is due to blood loss or a short red cell life span, this regulatory loop maximizes red cell production and constitutes a third important mode of compensation.

SIGNS AND SYMPTOMS OF ANEMIA

Patients with mild or moderate anemia are often asymptomatic. Many note breathlessness and/or fatigue only upon strenuous exercise. In severe anemia, dyspnea and fatigue are common complaints. These symptoms reflect limitations in the earlier-mentioned compensations for the tissue hypoxia imposed by a low red blood cell mass.

Physical findings also depend on the severity of the anemia and are best understood in terms of the Fick equation depicted in Figure 3-2. As mentioned earlier, pallor reflects a compensatory shunting of blood away from the skin to ensure adequate flow to vital organs. In individuals with deeply pigmented skin, pallor can be detected in nail beds as well as in membranes such as conjunctivae and the buccal mucosa. Those with severe anemia may have tachycardia at rest, owing to a compensatory increase in basal cardiac output. The hyperdynamic circulation in such patients often gives rise to a systolic "flow" murmur that is transmitted into the neck. In individuals with lesser degrees of anemia, the heart rate is normal at rest but, on exercise, increases more than normally. Anemic patients may have many other informative physical findings that depend on specific underlying pathophysiology. For example, those with hemolytic anemia often have splenomegaly, owing to trapping of defective or damaged red blood cells in the spleen, and jaundice, reflecting increased plasma bilirubin levels due to rapid destruction of red blood cells.

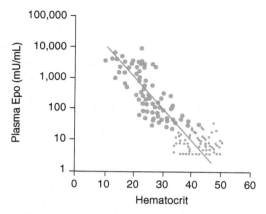

FIGURE 3-4 Plasma erythropoietin (Epo) levels in normal individuals (small symbols) and in patients with different types of anemia of varying severity (larger symbols). mU, milliunits.

BASIS OF ANEMIA: PRODUCTION VERSUS DESTRUCTION

The level of circulating red cells in the blood can be likened to the balance of cash in one's personal bank account. The balance is a function of how many dollars or cells are coming in each week versus how many are spent or lost. Thus, the anemias can be divided into three broad categories: decreased red cell production, increased red cell destruction, and blood loss. Often, the patient's history and physical examination provide information as to which process is going on. For example, the presence of blood loss is usually apparent from the history.

As mentioned earlier, physical findings such as jaundice and splenomegaly suggest hemolysis. Among the available laboratory tests, the reticulocyte count is

Anemia is due to:

Decreased
red cell production
or
Increased
red cell destruction
(hemolysis)
or
blood loss

the simplest and most reliable way to distinguish among the three major categories of anemia. This laboratory test is a measurement of the fraction of young red cells in the blood (<2.5 days old). In patients with impaired red cell production, the reticulocyte count will be inappropriately low. Despite elevated levels of plasma erythropoietin (Figures 3-2 and 3-4), the bone marrow is unable to respond to produce adequate numbers of new red cells. In contrast, the reticulocyte count is generally elevated in both hemolytic anemia and in acute blood loss.

ANEMIA DUE TO BLOOD LOSS

The loss of enough blood to cause significant anemia is usually due either to trauma, gastrointestinal hemorrhage, or uterine bleeding. The clinical presentation depends on both the rate and amount of blood loss. Relatively small amounts of hemorrhage are well-tolerated, owing to the compensatory mechanisms depicted in Figure 3-2. Donations at Red Cross or hospital blood banks are routinely 500 mL or 10% of the blood volume. Otherwise healthy individuals can lose up to 20% of their blood volume acutely without significant symptoms, owing to reflex vasospasm and redistribution of blood flow as described earlier. With greater blood loss, the patient develops the signs and symptoms of hypovolemia. Compensatory mechanisms such as redistribution of blood flow are no longer sufficient to maintain blood pressure. Postural hypotension, or a drop in systolic blood pressure when the patient goes from a supine to a sitting position, is a sign of significant hypovolemia. Even more extensive hemorrhage produces *hypovolemic shock*, which is denoted by altered mental status, cool clammy skin, tachycardia, hyperventilation, and hypotension in the supine position. Importantly, in patients with severe acute hemorrhage, the hematocrit and hemoglobin levels may initially be close to normal, owing to the concomitant loss of both red cells and plasma, such that the extent of the red cell loss becomes apparent only when the patient's plasma volume is restored, either spontaneously or by administration of intravenous fluids.

In patients with more gradual blood loss, the onset of the anemia is frequently insidious. Many patients develop non-specific symptoms and signs of anemia as described earlier in this chapter. These individuals are very likely to be or to become iron deficient.

The treatment of blood loss anemia depends on the extent and time frame of the hemorrhage. Patients in hypovolemic shock require both fluid and red cell replacement. Those with less severe blood loss may not require red cell transfusion. The rate of regeneration of new red blood cells may be enhanced by the administration of recombinant erythropoietin but is sometimes limited by lack of adequate iron stores. Thus, all patients with significant blood loss should receive enough therapeutic iron to replace the deficit from red cell loss. It is equally important to adequately monitor the patient to be sure blood loss is not continuing. Those with gastrointestinal blood loss need to have follow-up testing of stool specimens for the presence of blood.

ANEMIA DUE TO DECREASED RED CELL PRODUCTION

A wide variety of disorders result in anemia owing to inadequate production of red blood cells. However, these types of anemia have a number of features in common. The onset of symptoms is usually insidious. In individuals with a normal red cell life

In Underproduction Anemias:

Onset is usually insidious.
Retic count is inappropriately low.
Red cell indices are helpful.
Bone marrow exam is usually indicated.

span of 120 days, even if the production of red cells abruptly ceases, the drop in hemoglobin and hematocrit levels is quite gradual, and compensatory mechanisms may stave off the onset of symptoms until the anemia is quite severe. As mentioned earlier in this chapter, the reticulocyte count is inappropriately low. As shown in Figures 3-2 and 3-4, plasma erythropoietin levels rise quite markedly as patients become increasingly anemic. However, this highly specific and potent stimulus to erythropoiesis is ineffective in disorders in which there is a defect in red cell production. Some clinicians use the reticulocyte index as a more informative measure of red cell production. It is defined as the reticulocyte percentage times the hematocrit divided by the normal hematocrit (0.45). Normal individuals have a reticulocyte count of 1-2%, and, therefore, a reticulocyte index of 1 to 2. By comparison, a patient with a hematocrit of 0.15 and a reticulocyte count of 3% has a reticulocyte index of 1. Even though the reticulocyte count is slightly higher than normal, the reticulocyte index falls in the low normal range. Thus the patient's red cell production is stalled at a normal level even though the severe anemia is expected to induce a very high plasma erythropoietin level that, in a normal bone marrow, should enhance red cell production as much as 8-fold. This example illustrates the inappropriately low reticulocyte count in underproduction anemias.

The *red blood cell indices* are particularly helpful in determining the cause of anemia due to impaired red cell production. As mentioned in Chapter 1, these indices provide quantitative information about the average or mean red cell size or volume (MCV), mean red cell hemoglobin, and mean hemoglobin concentration within red cells. As shown in Table 3-1, the MCV is particularly useful in the classification of the underproduction anemias. Anemias associated with a low MCV are designated *microcytic*, and those with a high MCV are designated *macrocytic*. These two groups of anemias both involve defects in the maturation of erythroid cells in the bone marrow. The anemia-induced elevation of plasma erythropoietin produces a reactive hyperplasia of erythroid progenitors and precursors in the bone marrow, a feature that is readily detectable by microscopic examination of the bone marrow. However, impaired erythroid maturation suppresses the production of fully differentiated red cells to varying degrees, depending on the nature and severity of the underlying defect. As a result, patients with microcytic or macrocytic underproduction anemias have a disparate combination of erythroid hyperplasia in the marrow and a relatively low reticulocyte count in the peripheral blood. In fact, many erythroid precursors are so defective that they undergo programmed cell death (apoptosis) in the marrow and therefore cannot produce reticulocytes, a phenomenon referred to as *ineffective erythropoiesis*.

TABLE 3-1 Anemias Due to Decreased Red Cell Production

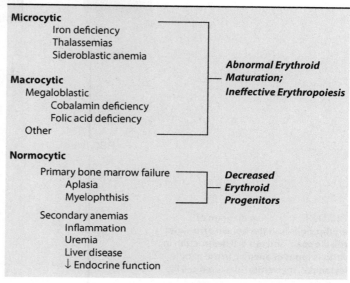

Microcytic
    Iron deficiency
    Thalassemias
    Sideroblastic anemia	

Macrocytic
    Megaloblastic
        Cobalamin deficiency
        Folic acid deficiency
    Other
	Abnormal Erythroid Maturation; Ineffective Erythropoiesis

Normocytic
    Primary bone marrow failure
        Aplasia
        Myelophthisis
	Decreased Erythroid Progenitors

Secondary anemias
        Inflammation
        Uremia
        Liver disease
        ↓ Endocrine function	

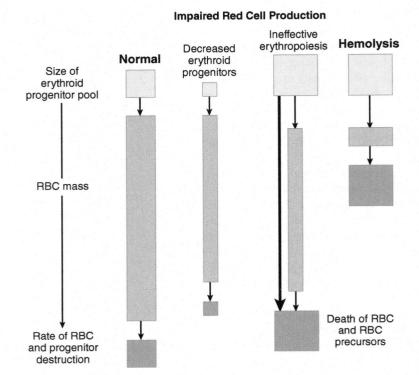

FIGURE 3-5 Flow diagram of erythropoiesis in the bone marrow, red cell life span, and red cell destruction in various types of anemia. In the middle rectangles, the vertical axis is red cell life span and the horizontal axis is red cells produced per day. Thus the area of the middle rectangle is a depiction of the red cell mass.

Ineffective erythropoiesis is a critically important component of the pathophysiology of a number of important underproduction anemias, including beta thalassemia major and intermedia, iron deficiency, sideroblastic and other myelodysplastic anemias, and the megaloblastic anemias. These entities are covered in detail in subsequent chapters.

Decreased red cell production is due either to a deficient number of erythroid progenitors or ineffective erythropoiesis. The dynamics of erythropoiesis, red cell survival, and red cell destruction in different types of anemias are depicted in Figure 3-5. Because the bone marrow is the site of erythropoiesis, microscopic examination of the bone marrow is particularly informative in the diagnosis of anemias of underproduction. Bone marrow biopsies are used to establish the overall cellularity of the marrow, whereas aspirate smears reveal the relative proportion of erythroid versus non-erythroid precursor cells as well as more subtle morphological features that often point to specific defects in erythroid maturation. Because these two procedures yield complementary information, both usually are performed at the time of marrow examination.

In *microcytic* anemias the small red cell volume is accompanied by a decrease in the mean red cell hemoglobin. As shown in Figure 3-6, microcytic anemia is due to a defect involving one of the three components of hemoglobin: iron, porphyrin (into which iron is inserted to make heme), or globin. The MCV is low when iron stores are depressed sufficiently to cause anemia and also in thalassemias, inherited mutations that impair the synthesis of either alpha or beta globin.

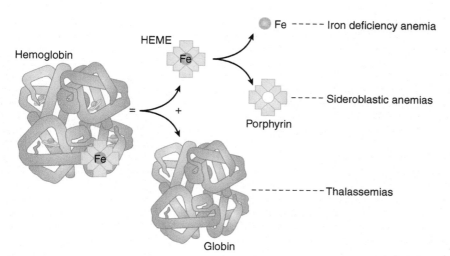

FIGURE 3-6 Components of hemoglobin that are deficient in the microcytic anemias.

In sideroblastic anemias caused by acquired or inherited defects in porphyrin synthesis, there is typically a much broader distribution of red cell sizes, but a prominent population of microcytic red cells is usually present.

Macrocytic red cells are encountered in a number of diverse causes of anemia. If the MCV exceeds 120 fL, the anemia is nearly always *megaloblastic*, a morphological appearance that reflects a defect in maturation due to impaired DNA synthesis. Megaloblastic anemias are most often caused by deficiency in vitamin B_{12} (cobalamin) or folate or by chemotherapy agents that block DNA synthesis, such as methotrexate. Lesser degrees of macrocytosis are encountered in hemolytic anemias, bone marrow failure, myelodysplastic syndromes, liver disease, alcoholism, and hypothyroidism.

Normocytic underproduction anemias also encompass a wide variety of disorders. Severe anemia associated with a normal MCV usually points to a primary marrow problem, either aplasia or marrow replacement by leukemia, metastatic tumor, fibrosis, or granulomas. The patient may have *pancytopenia*, defined as anemia associated with a concomitant reduction in the white blood cell count and the platelet count. Whenever the marrow is involved by infiltrative processes (e.g., tumor) or distorted by fibrosis, nucleated red cells and red cells with a tear-drop shape (Fig. 3-7) may appear in the peripheral blood. A bone marrow biopsy is essential to establish the diagnosis in such instances, because the marrow often cannot be aspirated, a clinical problem referred to as a "dry tap."

More commonly, normocytic anemias are secondary to an underlying systemic illness. Patients with cancer, long-standing infections, or connective tissue disorders such as rheumatoid arthritis have mild to moderate anemia, owing to chronic inflammation, which triggers abnormalities in iron homeostasis that impair erythropoiesis. The anemia of chronic inflammation is described in more detail in Chapter 7. Chronic liver disease and disorders of endocrine hypofunction also are associated with mild to moderate normocytic anemia. The anemia of renal insufficiency is the only secondary anemia that is commonly severe. These disorders are also covered in Chapter 7.

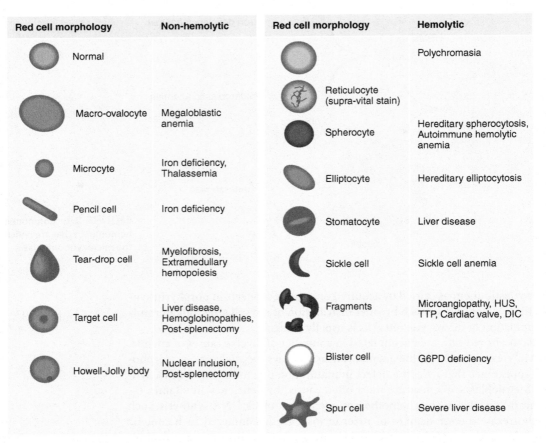

Red cell morphology	Non-hemolytic	Red cell morphology	Hemolytic
Normal			Polychromasia
Macro-ovalocyte	Megaloblastic anemia	Reticulocyte (supra-vital stain)	
Microcyte	Iron deficiency, Thalassemia	Spherocyte	Hereditary spherocytosis, Autoimmune hemolytic anemia
Pencil cell	Iron deficiency	Elliptocyte	Hereditary elliptocytosis
Tear-drop cell	Myelofibrosis, Extramedullary hemopoiesis	Stomatocyte	Liver disease
Target cell	Liver disease, Hemoglobinopathies, Post-splenectomy	Sickle cell	Sickle cell anemia
Howell-Jolly body	Nuclear inclusion, Post-splenectomy	Fragments	Microangiopathy, HUS, TTP, Cardiac valve, DIC
		Blister cell	G6PD deficiency
		Spur cell	Severe liver disease

FIGURE 3-7 Abnormalities of red cell morphology seen in different disorders. HUS, hemolytic uremic syndrome; TTP, thrombotic thrombocytopenic purpura; DIC, disseminated intravascular coagulation; G6PD, glucose-6-phosphate dehydrogenase.

In Hemolytic Anemias:

Reticulocyte count is elevated.
Examination of the blood smear is helpful,
Blood chemistries:
  ↑non-conj. bilirubin & LDH
  ↓haptoglobin
Specific tests establish the diagnosis:
  Coombs
  PNH screen
  Hb electrophoresis
  G6PD screen, etc.

ANEMIA DUE TO INCREASED RED CELL DESTRUCTION (HEMOLYSIS)

A wide range of structural, metabolic, immunologic, and mechanical defects can result in premature destruction of circulating red cells. However, irrespective of etiology, uncomplicated hemolytic anemias have a number of features in common. The capacity for efficient erythropoiesis is preserved, and indeed, in response to hypoxia-induced erythropoietin production (Fig. 3-1), red cell production is often markedly increased, an adaptive response that is reflected by an elevation of the reticulocyte count. Anemia accompanied by reticulocytosis of 5% or greater strongly suggests the presence of hemolysis. However, elevated reticulocyte counts also can be seen in nutritional anemias during the first two weeks of replacement therapy with iron, cobalamin (vitamin B_{12}), or folic acid. Acute hypoxia can also cause a transient elevation of the reticulocyte count. Finally, infiltrative bone marrow disorders such as metastatic cancer can also induce a modest sustained elevation of the reticulocyte count due to early release.

Microscopic examination of a carefully spread and well-stained blood smear is an important part of the evaluation of any unexplained anemia, but it is particularly informative in identifying the cause of hemolysis. A fascinating variety of red cell abnormalities can be observed in the different types of hemolytic anemia, many of which are shown in Figure 3-7. More details on the features and pathogenesis of these abnormal cells are provided in Chapters 9, 10, and 11, which cover specific types of hemolytic anemia.

In contrast to the value of examining the peripheral blood film, microscopic examination of the bone marrow is rarely helpful in identifying the cause of hemolytic anemia. The result that is nearly always obtained, erythroid hyperplasia, is predictable from the elevated reticulocyte count. A marrow examination is helpful only in exceptional instances such as the coexistence of lymphoma and immune hemolytic anemia and the presence of hypoplasia in paroxysmal nocturnal hemoglobinuria. These unusual but interesting exceptions to the rule are discussed in Chapter 11.

The presence of hemolysis can be further confirmed by readily available serum assays. These tests are based on the physiologic steps involved in the breakdown of red cells, as depicted in Figure 3-8. At the end of their life spans, both normal and abnormal red cells are engulfed by macrophages in the spleen, liver, and bone marrow. Here, globin, the protein in hemoglobin, undergoes proteolytic degradation. The heme is catabolized by heme oxygenase to biliverdin (a straight-chain tetrapyrole), carbon monoxide, and free iron. The biliverdin is then reduced to bilirubin, which exits the macrophage and binds to albumin in the plasma. The albumin-bound bilirubin is taken up by the liver, where it is conjugated to glucuronide, rendering it soluble in water. Conjugated bilirubin is excreted into the bile, enters the duodenum, and traverses the intestines. Bacteria in the gut mediate the conversion of conjugated bilirubin to urobilinogen, which in turn is converted to stercobilin, which causes the stool to be brown. In patients with hemolytic anemia, enhanced red cell breakdown and catabolism of heme result in an increase in the level of non-conjugated or "indirect" bilirubin in the plasma/serum. Patients with moderate or severe hemolytic anemia are often jaundiced (icteric). Chronic hemolysis puts patients at risk of developing bilirubin gall stones. If patients with hemolytic anemia have concomitant liver and biliary disease, serum levels of conjugated bilirubin will also be increased, and the total of non-conjugated and conjugated bilirubin may reach very high levels, resulting in much deeper jaundice.

Excess destruction of red cells, whether intravascular (within the blood) or extravascular (within macrophages), results in the leakage of hemoglobin and red cell enzymes into the circulation. Lactate dehydrogenase (LDH) is one easily measured enzyme, the levels of which increase above normal in proportion to the rate of hemolysis. It must be remembered, however, that even higher levels of LDH are seen in conditions such as megaloblastic anemia that are associated with severe, ineffective erythropoiesis. Free hemoglobin in the plasma binds with high affinity and specificity to haptoglobin, an abundant plasma protein, forming a hemoglobin-haptoglobin complex that is rapidly cleared from the circulation. As a result, haptoglobin is often completely absent from the plasma of patients with significant degrees of hemolysis.

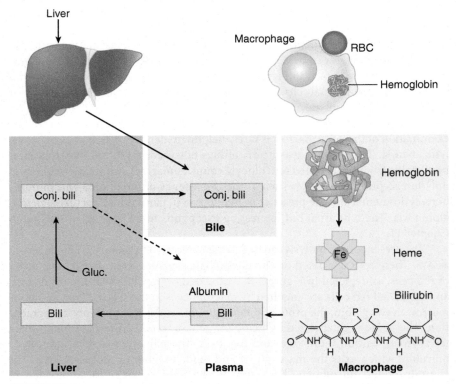

FIGURE 3-8 **Red cell breakdown.** At the top right, red cells, at the end of their life span, are engulfed by macrophages. Red cell hemoglobin is catabolized. The heme is broken down into bilirubin, which is exported into the plasma where it binds to albumin. This complex is taken up by the liver and the bilirubin is conjugated with glucuronide. Conjugated bilirubin is excreted in the bile. Normally the plasma contains very low amounts of conjugated bilirubin. In the presence of liver or biliary disease, increased levels of conjugated bilirubin will appear in the plasma (dashed arrow). RBC, red blood cell; Conj bili, conjugated bilirubin; Gluc, glucuronide; Fe, iron.

Most commonly, hemolysis occurs extravascularly within phagocytic macrophages. In patients with severe intravascular hemolysis, the amount of hemoglobin released from the lysed red cells exceeds the binding capacity of plasma haptoglobin. Free hemoglobin tetramers in the circulation ($\alpha_2\beta_2$) readily dissociate into $\alpha\beta$ dimers that are cleared by the renal glomeruli and reabsorbed by proximal tubule epithelial cells. Here, the hemoglobin is catabolized, and the heme iron is transferred to ferritin and hemosiderin (Chapter 5). Shedding of these cells results in the loss of iron, such that long-standing intravascular hemolysis can lead to iron deficiency. If the amount of filtered hemoglobin exceeds the reabsorptive capacity of the renal tubules, hemoglobin passes into the urine to produce a red-brown color (hemoglobinuria).

Once the presence of hemolysis is established, specific laboratory tests are available that, when used rationally in conjunction with relevant information from the history and physical examination, are very effective at homing in on specific causes. In planning the diagnostic workup, it is useful to draw on a coherent classification of the hemolytic anemias. Two different approaches, summarized in Table 3-2, are useful in considering these disorders. One approach groups hemolytic anemias according to whether the causative insult is an environmental factor versus a defect involving the cell membrane or the inside of the cell (hemoglobin or enzymes). A second approach distinguishes between inherited and acquired forms. These principles should be of value in understanding the different hemolytic anemias described in Chapters 9, 10, and 11.

TABLE 3-2 Classification of the Hemolytic Anemias

Environmental Factors
  Antibody: Immunohemolytic anemias
  Mechanical trauma: TTP, HUS, heart valve
  Toxins, infectious agents: Malaria, etc.
		Acquired

Membrane Defects
  Spur cell anemia
  Paroxysmal nocturnal hemoglobinuria
  Hereditary spherocytosis		

Defects of Cell Interior
  Hemoglobinopathies
  Enzymopathies
		Congenital

SELF-ASSESSMENT STUDY QUESTIONS

1. Which of the following laboratory tests would be least informative for establishing the presence of ineffective erythropoiesis in a patient with anemia?
   A. Serum lactate dehydrogenase level.
   B. Serum bilirubin level.
   C. Reticulocyte count.
   D. Serum erythropoietin level.
   E. Bone marrow examination.

2. Which of the following combinations of laboratory test values best supports the presence of hemolysis?
   A. Low lactate dehydrogenase, high unconjugated bilirubin, low haptoglobin.
   B. Low lactate dehydrogenase, high unconjugated bilirubin, high haptoglobin.
   C. High lactate dehydrogenase, high unconjugated bilirubin, low haptoglobin.
   D. High lactate dehydrogenase, high conjugated bilirubin, low haptoglobin.
   E. High lactate dehydrogenase, high conjugated bilirubin, high haptoglobin.

3. Which of the following provides the anemic patient with the most effective compensation for the deficit in red cell mass?
   A. Increased resting cardiac output.
   B. Increased red cell 2,3-diphosphoglycerate level and decreased red cell oxygen affinity.
   C. Increased red cell adenosine triphosphate level and increased red cell oxygen affinity.
   D. Increased plasma erythropoietin level.
   E. Increased arterial oxygen tension (pO_2).

4. What disorders are associated with small red cells (microcytosis)?

5. What disorders are associated with large red cells (macrocytosis)?

4

Anemias Due to Bone Marrow Failure or Infiltration

H. Franklin Bunn

LEARNING OBJECTIVES

After studying this chapter you should be able to:

- Establish a differential diagnosis of pancytopenia.
- Classify the primary bone marrow disorders.
- Explain the pathogenesis of aplastic anemia and the principles underlying its treatment.

It is clear from the information presented in Chapter 2 that the regulated production of circulating blood cells depends on the presence of an adequate number of functional multipotent hematopoietic stem cells. Accordingly, disease processes that either injure stem cells directly or compromise their environmental niche within the bone marrow result in a decrease in the numbers and sometimes the function of circulating blood cells. Thus, these bone marrow disorders often give rise to pancytopenia, a reduction in the numbers of circulating red cells, leukocytes, and platelets.

A variety of disorders can cause pancytopenia (Table 4-1). Because red cells, leukocytes, and platelets are all produced in the bone marrow, it is no surprise that microscopic examination of this organ by aspiration and biopsy is critical in evaluating patients with pancytopenia. As shown in the italicized portions of Table 4-1, this chapter will cover disorders involving injury to hematopoietic stem cells as well as those characterized by perturbation of the marrow microenvironment due to infiltration by cells that are extrinsic to the marrow (myelophthisis). Severe pancytopenia is a hallmark of marrow aplasia, whereas more variable degrees of cytopenia are encountered in myelophthisic disorders. Additional causes of pancytopenia listed in Table 4-1 are covered in other chapters of this book.

APLASTIC ANEMIA

ACQUIRED

Because over 95% of the cells in the bone marrow are progeny of hematopoietic stem cells, injury to these cells will result in a marked decrease in cellularity. Figure 4-1

TABLE 4-1 **Causes of Pancytopenia**

Category	Disorder
Hematopoietic stem cell injury	*Aplastic anemia**
	Idiopathic*
	Immune mediated*
	Secondary to drugs, toxins, irradiation, viruses*
	Fanconi anemia*
Clonal hematopoietic cell mutation	Acute leukemia (Chapter 21)
	Myelodysplasia (Chapter 20)
	Paroxysmal nocturnal hemoglobinuria (Chapter 11)
Myelophthisis (bone marrow infiltration)	*Metastatic cancer**
	Granulomatous disorders, tuberculosis*
	Lymphoma (Chapter 22)
	Myelofibrosis (Chapter 20)
Defective maturation	Megaloblastic anemias (Chapter 6)
Enhanced peripheral destruction	Hypersplenism (Chapter 1)
	Autoimmune disorders, systemic lupus erythematosus, etc.
	Hemophagocytic lymphohistiocytosis (Chapter 18)

*Discussed in this chapter.

compares a low-magnification view of normal bone marrow with that of bone marrow from a patient with severe aplastic anemia. In this specimen (Fig. 4-1B) it would be difficult to identify any cells of the erythroid, myeloid, or megakaryocyte lineages. The few cells that can be identified are a mix of lymphocytes, plasma cells, and marrow stroma that includes endothelial cells and fibroblasts.

Pathogenesis

Marrow aplasia is thought to arise from genetic alterations in hematopoietic stem cells, either spontaneous mutations or mutations induced by an extrinsic insult such as a drug, toxin, or viral infection. As shown in Figure 4-2, the genetic damage may either directly impair the stem cell's capacity for proliferation and differentiation or indirectly affect hematopoiesis by the induction of neoantigen expression in the stem cell and its progeny, which then triggers immune destruction via recruitment of cytotoxic T lymphocytes.

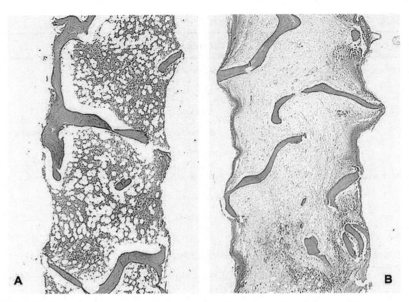

FIGURE 4-1   **Bone marrow biopsies.** A) Normal. B) Patient with aplastic anemia. (Courtesy of Dr. Stanley Schreier, American Society of Hematology Image Bank.)

Etiology

The most frequent cause of bone marrow aplasia is iatrogenic, due either to drugs or radiation therapy. Patients with malignancies are commonly treated with chemotherapeutic agents designed to kill tumor cells. Many of these interfere with DNA replication or with other critical aspects of cell growth and are therefore toxic to normal cells in the body that are continuously proliferating. Foremost among these are hematopoietic cells and gastrointestinal epithelial cells. Accordingly, patients treated with many of the commonly used cancer chemotherapy agents or with therapeutic ionizing radiation often develop pancytopenia, owing to bone marrow suppression. The myelosuppression that is induced is predictable, dose-related, and reversible. In contrast, certain drugs such as the antibiotic chloramphenicol can induce irreversible aplastic anemia in an idiosyncratic manner, affecting only an extremely small fraction of exposed individuals.

In evaluating patients with aplastic anemia, it is important to elicit a thorough history of exposure to toxic chemicals, particularly hydrocarbons and other industrial solvents. The most frequent offender is benzene. Viral infections, particularly non-A, non-B, and non-C hepatitis, can occasionally cause severe, irreversible marrow aplasia. It is not known whether the damage to hematopoietic stem cells is a direct consequence of the infection or is immune mediated. This is an exceedingly rare complication, whereas mild and fully reversible cytopenias are commonly seen in a wide variety of viral infections.

Patients with marrow aplasia not due to drugs, toxins, or viral infection are deemed to have idiopathic aplastic anemia. This is a rare disorder with an incidence of about two new cases per million people per year. By comparison, the incidences of acute leukemia and multiple myeloma are each about 15-fold higher.

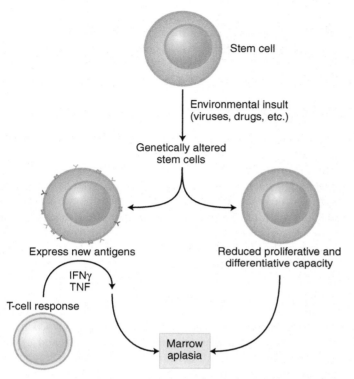

Stem cell

Environmental insult
(viruses, drugs, etc.)

Genetically altered
stem cells

Express new antigens

Reduced proliferative and
differentiative capacity

IFNγ
TNF

T-cell response

Marrow
aplasia

FIGURE 4-2 Pathogenesis of marrow aplasia. Damage to the genome of stem cells
may either cause defects that impair proliferation and differentiation or induce formation of
neoantigens that trigger immune destruction. (Red Blood Cell and Bleeding Disorders. In: Kumar V, Abbas, AK,
Fausto N, Aster JC, eds. *Robbins Pathologic Basis of Disease.* Philadelphia, U.S.A.: Elsevier; 2010: p. 663.)

As mentioned in the section on therapy on the following page, a substantial fraction of patients with idiopathic aplastic anemia respond to immunosuppressive
agents, but the mechanism underlying the immune attack on hematopoietic stem
cells has not been worked out.

Clinical Presentation and Diagnosis

The symptoms that bring these patients to the physician and the findings on physical examination are direct consequences of the severity of the cytopenias. Many
patients present with progressive fatigue and pallor, owing to anemia. Others have
petechiae or ecchymoses due to thrombocytopenia. Of most concern are patients
who present with fever and symptoms and signs of acute bacterial infection, as a
result of neutropenia. Of course many patients will have a combination of these
clinical findings. The physical examination usually reveals pallor, petechiae, perhaps ecchymoses, and often findings directly related to bacterial infection such as
an abscess or pneumonia. Lymph nodes and the spleen are not enlarged. A complete blood count usually will reveal marked pancytopenia. The average red cell
size or volume (MCV) is often modestly increased, and the reticulocyte percentage and absolute reticulocyte count are very low. The white cell differential count

shows neutropenia and monocytopenia, with relative preservation of lymphocyte numbers due to the long life spans of these cells. A bone aspirate and biopsy are essential for establishing the diagnosis. Histologic sections of a normal marrow generally reveal 35% to 50% cellularity (Fig. 4-1A), whereas in aplastic anemia the cellularity is usually below 10% (Fig. 4-1B).

Therapy, Clinical Course, and Prognosis

Once the diagnosis of aplastic anemia is made, attention should immediately focus on discontinuing any exposure to drugs or toxins that could be myelosuppressive. In the past, the treatment of aplastic anemia was entirely supportive: administration of red cell and platelet transfusions as needed to correct the anemia and prevent bleeding from thrombocytopenia, along with antibiotics to treat infections. Despite these interventions, the vast majority of patients with severe disease died, generally from overwhelming sepsis. Meticulous supportive care continues to be critically important. However, the majority of patients with severe aplastic anemia can now be brought into remission and many cured with either hematopoietic stem cell transplantation or immunosuppressive therapy.

Historically, the first patients treated with stem cell transplantation were those with aplastic anemia. The initial results were sufficiently encouraging that this therapy was extended to patients with other hematologic disorders (discussed in Chapter 26). During the last 30 years, advances in transplantation regimens and supportive care have produced higher rates of engraftment and lower incidences of graft-versus-host disease and opportunistic infections, leading to a marked improvement in disease-free survival. Currently, about 75% of patients age 20 or younger receiving stem cells from HLA-matched sibling donors go into long-term, stable hematologic remissions and can be considered cured. In patients older than 40, this figure drops to about 40%. The results are less impressive with transplants from unrelated donors.

Patients who lack a suitable stem cell donor or who are too old to undergo transplantation are treated with immunosuppressive therapy, generally consisting of a combination of a calcineurin inhibitor such as cyclosporine and antithymocyte or antilymphocyte globulin. The fact that nearly three-fourths of patients with idiopathic aplastic anemia respond suggests that immune-mediated destruction of hematopoietic progenitors plays a major role in its pathogenesis (Fig. 4-2). Compared with stem cell transplantation, immunosuppressive therapy is less expensive and has less immediate toxicity. However, remissions are less stable and nearly a third of patients eventually develop a clonal hematologic disorder such as myelodysplasia, acute leukemia, or paroxysmal nocturnal hemoglobinuria. These dreaded late complications are much less often seen in patients treated with stem cell transplantation.

Pure Red Cell Aplasia

Rarely, a patient may present with severe anemia and virtual absence of reticulocytes but normal platelet, white cell, and differential counts. As shown in Figure 4-3, the bone marrow reveals normal cellularity and normal megakaryocytes and myeloid precursors but a virtual absence of erythroid precursors. An immune-mediated pathogenesis is suggested by the presence of thymoma (a tumor of thymic epithelial

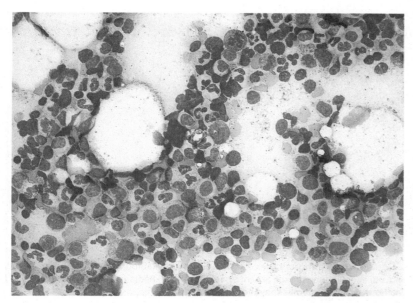

FIGURE 4-3 Bone marrow aspirate smear of a patient with pure red cell aplasia. Note the absence of erythroid precursor cells. (Courtesy of Dr. Peter Maslak, American Society of Hematology Image Bank.)

cells), lymphoma, or an autoimmune disorder in about a third of patients, as well as frequent and long-lasting responses to immunosuppressive therapy. On rare occasions, pure red cell aplasia can occur in a patient treated with recombinant erythropoietin, due to development of an autoantibody that inactivates both the pharmacologic erythropoietin and the patient's endogenous erythropoietin.

Acute, transient suppression of erythropoiesis can be caused by infection with parvovirus B19, which has specific tropism for erythroid precursor cells. In normal individuals, parvovirus B19 infection causes an erythemic rash (fifth disease) and no more than a modest drop in hemoglobin levels. However, patients with underlying chronic hemolytic anemias such as sickle cell disease develop a sudden and marked drop in hemoglobin, owing to a combination of acute suppression of erythropoiesis and ongoing rapid destruction of circulating red cells.

CONGENITAL

Bone marrow failure can be encountered in newborns and infants as a feature of a number of rare genetic disorders, many with complex phenotypes. Here we will consider only two: Fanconi anemia, the most often encountered and best characterized of the congenital causes of bone marrow failure, and Diamond-Blackfan anemia, a congenital disorder that closely parallels acquired pure red cell aplasia.

Fanconi anemia

This rare, autosomal recessive disorder has an incidence of about three per one million births. Fanconi anemia is characterized by progressive bone marrow failure along

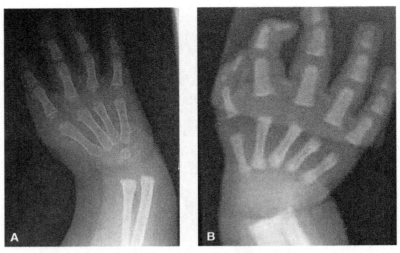

FIGURE 4-4 **Hand abnormalities, Fanconi anemia.** A) Radiograph of the hand of a child with Fanconi anemia, showing the absence of the thumb. B) Radiograph of the hand of a child with Diamond-Blackfan anemia, showing a triphalangeal thumb.

with a heterogeneous group of congenital anomalies, particularly abnormal skin pigmentation (café au lait spots), short stature, and skeletal, gonadal, and renal defects. Figure 4-4A shows a patient lacking a thumb, a relatively common skeletal defect in Fanconi anemia. Affected individuals have a defect in one or another of the components of a multiprotein complex that plays a key role in DNA repair. About 10% of patients with Fanconi anemia develop acute myeloid leukemia. Patients may enter prolonged remissions following stem cell transplantation.

Diamond-Blackfan anemia

Diamond-Blackfan anemia is a rare disorder (about five per million births) that is both genetically and clinically heterogeneous. Anemia is usually detected either at birth or within the first year of life but occasionally may appear later in life. Affected babies often have underlying skeletal (particularly thumb [Fig. 4-4B]), renal, craniofacial, or cardiac anomalies. Short stature is common. Similar to that in acquired pure red cell aplasia, the bone marrow in Diamond-Blackfan anemia has a paucity of erythroid precursors, whereas myeloid precursors and megakaryocytes are normal, giving rise to normal peripheral white cell and platelet counts. Like children with Fanconi anemia, those with Diamond-Blackfan anemia are at increased risk of developing malignancies. About half of children with the Diamond-Blackfan anemia clinical phenotype are heterozygotes with a mutation in one of the proteins of the small or large ribosome subunit. In addition, red cells of affected individuals often have markedly increased activity of adenosine deaminase, an enzyme in the purine salvage pathway, which can be used to support the diagnosis. It is not yet clear how either the defect in a ribosomal protein or the enhanced adenosine deaminase activity contributes to the pathogenesis and clinical phenotype. Nor is it clear why most patients respond to steroid therapy.

MYELOPHTHISIC ANEMIA

Patients may develop anemia often accompanied by thrombocytopenia and occasionally leukopenia when the bone marrow space is secondarily invaded by one of several different types of disease processes, a phenomenon referred to as *myelophthisis*. The most frequent cause of myelophthisic anemia is metastatic cancer. Breast, lung, and prostate carcinomas are particularly frequent culprits. Metastatic cancers not only replace the marrow but also often activate marrow fibroblasts, leading to extensive deposition of collagen. This reactive fibrosis distorts the marrow microenvironment, disrupting the production of hematopoietic cells and leading to the release of immature marrow elements. These deleterious effects on marrow function are reflected in peripheral blood films (Fig. 4-5), which generally show prominent tear-drop red cells and the presence of nucleated red cells, sometimes accompanied by immature myeloid forms. The tumor cells often appear in large clumps in marrow aspirates and can usually be readily distinguished from normal hematopoietic cells. Figure 4-6 shows clumps of tumor cells in the marrow of patients with rhabdomyosarcoma (A) and bladder carcinoma (B). In some instances the tumor cells cannot be recovered in bone marrow aspirates because of the marrow fibrosis and are seen only in biopsies. At the point at which myelophthisic anemia emerges, cancers have advanced to the point at which therapy seldom induces remission.

Myelophthisic anemia also occurs in hematologic malignancies—both lymphomas and leukemias—but in these settings the patient's anemia is less likely to be accompanied by the peripheral blood morphology shown in Figure 4-5, probably because in most instances the degree of marrow fibrosis is less than that seen with metastatic cancers. Other causes of myelophthisic anemia are myeloproliferative

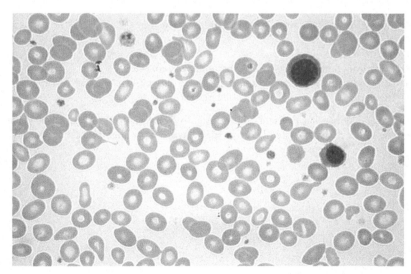

FIGURE 4-5   Peripheral blood film from a patient with myelofibrosis. Note the tear-drop cells and nucleated red cells. (Diseases of White Blood Cells, Lymph Nodes, Spleen And Thymus. In: Kumar V, Abbas, AK, Fausto N, Aster JC, eds. *Robbins Pathologic Basis of Disease.* Philadelphia, U.S.A.: Elsevier; 2010: p. 631.)

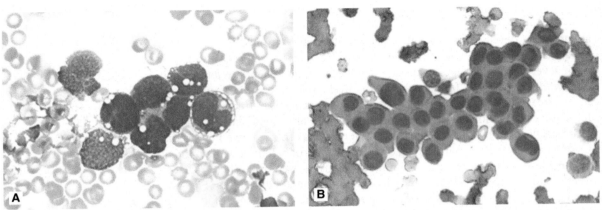

FIGURE 4-6 **Bone marrow aspirate smears showing the presence of clumps of tumor cells.** A) Rhabdomyosarcoma. B) Bladder carcinoma. (Image B Courtesy of Dr. Peter Maslak, American Society of Hematology Image Bank.)

disorders associated with reactive marrow fibrosis, particularly primary myelofibrosis (Chapter 20), and disseminated granulomatous diseases such as miliary tuberculosis.

SELF-ASSESSMENT STUDY QUESTIONS

1. What is the best evidence that idiopathic aplastic anemia is an autoimmune disorder?
    A. The presence of serum antibodies against red cells, neutrophils, and platelets.
    B. The presence of increased cytotoxic T lymphocytes in bone marrow.
    C. The presence of infiltrates of B lymphocytes in bone marrow.
    D. Splenomegaly.
    E. Reversal of aplasia with immunosuppressive therapy.

2. Patients with Fanconi anemia have a congenital defect in:
    A. Synthesis of DNA.
    B. Repair of DNA.
    C. The production of pluripotent hematopoietic stem cells.
    D. The production of an important hematopoietic cytokine–stem cell factor.
    E. The homing of stem cells to the bone marrow.

3. A 67-year-old man has prostate cancer. Recently he developed severe anemia. What finding in the peripheral blood is most suggestive that the anemia is caused by metastases to the bone marrow?
    A. Thrombocytopenia.
    B. Neutropenia.
    C. Leukocytosis.
    D. Thrombocytosis (increased platelet count).
    E. The presence of nucleated red blood cells.

Iron Homeostasis: Deficiency and Overload

H. Franklin Bunn and Matthew M. Heeney

LEARNING OBJECTIVES

After studying this chapter you should be able to:

- Construct a flow diagram depicting iron homeostasis: absorption from the gut, transport in the plasma, incorporation into erythroid precursors, release from senescent red cells, and return to the plasma.
- Explain the important role of hepcidin in iron absorption from the gut and release of iron from macrophages.
- Name and prioritize the causes of iron deficiency.
- Describe the key laboratory features of iron deficiency.
- Identify the causes of iron overload and its clinical manifestations.

In all organisms from bacteria to man, iron is by far the most important metallic element. Its outer shell of electrons is ideally poised for complex coordination chemistry, enabling the binding of ligands such as oxygen as well as participation in critical oxidation-reduction reactions. Iron is essential not only for the biological activity of heme proteins such as hemoglobin, myoglobin, and cytochromes but also as a key cofactor in a number of enzymes spanning a wide range of metabolism. However, because of iron's high degree of reactivity, it can catalyze the generation of oxygen free radicals and other toxic species, leading to cellular and tissue injury by way of protein cross-links, lipid peroxidation, and damage to DNA. Therefore, in order for iron to safely fulfill its biological functions, an exquisite degree of control is required. In this chapter we will review the basic elements of iron homeostasis: absorption, transport, utilization, recycling, and excretion. During the last decade, understanding of these processes has been enormously enhanced by the molecular cloning and characterization of critical genes, some of which were discovered by investigation of mutant mice and zebra fish whose phenotypes suggested perturbed iron metabolism.

This chapter will begin with an overview of iron homeostasis, as this information is essential for understanding the pathogenesis, clinical features, and treatment of iron deficiency and iron overload.

NORMAL IRON HOMEOSTASIS

Safe and effective transport and utilization of iron are achieved by tight regulation at the level of both individual cells and the organism as a whole. The expression of a number of proteins that play critical roles in iron metabolism is regulated by the intracellular concentration of iron. This is achieved through a consensus stem loop sequence in the messenger ribonucleic acids (mRNAs) that encode these proteins. When iron is scarce, two iron regulatory proteins (IRPs) bind specifically to this stem loop and modify either the stability or rate of translation of the mRNAs, whereas when intracellular iron is abundant, the IRPs assume a conformation that precludes mRNA binding. Systemic iron metabolism is regulated by the circulating polypeptide hormone *hepcidin*, which controls both dietary iron absorption from the gut and release of recycled iron from macrophages. These two modes of regulation are described in detail later in this chapter.

IRON ABSORPTION

The dietary sources of iron vary considerably according to geographic location, cultural tastes, and economic status. Iron in food consists of inorganic salts and organic complexes derived from plants as well as heme from animal sources. Digestion of grains, vegetables, and fruits in the stomach and duodenum results in the release of ferric iron. As depicted in Figure 5-1, normal individuals absorb only 1 to 2 mg of iron per day, primarily at the villous tips of duodenal enterocytes. A ferrireductase at this site reduces the iron to its ferrous form, allowing it to enter the cell through a luminal transmembrane channel, the divalent metal transporter DMT1 (Fig. 5-2). A portion of the iron that has entered the enterocyte may be stored within a porous multimeric protein cage called *ferritin*. Ferrous iron exits from the cell through the transport protein ferroportin, which is localized within the plasma membrane on the abluminal or basolateral side of the enterocyte. Here the iron is rapidly oxidized to the ferric form that binds transferrin, the plasma protein responsible for iron transport throughout the circulation. As shown in Figure 5-2, the export of iron from the duodenal enterocyte can be suppressed by hepcidin, a small polypeptide hormone produced in the liver. The binding of hepcidin to its receptor, ferroportin, triggers the latter's internalization and subsequent degradation. As a result, the rate of egress of iron from the enterocyte is markedly dampened.

Among individuals from North and South America as well as Europe, a substantial portion of dietary iron is in the form of hemoglobin and myoglobin within meat and other animal sources. Following proteolytic degradation of these proteins in the stomach and proximal intestine, heme is released and absorbed intact into the enterocyte, where it is degraded by heme oxygenase, resulting in the release of iron that is either stored as ferritin or exits from the cell via ferroportin. The luminal heme channel/importer has not yet been identified.

IRON TRANSPORT

The plasma protein transferrin binds ferric iron at two sites with extraordinarily high affinity. As a result of such tight binding, the concentration of free iron in the plasma is too low to be easily measured. Thus transferrin effectively protects tissues and

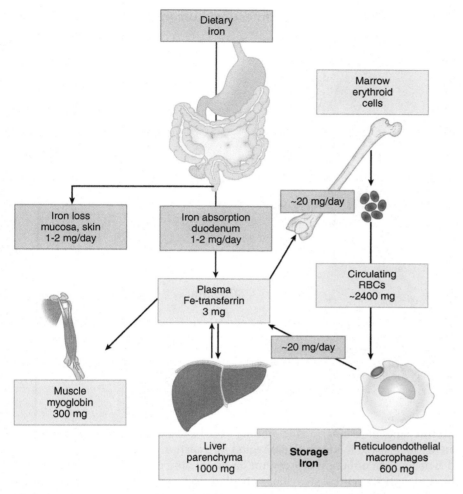

FIGURE 5-1 **Iron homeostasis and distribution within the body: absorption, transfer to Fe-transferrin, incorporation into heme in red cell hemoglobin and muscle myoglobin, storage in the liver and reticuloendothelial system, and reutilization.** These values pertain to a 70-kg adult male.

cells from the toxicity of "free" iron. As shown in Figure 5-1, transferrin picks up iron either from duodenal enterocytes or from macrophages, which (as discussed later in the "Iron Recycling" section) accumulate iron recycled from hemoglobin in senescent red cells.

IRON ENTRY INTO CELLS

All cells except the duodenal enterocyte take up iron via the binding of Fe-transferrin to transferrin receptors on the plasma membrane. In keeping with their obligation to produce high levels of hemoglobin, erythroid precursor cells express much higher levels of transferrin receptors than do other cells. As illustrated in Figure 5-3, the expression of transferrin receptor is regulated in an

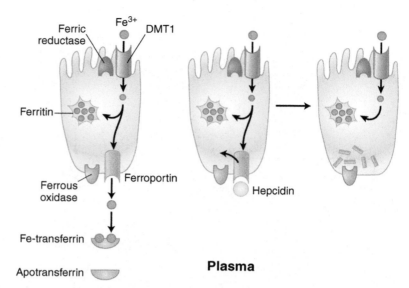

FIGURE 5-2 Absorption and egress of iron in the duodenal enterocyte. Iron (Fe^{3+}) within the duodenal lumen is reduced to Fe^{2+} which enters the cell through divalent metal transporter (DMT1) and exits the cell on the other (abluminal) side through ferroportin and is oxidized to Fe^{3+}. The binding of the master regulator hepcidin to ferroportin (*middle*) causes rapid internalization and degradation (*right*) of ferroportin, thereby blocking further egress of iron from the cell.

iron-dependent manner by the binding of IRPs to earlier-mentioned consensus stem loops at the 3′ untranslated region of transferrin receptor mRNA. In iron deficiency, when there is a premium on optimizing entry of iron into cells, the binding of IRPs to these stem loops greatly enhances the stability of the transferrin receptor mRNA and thereby increases protein expression. Up-regulation of the transport protein DMT1 in iron deficiency also depends on enhanced mRNA stability via binding of IRPs to 3′ mRNA stem loops.

Transferrin molecules loaded with two iron atoms have much greater affinity for the receptor than do those with either a single atom or none. As shown in Figure 5-4, the iron-transferrin/transferrin receptor complex is rapidly internalized as a plasma membrane microvesicle that includes the iron transport protein DMT1. A proton pump docks onto this microvesicle and acidifies its interior, thereby releasing iron, which then exits via DMT1. Once in the cytosol, this iron either goes to mitochondria for heme biosynthesis or is stored as ferritin.

IRON UTILIZATION IN ERYTHROPOIESIS

In vivo studies using radiolabeled iron have shown that more than 90% of transferrin-bound iron in the plasma goes to erythroid cells in the bone marrow and is incorporated into heme in hemoglobin. Normally, this process is very efficient. In contrast, in patients with ineffective erythropoiesis or marrow hypoplasia, only

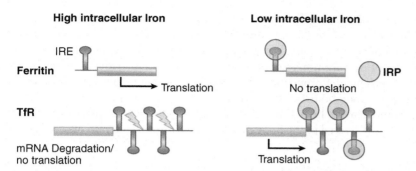

FIGURE 5-3 Iron-dependent regulation of the rate of translation of ferritin messenger ribonucleic acid (mRNA) and the stability of transferrin receptor (TfR) mRNA. When the intracellular iron level is low, iron regulatory proteins (IRPs) bind to a consensus stem loop iron regulatory element in the respective mRNAs, resulting in enhancement of transferrin receptor mRNA levels and suppression of ferritin translation. When the intracellular iron level is high, the IRPs do not bind to the stem loops. Transferrin receptor mRNA is degraded (*yellow arrows*), and translation of ferritin is unimpeded.

a small proportion of circulating Fe-transferrin is incorporated into circulating red cells.

IRON RECYCLING

Normal red cells survive in the blood for about 120 days. When they reach their dotage, they are recognized and taken up primarily by splenic macrophages (Fig. 5-1), where

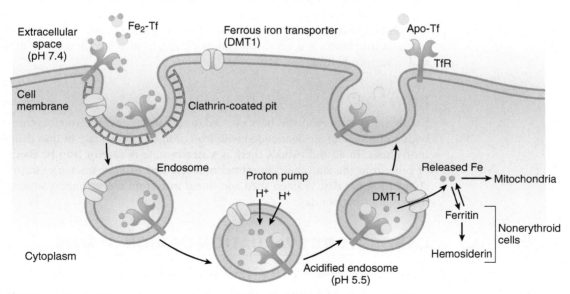

FIGURE 5-4 The uptake of transferrin-bound iron (Fe₂-Tf) into a cell via the transferrin receptor (TfR). Microvesicles containing the Fe₂-Tf/TfR complex fuse with a proton pump, which acidifies the interior of the microvesicle, triggering the release of iron, which then exits via divalent metal transporter (DMT1). Once the iron atoms are released, the TfR releases apotransferrin (Apo-Tf). When the vesicle fuses with the plasma membrane, apotransferrin is returned to the plasma.

the hemoglobin is degraded with the release of its iron into ferritin stores. Similar to the mechanism of its exit from the duodenal enterocyte (Fig. 5-2), iron exits from the macrophage via ferroportin and is bound to transferrin in the plasma. The flux of iron from macrophages back to the bone marrow is about 20 mg per day, a much greater proportion of the daily utilization than the influx of iron from the duodenum (about 1-2 mg/day). Thus *in vivo* iron homeostasis invests heavily in a high-capacity, high-throughput cycle in which iron derived from senescent red cells is delivered to the bone marrow for incorporation into new red cells.

IRON STORAGE

Because free iron is so toxic to cells and tissues, it is important that whatever iron is not being used for synthesis of heme or for other purposes is sequestered within the cell as a storage depot that can be tapped as needed. The challenge of safe and highly bioavailable dynamic storage of iron is met by ferritin, a protein that assembles into a 24-subunit cage surrounding an inner core of iron hydroxide. The production of ferritin is exquisitely attuned to the cell's needs. As shown in Figure 5-3, when iron is scarce, ferritin production is halted because the binding of IRPs to the stem loop iron in the 5′ end of ferritin mRNA blocks translation. In contrast, when iron is abundant, the IRPs can no longer bind to the stem loop, and translation is unimpeded. With increasing accumulation of cellular iron, some of the ferritin becomes denatured and is converted to hemosiderin, from which iron is less readily mobilized. The preponderance of body iron is stored as ferritin and hemosiderin in two sites shown in Figure 5-1: about 600 mg in reticuloendothelial macrophages that include hepatic Kupffer cells and about 1000 mg in hepatic parenchymal cells. These estimates pertain to men of all ages. Women in the childbearing age group have less stored iron because of blood loss from menses and iron usurpation by the fetus during pregnancy. Because the accumulation of iron stores is a very slow process, children also have low levels of liver and macrophage iron.

IRON LOSS

No physiologic mechanisms have evolved to enhance the rate of iron loss from the body in those who are overloaded with iron or to retard this rate in iron deficient individuals. In all individuals there is a steady-state release of iron by shedding of cells from the skin, hair, intestinal mucosa, and urinary tract, amounting to about 1 mg per day. Women shed additional iron from menstruation amounting to roughly 1 mg per day.

LABORATORY EVALUATION OF IRON STATUS

SERUM IRON AND TRANSFERRIN SATURATION

Except in patients with iron overload, virtually all of the iron in plasma and serum is bound to transferrin. The interpretation of serum Fe-transferrin levels is considerably enhanced by concurrent measurement of total transferrin in serum, thereby providing an index of the fractional saturation of transferrin with iron.

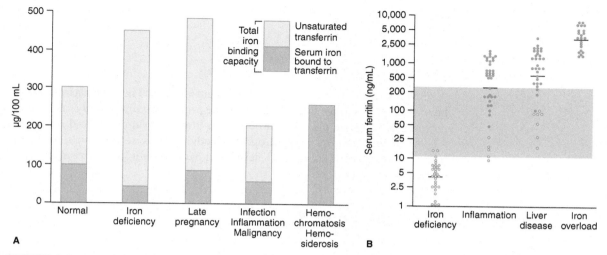

FIGURE 5-5 Laboratory assessment of iron status. A) Serum iron and transferrin saturation in different disorders. B) Serum ferritin in different disorders. Note that the Y-axis in this panel is on a log scale. The open circles represent iron deficiency either uncomplicated (left) or in association with inflammation or liver disease. (Image B was adapted from Lipschitz DA, Cook JD, and Finch CA. A clinical evaluation of serum ferritin as an index of iron stores. N Eng J Med 1974;290:1213-6. Copyright © 1974 Massachusetts Medical Society, all rights reserved)

As shown in Figure 5-5A, patients with iron deficiency have both low serum iron and elevated total transferrin levels and therefore very low fractional saturation. The level of total transferrin in the plasma is also elevated during pregnancy and in women taking oral contraceptives. Patients with inflammatory disorders, discussed in Chapter 7, have both low serum iron levels and low levels of total transferrin. Accordingly, fractional transferrin saturation is often normal. Patients with iron overload usually have elevated serum iron levels, but, importantly, fractional saturation of transferrin is very high.

SERUM FERRITIN

A small fraction of ferritin subunits are released from iron storage depots in macrophages and the liver and enter the plasma, unattached to iron. Measurement of serum ferritin is an accurate surrogate index of iron stores in the body. Thus, as shown in Figure 5-5B, serum ferritin levels are low in iron deficiency and elevated not only in patients with iron overload but also in those with inflammation, tissue damage (e.g., cancer, trauma), and liver disease. In patients with concurrent iron deficiency and either inflammation or liver disease, serum ferritin levels are usually in the normal range.

BONE MARROW AND LIVER IRON STORES

The most direct way to assess iron stores in macrophages is by staining of a bone marrow aspirate with Prussian blue, which is specific for iron. Iron stores in the liver can be assessed in biopsies qualitatively by Prussian blue staining of tissue sections or quantitatively by direct measurement of iron. Some medical centers are equipped to assess liver iron stores non-invasively by means of magnetic resonance imaging.

SERUM TRANSFERRIN RECEPTOR

A small fraction of transferrin receptor protein is released into the plasma and can be measured in serum. Because a very large proportion of the body's transferrin receptor is expressed on erythroid cells, the level of serum erythroid receptor is a good surrogate index of erythropoietic activity. Thus, serum levels are low in patients with marrow aplasia and elevated in patients with ineffective erythropoiesis and hemolysis.

IRON DEFICIENCY

ETIOLOGY

Iron deficiency is the most prevalent cause of anemia worldwide. In the vast majority of cases, it is due to blood loss. Heavy menstrual blood flow (menorrhagia) and pregnancy frequently lead to iron deficiency in women in the childbearing age group. Gastrointestinal bleeding is commonly encountered in males and females of all age groups, owing to a variety of lesions including esophageal varices, gastritis, peptic ulcer, diverticula, polyps, cancer, and hemorrhoids. In parts of the world where intestinal parasites such as hookworm are endemic, iron deficiency anemia is particularly widespread and severe. Patients with upper intestinal malabsorption, such as celiac disease, develop anemia because of impaired uptake of iron from the duodenum. Infants whose diets consist primarily of cow's milk often become iron deficient. However, the prevalence has been lessened by increased breast feeding and the widespread use of iron-fortified formulas. Although inadequate diet is an uncommon cause of iron deficiency, adolescents are at risk if their nutrition consists primarily of non-nutritious snack foods. Because the efficiency of iron absorption is enhanced by low gastric pH, elderly people with achlorhydria are at increased risk of becoming iron deficient.

CLINICAL FEATURES

The signs and symptoms of iron deficiency are primarily based on the degree of anemia, as discussed in Chapter 3. However, there are clinical features associated specifically with iron deficiency. Both children and adults may evince pica, a peculiar need to chew or gnaw on non-digestible substances such as clay (geophagia) or ice (pagophagia). Much less commonly, patients with severe iron deficiency may have concave nail beds (spoon nails or koilonychia), fissures at the angles of the mouth, or a thin membrane web in the esophagus that can cause dysphagia. There is evidence that iron deficient children may have impairment in cognition and learning that cannot be explained by the degree of anemia. It is less certain whether adults have compromised mental or physical performance due to iron deficiency per se.

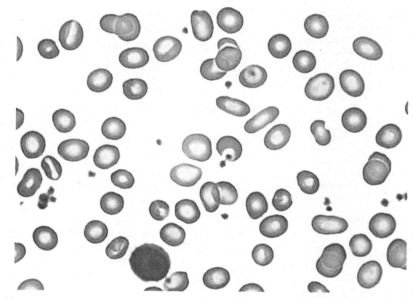

FIGURE 5-6   Blood smear from a patient with severe iron deficiency anemia. Note the microcytosis and hypochromia of the red cells and the presence of "pencil" cells and target cells. Normal red cells are the size of the small lymphocyte in the bottom of the field.

HEMATOLOGICAL FEATURES

The development of iron deficiency can be tracked quite accurately by changes in laboratory results. Incipient iron deficiency is characterized by normal hemoglobin, hematocrit, red cell indices, and serum iron level but absence of iron stores in the liver and in macrophages. As the deficiency becomes more severe, the mean red cell volume falls, followed by a decrease in hematocrit and hemoglobin concentrations. During this time, serum ferritin and iron levels fall, whereas serum iron binding capacity (total transferrin) rises. With further worsening of the deficiency, the patient becomes increasingly anemic, and microcytosis is then accompanied by hypochromia, a decrease in mean red cell hemoglobin concentration. The blood smear reveals small red cells with an increase in central pallor, along with abnormalities in red cell shape, including pencil forms and a wide range in cell size. These morphologic changes are illustrated in Figure 5-6. The white blood cell count is normal, but the platelet count is often elevated for unclear reasons.

TREATMENT

Oral administration of iron salts, particularly ferrous sulfate, has been standard therapy for nearly a century. However, most patients have difficulty tolerating oral iron, owing to gastrointestinal symptoms such as heartburn and constipation. Recently developed preparations of soluble iron-carbohydrate complexes have proven to be safe and effective when administered intravenously, and they offer assurance of full iron replacement without dependence on patient compliance.

TABLE 5-1 Laboratory Evaluation of Iron Status

	Deficiency	Overload
Serum iron	↓	↑-↑↑
Total iron binding capacity	↑	normal
Transferrin saturation	↓-↓↓	↑-↑↑
Serum ferritin	↓	↑-↑↑
Serum transferrin receptor	↑	normal
Bone marrow iron	0-↓	normal-↑↑
Liver iron	0-↓	↑-↑↑↑

Patients with uncomplicated iron deficiency anemia respond with a burst of reticulocytes, peaking about a week after initiation of iron therapy. During the ensuing weeks, the hematocrit and mean red cell volume gradually return to normal levels. The importance of iron replacement therapy is matched by the need to establish the cause of the deficiency. All patients should be evaluated for gastrointestinal blood loss. Unless there is a convincing explanation for iron deficiency such as menorrhagia, frequent blood donations, or upper intestinal malabsorption, the diagnostic inquiry should extend beyond testing the stool for occult blood to radiologic/endoscopic evaluation of the gastrointestinal tract.

IRON OVERLOAD

As mentioned earlier in this chapter, molecular adaptation has provided a number of safeguards to protect the body against oxidative damage from free iron. However, there are both inherited and acquired disorders in which these safeguards are not adequate to prevent morbidity and mortality resulting from excess iron. Irrespective of etiology, patients with significant iron overload share a number of clinical and laboratory features. The target organs vulnerable to damage include the heart, liver, and endocrine glands, particularly pituitary, gonads, and pancreatic islets. Not surprisingly, as shown in Table 5-1, laboratory results in disorders of iron overload are the mirror opposite of those in iron deficiency.

HEREDITARY HEMOCHROMATOSIS

Inherited disorders of iron overload involve defects either in hepcidin expression or in its receptor ferroportin. The most commonly encountered form of hereditary hemochromatosis is due to a single missense mutation (C282Y[1]) in the gene *HFE*, which encodes a transmembrane protein that is homologous to major histocompatibility class 1 proteins and, like them, binds to beta-2 microglobulin. This mutation is encountered in about 10% of individuals of European ancestry. Thus, about 1 in 400 people of European lineage are homozygotes. Heterozygotes have no clinical manifestations of hemochromatosis. The penetrance of the defect in homozygotes is low; only about 10% of homozygotes are at risk for developing organ damage from iron overload. In those affected, the signs and symptoms are not apparent until middle age in men and even later in women, owing to iron loss from menstruation and pregnancy. In addition to findings that are a direct consequence of damage to the heart, liver, and endocrine glands, patients with hereditary hemochromatosis often have increased skin pigmentation and complain of fatigue and arthralgia.

[1]Replacement of cysteine by tyrosine at amino acid 282 in HFE.

Much less commonly, adult-onset hereditary hemochromatosis can be caused by mutations in transferrin receptor 2 and ferroportin. In addition, there are rare kindreds with juvenile hemochromatosis who develop iron-induced organ damage early in life as a result of mutations in either hepcidin or a protein called hemojuvelin. The molecular pathogenesis of hereditary hemochromatosis has been dramatically clarified by the discovery of hepcidin and its key role in regulating iron homeostasis. HFE, transferrin receptor 2, and hemojuvelin all participate in the up-regulation of hepcidin transcription. Thus, inactivating mutations of these genes as well as of hepcidin deprive cells of this key regulator and result in iron overload due to enhancement of absorption from the gut and egress from macrophages.

Serum transferrin saturation is the best screening test for detecting patients with iron overload. The diagnosis of hereditary hemochromatosis often can be validated by demonstration of homozygosity of the C282Y *HFE* mutation. If this test is negative, a liver biopsy and/or further genetic analysis may be required.

Adults with hereditary hemochromatosis generally respond quite well to regular phlebotomies to lower their iron stores. If begun prior to the development of organ damage, this intervention has proven effective in preventing diabetes, cardiac failure, and cirrhosis.

SECONDARY HEMOSIDEROSIS

As mentioned earlier in this chapter, the only way the body excretes iron is by the constant and unregulated shedding of epithelial cells (about 1-2 mg Fe/day). Anemic patients who are dependent on transfusions have a marked increase in the intake of iron. One unit of whole blood or packed red cells contains about 250 mg of iron. Thus, a patient who receives two units per month has an additional intake of 500 mg of iron, whereas the amount of iron excreted remains around 50 mg per month. Accordingly, heavily transfused patients inexorably develop iron overload. In certain anemic patients this problem is compounded by a second independent process. Patients with anemia due to ineffective erythropoiesis, such as β-thalassemia major and intermedia (Chapter 8) or sideroblastic anemia (described below) have an inappropriate and maladaptive enhancement of iron absorption from the gut, owing to suppressed hepcidin levels. It follows then that patients with ineffective erythropoiesis who are transfusion-dependent have a very high rate of iron accumulation.

Like patients with hereditary hemochromatosis, those with secondary hemosiderosis are at risk of damage to the heart, liver, and endocrine glands. Because all of these patients are anemic, the contribution of iron overload to fatigue and skin color is much harder to assess. Moreover, they are much less likely to complain about arthralgia than those with hereditary hemochromatosis.

Because all patients with secondary hemosiderosis are anemic, therapeutic phlebotomy is not an option. They must be treated with iron chelation, the details of which are presented in Chapter 8.

SIDEROBLASTIC ANEMIA

Normally, as shown in Figure 5-1, each day a large amount of iron (about 20 mg) enters erythroid precursors in the marrow, where it is rapidly and efficiently incorporated into hemoglobin. The insertion of iron into protoporphyrin IX to make heme takes place in mitochondria. In certain congenital and acquired anemias, there is a block in the incorporation of iron into heme in erythroid cells and a buildup of iron in mitochondria. This results in the appearance of ringed sideroblasts, erythroid precursors with iron-laden mitochondria that can be detected with a Prussian blue stain (see Fig. 20-8C, Chapter 20). Hemoglobin production tends to be defective in sideroblastic anemias, sometimes giving rise to a population of microcytic red cells.

Congenital sideroblastic anemia is very uncommon. Most affected individuals are males who have inherited a mutation in the X-linked gene encoding erythroid-specific δ-aminolevulinic acid synthase, the rate-limiting step in heme biosynthesis.

In contrast, acquired sideroblastic anemias are quite often encountered. In some patients there is a transient and reversible dysregulation of erythropoiesis following exposure to a toxic substance, most commonly ethanol but occasionally a drug such as the antibiotic chloramphenicol. Ringed sideroblasts are also frequently seen in patients with myelodysplastic syndromes (Chapter 20), a relatively common cause of anemia in the elderly.

SELF-ASSESSMENT STUDY QUESTIONS

1. In combination with low mean cell volume (MCV), which of the following laboratory test findings are most consistent with iron deficiency?
   A. Normal mean cell hemoglobin concentration (MCHC), low serum iron level, low iron binding capacity, low serum ferritin level.
   B. Low MCHC, low serum iron level, high iron binding capacity, low serum ferritin level.
   C. Low MCHC, low serum iron level, low iron binding capacity, low serum ferritin level.
   D. Low MCHC, low serum iron level, high iron binding capacity, high serum ferritin level.
   E. Normal MCHC, low serum iron level, high iron binding capacity, high serum ferritin level.

2. In normal individuals, what is the major source of iron bound to serum transferrin?
   A. Absorption of inorganic iron from the duodenum.
   B. Absorption of heme iron from the duodenum.
   C. Breakdown of senescent red blood cells.
   D. Release of iron from hepatocytes.
   E. Release of iron from muscle myoglobin.

3. What is the common denominator in the pathogenesis of hereditary hemochromatosis?
   A. Impaired expression of hepcidin.
   B. Enhanced expression of transferrin receptor.
   C. Enhanced expression of ferritin.
   D. Impaired expression of transferrin.
   E. Enhanced expression of ferroportin.

Megaloblastic Anemias

H. Franklin Bunn and Matthew Heeney

LEARNING OBJECTIVES

After studying this chapter you should be able to:

- Draw a simple scheme outlining the key biochemical reactions involving cobalamin (vitamin B_{12}) and folate.
- Understand how cobalamin and folate are absorbed from the gut and transported in plasma.
- Explain the mechanisms that cause megaloblastic morphology in the bone marrow and blood and describe these features.
- List the causes of cobalamin deficiency.
- List the causes of folate deficiency.

Hematopoiesis depends upon orderly cell division for the logarithmic expansion of progenitor cells into large numbers of circulating blood cells. In the megaloblastic anemias, DNA synthesis is impaired, leading to slowing or arrest of cellular division during the DNA synthesis phase of the cell cycle (S phase). A high fraction of cells suffering from such defects undergo programmed cell death (apoptosis). In the bone marrow, the decreased survival of hematopoietic progenitors leads to reduced production of circulating cells (ineffective hematopoiesis). Because RNA synthesis and cytoplasmic differentiation are relatively unaffected, progenitors and progeny that survive are enlarged (macrocytic). The main cause of megaloblastic anemias is deficiency of either cobalamin (vitamin B_{12}) or folic acid, vitamins that are essential for DNA replication and repair. In addition, chemotherapeutic drugs that inhibit DNA synthesis can result in findings similar to those seen in cobalamin or folate deficiency. It is not surprising that the clinical phenotype extends to other tissues that rely on continuous and robust cellular proliferation and differentiation, particularly the gastrointestinal tract.

Understanding the pathophysiology of the megaloblastic anemias requires knowledge about the absorption, transport, and utilization of folate and cobalamin as well as familiarity with the key chemical reactions in which these vitamins are essential cofactors.

PHYSIOLOGY OF COBALAMIN AND FOLATE

Cobalamin is a complex organic molecule consisting of a tetrapyrole corrin ring, similar in structure to heme except that the divalent metal atom in the center of the ring is cobalt rather than iron. Like heme iron, the cobalt atom in the corrin ring binds to two axial ligands. One is a benzimidazole nucleotide, whereas the other can be either a methyl group (methylcobalamin) or an adenosyl group (adenosylcobalamin). Cobalamin is found in all foods of animal origin including meat, fish, and dairy products. Food cobalamin is tightly bound to proteins. Following ingestion, some cobalamin in food is transferred to human haptocorrin in saliva. As depicted in Figure 6-1, the acidic environment of the stomach enables efficient release and transfer of the remaining food cobalamin to haptocorrin in gastric juice. After transit to the duodenum, the increase in pH enables the transfer of cobalamin from haptocorrin to intrinsic factor, a transport protein secreted by gastric parietal cells. The cobalamin-intrinsic factor complex resists digestion and travels down the gut until it encounters epithelial cells in the distal ileum that express cubilin, a receptor with specificity for this bimolecular complex. The cobalamin that is absorbed in the ileum exits the basolateral side of the mucosal epithelial cell into the plasma where it traverses the portal circulation into the liver. Here cobalamin binds transcobalamin, a plasma transport protein that is functionally analogous to transferrin, the transport protein for iron. As in iron homeostasis, the liver is the principal storage site for cobalamin. The uptake of the circulating transcobalamin-cobalamin complex by receptors on plasma membranes is the principal and probably the only way that the

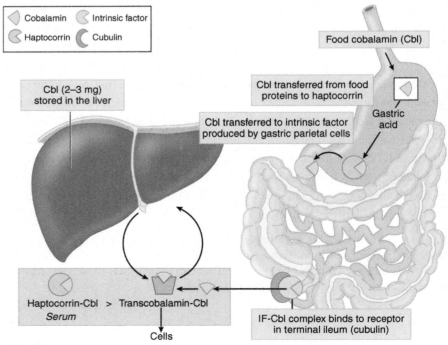

FIGURE 6-1 The absorption, utilization, and storage of cobalamin.

vitamin is taken into cells other than liver cells. In keeping with the broad importance of cobalamin for the biochemical reactions described below, transcobalamin
receptors are expressed on a wide variety of cells.

The transcobalamin-cobalamin complex makes up only a minority of the
cobalamin in plasma. About 70% to 90% is bound to haptocorrin, derived primarily from leukocytes of the myeloid lineage. Haptocorrin is secreted into a number
of bodily fluids including saliva and gastric juice, as mentioned earlier. Its biologic
function is unclear.

Folic acid, commonly designated *folate*, refers to a group of compounds consisting of a tricyclic pteroyl group linked to one or more glutamic acid residues.
Food sources include fruits, vegetables, liver, and meat, in all of which folate exists
primarily as polyglutamate conjugates. The bioactivity of folate in food may be
attenuated or destroyed by prolonged cooking. As shown in Figure 6-2, during
transit in the gut, folate polyglutamates are hydrolyzed to the monoglutamate
derivative, which is readily absorbed by a specific transmembrane channel into the
enterocytes of the duodenum and jejunum. It is further metabolized in enterocytes
into N5-methyl tetrahydrofolate (N5-methyl THF), which exits these cells and circulates freely in the plasma. Several types of folate receptors have been identified
on cell surfaces, but their role in mediating uptake has not been explained. Like
cobalamin and iron, folate is stored mainly in the liver.

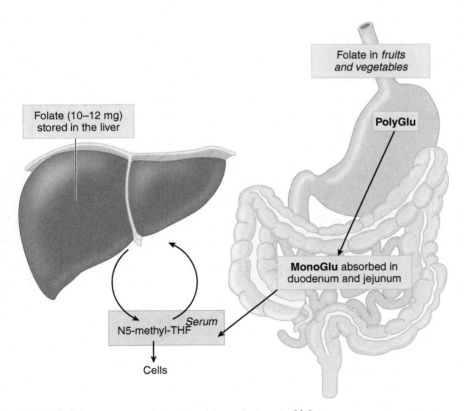

FIGURE 6-2 **The absorption, utilization, and storage of folate.**

BIOCHEMISTRY OF COBALAMIN AND FOLATE

These cofactors participate in a series of reactions involved in the biosynthesis of a variety of products including amino acids, metabolic intermediates, purines, and nucleotides. As summarized in Figure 6-3, the two forms of cobalamin mentioned earlier participate in different reactions.

Adenosylcobalamin is required for the conversion of methylmalonyl-coenzyme A (CoA) to succinyl-CoA. As discussed later in this chapter, measurement of methylmalonate in the serum is a useful test for identifying individuals with cobalamin deficiency. As shown in Figures 6-3 and 6-4, *methylcobalamin* is required for the conversion of homocysteine to methionine.

After N5-methyl THF enters the cell from the plasma, it is conjugated to polyglutamate, which prevents egress back into the plasma. Transfer of the methyl group from N5-methyl THF to methionine results in the formation and maintenance of adequate intracellular levels of THF. This reaction exemplifies the primary function of folate as a conduit for the addition of one-carbon moieties such as methyl and formyl groups to organic compounds. The conversion of the amino acid serine to glycine enables the transfer of a methyl group to THF to form N5,10-methylene THF, which is then used for both de novo purine biosynthesis and for the conversion of deoxyuridylate to deoxythymidylate. Thus cobalamin and folate play critical roles in production of the building blocks for DNA synthesis. As discussed in detail in the next section, deficiency in either of these two vitamins results in impairment of cell division, with adverse consequences particularly in proliferating cells such as in the bone marrow and gastrointestinal epithelium.

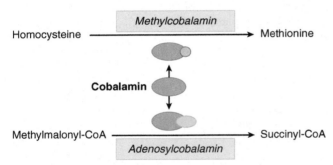

FIGURE 6-3 **Cobalamin-dependent chemical reactions.**

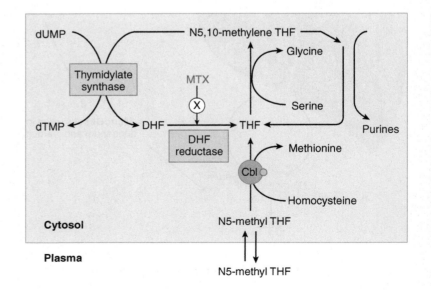

FIGURE 6-4 **Entry of folate into the cell and the principal biochemical pathway by which folate transfers one-carbon fragments for synthesis of methionine, purines, and thymidylate (dTMP).** THF, tetrahydrofolate; DHF, dihydrofolate; MTX, methotrexate, which inhibits DHF reductase.

PATHOPHYSIOLOGY AND FEATURES OF MEGALOBLASTIC ANEMIA

The impairment in DNA synthesis imposed by cobalamin or folate deficiency results in striking morphologic abnormalities in the bone marrow and peripheral blood, often referred to as *megaloblastic changes*. The bone marrow reveals increased cellularity and hyperplasia of erythroid precursors. The model diagram at the bottom of Figure 6-5 compares the maturation of normal and megaloblastic erythroid cells. Throughout the stages of erythroid development, the megaloblastic cells are larger. Although cytoplasmic differentiation, as assessed by increasing hemoglobin production, is normal, nuclear maturation is retarded, a phenomenon called *nuclear-cytoplasmic dyssynchrony*. Megaloblastic cells may acquire non-clonal chromosomal abnormalities, owing to incomplete DNA repair. These erythroid precursor cells are defective and vulnerable to destruction within the bone marrow prior to their maturation and release into the peripheral circulation as reticulocytes. Thus, erythropoiesis is ineffective.[1] Myeloid precursors reveal similar abnormalities: increased size and retarded nuclear maturation. The increased rate of apoptosis of erythroid precursor cells results in a slight increase in the level of non-conjugated bilirubin in the serum and a marked increase in serum lactate dehydrogenase (LDH).

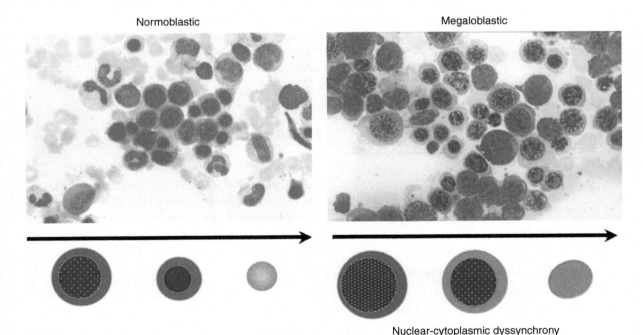

Normoblastic   Megaloblastic

Nuclear-cytoplasmic dyssynchrony

FIGURE 6-5 Comparison of normal (normoblastic) and megaloblastic maturation. Below the bone marrow smears is a diagram contrasting the differences between normal and megaloblastic erythroid maturation in cell size and in nuclear development. (This figure was prepared by Dr. Mark Fleming.)

---

[1] See Chapter 3 for general coverage of ineffective erythropoiesis.

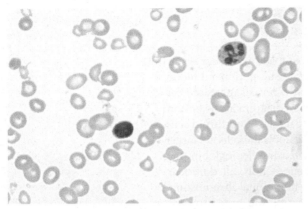

FIGURE 6-6 Peripheral blood smear from a patient with megaloblastic anemia. Note increased variation in red cell size, macrocytosis, macro-ovalocytes, and a hypersegmented neutrophil.

The peripheral blood smear reveals striking variation in red cell size (anisocytosis) and frequent large oval red cells (macro-ovalocytes), placing megaloblastic anemias in the differential diagnosis of macrocytic anemias (see Chapter 3). The mean cell volume (MCV) increases progressively as the hemoglobin falls. An MCV of >110 fL generally indicates megaloblastic maturation. Less marked degrees of "non-megaloblastic" macrocytosis can be seen in patients with hemolysis, marrow aplasia or myelodysplasia, liver disease, and alcoholism. The reticulocyte count is low in megaloblastic anemia, in keeping with ineffective erythropoiesis. In severe megaloblastic anemia, the white count and platelet count also often are decreased but rarely to levels that put the patient at risk of infection or bleeding. Of greater diagnostic value is the presence of neutrophils that have an increased number of lobes, often called *hypersegmented polys*, shown in Figure 6-6. The mechanism underlying this finding is unclear. Abnormalities in bone marrow and blood cell morphology and in cell numbers are the same in cobalamin deficiency and folic acid deficiency. Morphologic abnormalities, including increased cell size and megaloblastic nuclei also are seen in epithelial cells that line the gastrointestinal tract.

Similar morphologic changes in the bone marrow and gastrointestinal tract are commonly seen following administration of chemotherapy drugs that inhibit DNA replication and cell division. A good example is the drug methotrexate (shown in Fig. 6-4 as MTX), which inhibits the enzyme dihydrofolate reductase.

TABLE 6-1 Causes of Cobalamin Deficiency

Malabsorption
Intrinsic factor deficiency
Pernicious anemia-*common*
Total gastrectomy
Food cobalamin malabsorption-*common*
Disease of distal ileum: sprue, ileitis, resection
Competition from parasites
Bacteria: "blind loop"; intestinal diverticulum
Fish tapeworm
Much less common:
Inadequate dietary intake
Nitrous oxide

COBALAMIN DEFICIENCY

ETIOLOGY

The causes of cobalamin deficiency are listed in Table 6-1. The vast majority of affected individuals have some type of gastrointestinal malabsorption. In the United States and in other areas with temperate climate, most patients have either pernicious anemia or food cobalamin malabsorption.

Pernicious anemia is an autoimmune disorder that destroys the parietal cells in the gastric mucosa. These cells are the site of both intrinsic factor production and the pumping of protons into the gastric lumen. A gastric biopsy may reveal an infiltrate of lymphocytes and plasma cells in the lamina propria. With time, the mucosa atrophies, and the gastric wall becomes thin. Some studies have suggested that the autoimmune attack on gastric parietal cells is a consequence of inflammation induced by *Helicobacter pylori* infection. As shown in Figure 6–1, the absence of intrinsic factor prevents cobalamin from being absorbed in the distal ileum. Normally, 2 to 3 mg of cobalamin is stored in the liver. With loss of intrinsic factor, cobalamin can no longer be absorbed; after 2 to 5 years, the stores in the liver are exhausted, and the patient is at risk of developing severe deficiency.

An even more common cause of cobalamin deficiency is malabsorption due to the absence of gastric acid that is necessary for the transfer of cobalamin in food to haptocorrin (Fig. 6-1). The prevalence of gastric achlorhydria increases sharply with age, affecting 40% of individuals over age 80. Cobalamin deficiency is also encountered among younger individuals following long-term administration of proton pump inhibitors for treatment of various disorders of the upper gastrointestinal tract. Because intrinsic factor is present, the impairment in cobalamin absorption is less marked than in pernicious anemia. Accordingly, the deficiency takes longer to develop and is usually less severe.

Because intrinsic factor is produced only in the stomach, it follows that total gastrectomy will lead to malabsorption of cobalamin. By the same token, surgical resection of the terminal ileum, where cobalamin is absorbed, has the same effect. However, these surgeries are seldom performed and are therefore uncommon causes of cobalamin deficiency. In contrast, deficiency of both cobalamin and folate is often encountered in certain parts of the world near the equator including Puerto Rico and Haiti, owing to a chronic malabsorption condition known as tropical sprue. The cause of this disorder is unclear, but the fact that patients respond to antibiotic therapy offers a clue to pathogenesis. Other chronic inflammatory diseases of the ileum such as regional enteritis (e.g., Crohn disease) also can lead to cobalamin malabsorption. Deficiency of cobalamin also may arise because of competition from organisms within the gastrointestinal tract. Anatomical stasis due to diverticula, stricture, or surgically created "blind loops" can lead to overgrowth of bacteria that usurp cobalamin-intrinsic factor complexes that are *en route* to the ileum. In Scandinavia, infestation with the fish tapeworm results in a similar parasitic confiscation of cobalamin.

Two other rare causes of cobalamin deficiency deserve mention. Individuals who are strict vegans and ingest no animal products at all (including dairy products) may, over a protracted time period, become deficient. In contrast, acute cobalamin deficiency is occasionally encountered in individuals following prolonged exposure to the anesthetic agent nitrous oxide, which can combine chemically with cobalamin and abolish its biological activity.

CLINICAL PRESENTATION

Patients with cobalamin deficiency come to medical attention because of anemia and/or neurological symptoms. They tend to be elderly. Those with pernicious anemia may have other autoimmune manifestations such as vitiligo or antibody-mediated endocrinopathies. The onset of the anemia is insidious, with symptoms and signs no different than those seen in other causes of chronic anemia. The anemia is often severe. It is not unusual for a patient with cobalamin deficiency to present with a hemoglobin level as low as 5 g/dL. In addition to pallor, a patient's skin may have a lemon tinge, and there may be slight scleral icterus, owing to

Cobalamin Deficiency:

Hematologic-*common*:
Anemia > ↓ WBC, ↓ Plts
Gastrointestinal-*rare*:
Glossitis, malabsorbtion
Neurologic-*common*:
Neuropathy > spinal
disease > dementia

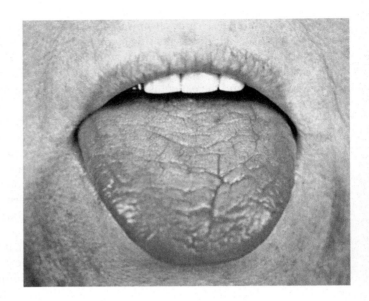

FIGURE 6-7 Atrophic glossitis in a patient with pernicious anemia. The smooth surfaces on the periphery of the tongue reflect loss of papillae.

increased levels of bilirubin in the plasma arising from destruction of erythroid cells in the bone marrow (ineffective erythropoiesis).

Although cobalamin deficiency can impair proliferation of mucosal cells in the gastrointestinal tract, this seldom causes symptoms. Some patients develop a sore, beefy red, smooth tongue (glossitis) due to atrophy of the papillae (Fig. 6-7). Cobalamin deficiency can also cause blunting of the mucosal villi in the small intestine and mild malabsorption. These findings are normalized by treatment.

Neurological manifestations are an important and sometimes overlooked consequence of cobalamin deficiency. They are generally associated with severe anemia. However, patients may present with significant neurological findings without anemia or even macrocytosis. Most patients complain of numbness or tingling, generally in the legs. Less often patients develop ataxia and loss of proprioception as a result of damage to the posterior columns of the spinal cord. They also may have muscle weakness and spasticity as a result of damage to the lateral columns (Fig. 6-8). Dementia may be observed in patients with severe cobalamin deficiency. As a rule of thumb, *any patient who presents with neurological manifestations of peripheral neuropathy, ataxia, or dementia should be evaluated for cobalamin deficiency, even in the absence of concurrent anemia or macrocytosis.*

LABORATORY EVALUATION

The hematologic features of the megaloblastic anemias are described earlier and do not distinguish in any way between cobalamin and folate deficiency. Demonstration of a low serum cobalamin level is a useful initial step in establishing a diagnosis. However, if the result is at the lower end of the normal range, cobalamin deficiency can be verified by an elevation in the serum levels of methylmalonate and homocysteine, which are the substrates for the respective adenosylcobalamin

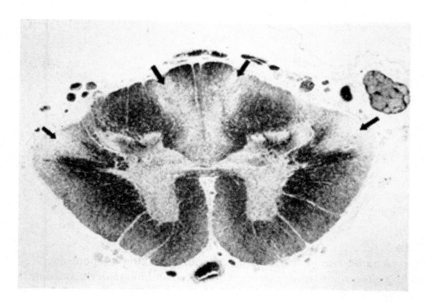

FIGURE 6-8 **Spinal cord section showing demyelination of the posterior and lateral columns (arrows) in a patient with pernicious anemia.**

and methylcobalamin reactions (Fig. 6-3). Once cobalamin deficiency is documented, its cause should be investigated. About half of patients with pernicious anemia will have antibodies in the serum against intrinsic factor. Gastric achlorhydria will be found in all those with either pernicious anemia or food cobalamin malabsorption. If stomach acid is present, it is likely that the patient has either bacterial overgrowth or malabsorption in the terminal ileum.

TREATMENT

In all patients with cobalamin deficiency, replacement therapy results in complete cure of the hematologic abnormalities, unless there is a second process that independently suppresses erythropoiesis. Unfortunately, therapy is much less effective in reversing the neurological complications. It is important to establish a diagnosis prior to instituting a treatment plan because the administration of folate to a cobalamin-deficient patient will partially correct the anemia but (for unknown reasons) may exacerbate the neurological manifestations.

Patients with severe anemia are at risk of becoming hypokalemic immediately following initiation of therapy, owing to the anabolic burst of orderly cell division. Moreover, these patients, particularly the elderly, may be at the brink of cardiac decompensation. Therefore, sudden expansion of blood volume should be carefully avoided. Typically, these patients mount a brisk hematologic recovery, and red cell transfusions should be avoided unless the patient evinces symptoms or signs of ischemic damage to vital organs such as the brain or heart.

Because the vast majority of cobalamin deficiency is due to malabsorption, replacement therapy is given parenterally. Regular injections of cobalamin (initially weekly, then monthly) are effective in keeping patients in hematologic remission. A typical response following the initiation of treatment is shown in

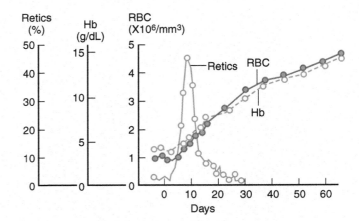

FIGURE 6-9 Response of a patient with pernicious anemia to cobalamin therapy. Note the brisk reticulocyte response during the first week of therapy and the subsequent rise in hemoglobin (Hb) and red cell count (RBC). Note also the shift in the ratio of (Hb) to RBC, reflecting the gradual reduction in mean cell volume during therapy.

Figure 6-9. A rapid rise in the reticulocyte count, peaking at about day 7, is followed by a slower but steady rise in hemoglobin and hematocrit concentrations, accompanied by a decline in the MCV to normal. Oral administration of cobalamin can be equally effective when given in doses high enough to penetrate the intestinal mucosal barrier by mass action. However, because many patients (particularly the elderly) fail to take their medications regularly, most physicians favor parenteral administration.

FOLATE DEFICIENCY

ETIOLOGY

In contrast to cobalamin deficiency, which is generally isolated, folate deficiency is usually accompanied by deficits in other nutrients. As indicated in Table 6-2, there are three major causes of folate deficiency: malnutrition, malabsorption, and increased requirements.

As mentioned earlier, folate is present primarily in fruits, vegetables, liver, and certain meat products and can be inactivated by prolonged cooking. Unlike cobalamin deficiency, which is rarely due to an inadequate diet, decreased intake of folate is quite common, particularly among certain population groups. Infants who are fed goat milk exclusively become markedly folate deficient. Also at risk are adolescents who subsist on "junk" food. In these two instances, the deficiency is the result of a combination of inadequate intake and the increased demand imposed by rapid growth. Indigent and house-bound people are also prone to folate deficiency because of the expense and difficulty in obtaining fresh food. Alcoholics commonly become folate deficient, owing to poor diet along with ethanol-induced suppression of folate absorption and impaired enterohepatic circulation.

TABLE 6-2 Causes of Folic acid Deficiency

Decreased intake:
Infancy
Poor diet
Alcoholism
Impaired absorption:
Sprue, etc.
Increased requirements:
Growth spurts: infancy, adolescence
Pregnancy
Marrow hyperplasia
Bulky tumors

Folate malabsorption can be caused by a variety of gastrointestinal disorders, particularly those that affect the mucosa of the duodenum and jejunum. Of particular importance are celiac disease and tropical sprue. As mentioned earlier, the latter also can cause cobalamin deficiency. Finally, folate deficiency often is encountered in conditions in which growth or pathologic cell proliferation leads to an increased demand for folate. Infancy and adolescence already have been mentioned. In the past, folate deficiency was commonly encountered in pregnant women, particularly those who were indigent and malnourished. Now folate is administered as part of an iron-vitamin supplement given routinely to all expectant mothers. Occasionally folate deficiency is seen in patients with disorders associated with enhanced cell proliferation. Those with chronic hemolytic anemias such as sickle cell disease are commonly given prophylactic folate to satisfy the enhanced demand of the hyperplastic erythroid progenitors. In like manner, patients with rapidly growing tumors are prone to folate deficiency, particularly if they are not maintaining a good diet.

CLINICAL PRESENTATION

The hematologic and gastrointestinal manifestations of folate deficiency are identical to those of cobalamin deficiency. Both have megaloblastic maturation and identical morphologic features. However, the conditions differ in one important respect: patients with folate deficiency rarely, if ever, develop neurologic manifestations.

> **Folate Deficiency:**
>
> Hematologic-*common*:
>   Anemia > ↓WBC, ↓Plts
> Gastrointestinal-*rare*:
>   Glossitis, malabsorbtion

If a pregnant woman is folate deficient during the first trimester, there is increased risk that the baby will be born with a neural tube defect such as spina bifida. Why folate deficiency leads to these particular defects is not understood; it may be related to a requirement for folate in the biochemical reactions that lead to DNA methylation, a modification that controls gene expression. Whatever the mechanism, the risk of neural tube defects is obviated by administration of folic acid early in pregnancy. Since 1998, fortification of flour and other grains with folate has been compulsory in the United States and has resulted in a marked decrease in the incidence of these birth defects.

Because the turnover of folate in the body is much more rapid than that of cobalamin, the 10 to 12 mg stores of folate in the liver can be exhausted in a few months under circumstances in which intake or absorption is abruptly curtailed.

LABORATORY EVALUATION

In folate deficiency, blood cell counts as well as marrow and peripheral blood morphology are indistinguishable from those of cobalamin deficiency. Both conditions cause megaloblastic maturation. The standard diagnostic test is measurement of serum folate, which is usually low in patients who are deficient. However, serum levels can change quite rapidly with alterations in diet. In contrast, red cell folate is stable over a period of several days and therefore can provide a more accurate index of deficiency. As predicted from the chemical reactions shown in Figure 6-3, in folate deficiency, the serum homocysteine level is elevated (as in cobalamin deficiency), and the serum methylmalonate level is normal (in contradistinction to cobalamin deficiency).

TREATMENT

Oral folic acid, 1 mg/day, is remarkably safe, inexpensive and effective therapy. The hematologic response is identical to that with cobalamin deficiency. Because folate deficiency is often accompanied by deficits in other vitamins and nutrients, a full nutritional evaluation should be done.

SELF-ASSESSMENT STUDY QUESTIONS

1. A 61-year-old man has just had surgical resection of his entire stomach because of cancer. This type of surgery puts him at risk for a nutritional anemia because of the lack of:
   A. Cubilin.
   B. Transcobalamin.
   C. Haptocorrin.
   D. Intrinsic factor.
   E. Gastrin.

2. A 25-year-old woman comes to you for a Papanicolaou smear test. She says she is hoping to get pregnant and is going to discontinue using her birth control pills. You do routine laboratory tests and find that she has an elevated mean cell volume, normal serum iron level, and normal serum ferritin level. Which nutritionally related health risk to her offspring should you be most concerned about at this point?
   A. Neural tube defects.
   B. Stunted growth.
   C. Pernicious anemia.
   D. Malabsorption.
   E. Decreased learning ability.

3. Which laboratory test result is most indicative of cobalamin deficiency?
   A. Elevated serum methylmalonate.
   B. Elevated serum homocysteine.
   C. The presence in serum of antibodies against gastric parietal cells.
   D. Neutral pH of gastric fluid (achlorhydria).
   E. Hypersegmented neutrophils.

Anemias Associated With Chronic Illness

H. Franklin Bunn

All of the different types of anemia covered in preceding chapters (4-6) as well as those that follow this one (Chapters 8-11) are *primary* hematologic disorders arising because of an inherited or an acquired defect that directly lowers the red cell mass by impairing erythropoiesis or shortening cell survival. The importance of these disorders notwithstanding, it is worth stressing that among the most common anemias and the ones most prevalent in patients hospitalized on a medical or pediatric service are those *secondary* to an underlying chronic illness (summarized in Table 7-1).

ANEMIA OF CHRONIC INFLAMMATION

A chronic systemic inflammatory disorder persisting more than a month is nearly always accompanied by anemia. As indicated in Table 7-1, the chronic inflammation is usually due to infection, tumor, or a connective tissue disorder. A wide array of infections may be responsible, including subacute bacterial endocarditis, tuberculosis, lung abscess, osteomyelitis, and pyelonephritis. In some types of chronic infections, the pathogenesis is more complex. For example, in AIDS the HIV virus can directly infect hematopoietic progenitor cells. In malaria and babesiosis, the parasite infects and destroys circulating red cells.

Tumors vary considerably in their ability to trigger an inflammatory response. Some secrete inflammatory cytokines as part of their profiles of aberrant gene expression. In others, impairment of oxygen or nutrient supply to the interior of the tumor can result in necrosis and an inflammatory response. In some tumors, such as the leukemias and lymphomas and those that have metastasized to bone, red cell production is further compromised by marrow invasion.

TABLE 7-1 Anemia of Chronic Illness

Anemia of chronic inflammation

   Infection

   Cancer

   Connective tissue disorders

Anemia of renal insufficiency

Anemia of chronic liver disease

Anemia of endocrine hypofunction

Anemia is encountered in a wide variety of inflammatory disorders not associated with either infection or cancer. In many of these conditions, autoimmune attack on the patient's cells and tissues is accompanied by a robust inflammatory response. Rheumatoid arthritis is the most prevalent connective tissue disorder and a prototypical cause of anemia of chronic inflammation. Polymyalgia rheumatica/temporal arteritis is associated with even more intense inflammation and accordingly more severe anemia. In anemia due to systemic lupus erythematosus, the deleterious impact of inflammation is often compounded by increased red cell destruction (due to the presence of autoantibodies) and the anemia of renal insufficiency (described in the following section).

PATHOGENESIS AND LABORATORY FINDINGS

It has been long appreciated that the anemia of chronic inflammation is associated with a systemic derangement of iron homeostasis. Increased amounts of iron are stored in macrophages in the bone marrow, liver, and spleen, as reflected by elevated levels of ferritin in serum (Chapter 5, Fig. 5-5B). However, there is a block in the transfer of this excess iron to the plasma, resulting in low levels of serum iron (Chapter 5, Fig. 5-5A). For unclear reasons, the level of total transferrin in the serum is also low. Because of this limitation in iron availability, erythropoiesis is somewhat "iron deficient." Erythroid precursors in the bone marrow have decreased amounts of cytoplasmic iron, and the red cells that enter the circulation are slightly smaller than normal. The suppression of red cell production results in a low reticulocyte index. Because this block in iron utilization is subtle, the degree of anemia in patients with chronic inflammation is rarely severe. If a patient with one of the disorders listed previously has a hemoglobin level of less than 8 g/dL, it is essential to look for additional contributors such as bleeding or hemolysis.

In the last 5 years, the pathogenesis of the anemia of chronic inflammation has been greatly clarified by the realization that plasma hepcidin levels are markedly increased, as a direct result of induction of transcription by inflammatory cytokines. As shown in Figure 7-1, hepcidin blocks both iron absorption from the gut and the egress of iron from macrophages, thus explaining both increased storage iron and reduced levels of serum iron.

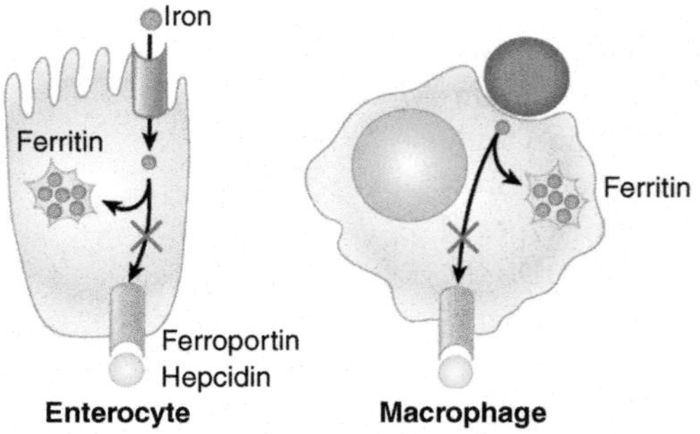

FIGURE 7-1 Pathogenesis of abnormal iron homeostasis in anemia of chronic inflammation. The induction of plasma hepcidin by inflammatory cytokines results in inactivation of ferroportin and consequent suppression of iron egress from the duodenal enterocyte and from the macrophage.

TREATMENT

Patients with anemia of chronic inflammation seldom require red cell transfusions. As mentioned in the next section, selected patients may benefit from recombinant erythropoietin therapy. The anemia can be cured only by correction of the underlying disease.

ANEMIA OF RENAL INSUFFICIENCY

Chronic renal insufficiency is accompanied by suppression of erythropoiesis. The degree of anemia is roughly proportional to the loss of functional nephrons. Unlike the other secondary anemias covered in this chapter, anemia due to chronic kidney disease is often severe, and some patients require red cell transfusions. The red cell indices are normal, and the reticulocyte index is low. The red cell morphology is usually normal, but some patients with uremia have burr-shaped red cells with evenly scalloped borders. In some uremic patients, the anemia is aggravated by gastrointestinal bleeding due in part to impaired platelet function (see Chapter 14). Although red cell survival is nearly normal in most uremic patients, brisk intravascular hemolysis accompanied by the presence of schistocytes is seen in those with hemolytic uremic syndrome and thrombotic thrombocytopenic purpura (Chapters 11 and 14).

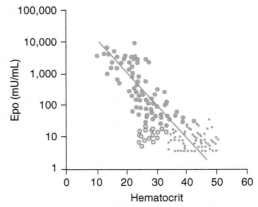

FIGURE 7-2 Plasma erythropoietin (Epo) levels in patients with different degrees of anemia. The subset of anemia patients with chronic renal disease (*large, green dots*) have much lower plasma erythropoietin levels than those with other types of anemia (*large, blue dots*). Normal individuals are represented as small, blue dots. mU, milliunits.

The primary mechanism responsible for the anemia of renal failure is the inability of the diseased kidneys to secrete adequate amounts of erythropoietin (Epo) into the plasma. As mentioned in Chapters 2 and 3, the kidney is the major site of Epo production. As shown in Figure 7-2, plasma erythropoietin levels are considerably lower in patients with renal failure than in non-uremic patients with a comparable degree of anemia.

The importance of erythropoietin in the pathogenesis of the anemia of renal failure has been proven by the dramatic efficacy of recombinant human erythropoietin (rhEpo) therapy. Figure 7-3 shows one of the first cases treated with rhEpo. The patient had developed progressive loss of renal function and then underwent bilateral nephrectomy for control of hypertension. The patient required hemodialysis for excretion of urinary waste products and frequent blood transfusions in order to maintain hematocrit levels in the low 20s. Shortly after initiation of rhEpo therapy, the hematocrit concentration approached normal, necessitating a reduction in dose. Prior to rhEpo treatment, this patient was overloaded with iron as documented by full saturation of serum transferrin and increased serum ferritin. The marked increase in red cell mass following treatment was accompanied by enhanced utilization of iron stores, as reflected in a decline in serum iron and serum ferritin levels. Other patients who have normal or low iron stores prior to rhEpo therapy need concomitant administration of iron in order to achieve an optimal erythropoietic response.

As the case in Figure 7-3 demonstrates, the anemia of chronic renal failure can be cured by rhEpo therapy. Several million patients around the world have benefited from treatment. However, a number of large studies have signaled a note of caution; doses that push the hemoglobin level above 12 g/dL are associated with a slight but significant increase in the risk of thrombosis and cardiovascular mortality.

As shown in Table 7-2, rhEpo is effective in other types of anemia. Treatment can lower transfusion requirements in patients with cancer or HIV infection in whom anemia has been aggravated by chemotherapy. Compared with doses used

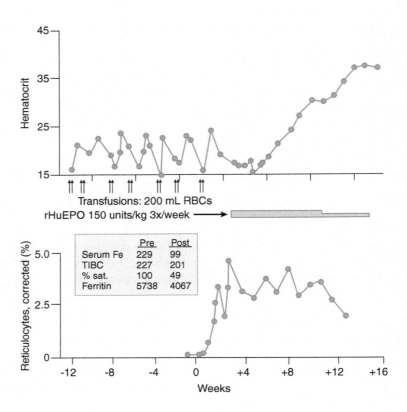

FIGURE 7-3 **Response of an anephric patient to recombinant human erythropoietin (rHuEpo) therapy.** Note that prior to therapy the patient was severely anemic and transfusion dependent. Treatment with rhEpo resulted in reticulocytosis followed by a progressive increase in the hemoglobin level. The dose of rhEpo had to be lowered to prevent the hemoglobin from rising too high. Prior to rhEpo therapy, the patient was severely iron overloaded. The marked increase in red cell mass following therapy was accompanied by a significant reduction in iron stores. RBC, red blood cell; TIBC, total iron binding capacity; sat, saturation.

TABLE 7-2	Clinical Uses of rhEpo
Anemia of renal failure	
Anemia of chronic inflammation	
Cancer	
HIV Infection	
Primary bone marrow disorders	
Surgery	

in patients with renal failure, higher doses are required for cancer and AIDS patients to achieve the same increment in red cell mass, and, therefore, they may be at even greater risk of developing thromboses. Treatment with rhEpo also has been effective in some patients with primary bone marrow disorders, particularly myelodysplasia (Chapter 20). Short-term administration of rhEpo may lower transfusion requirements in surgical patients, both preoperatively and perioperatively. Treatment also may be of benefit in rare patients who are unable to receive blood transfusions, either because of antigen incompatibility or religious convictions.

ANEMIA OF CHRONIC LIVER DISEASE

Most patients with hepatocellular liver disease, regardless of etiology, have mild or moderate anemia that is normocytic or slightly macrocytic. Red cell morphology is normal except for the presence of target cells (Chapter 3, Fig. 3-7). Target cells are formed because of abnormalities in plasma lipids that lead to the passive uptake of cholesterol and phospholipids into the lipid bilayer of the red cell membrane, thereby increasing the surface-to-volume ratio of the cell. The reticulocyte index is low, reflecting a failure of erythropoiesis to compensate for a modest shortening of red cell life span. The anemia persists as long as hepatic function is defective. The mechanism underlying the anemia of chronic liver disease is not understood.

Patients with alcoholic liver disease have more severe anemia, owing to several additional factors. Alcohol is a direct suppressor of hematopoiesis and therefore can cause pancytopenia. In alcoholics who have continued to drink up to the time of clinical evaluation, the bone marrow often reveals vacuoles in the cytoplasm of red and white blood cell precursors. In addition, ring sideroblasts may be observed, particularly in patients who are malnourished. Alcoholics are often deficient in folate because of both inadequate intake and impaired utilization. Furthermore, the anemia in alcoholics may be aggravated by hemorrhage from gastritis, esophageal varices, or duodenal ulcer. The risk of gastrointestinal bleeding is further increased by thrombocytopenia and/or deficiencies in soluble clotting factors. Chronic blood loss often leads to iron deficiency. Rarely, patients with alcoholic cirrhosis or forms of obstructive liver disease develop severe hemolytic anemia accompanied by the appearance of rigid red cells with irregular borders, called *spur cells* (Chapter 3, Fig. 3-7). This entity is discussed in Chapter 11.

ANEMIA OF ENDOCRINE HYPOFUNCTION

A number of hormones, including thyroxine, glucocorticoids, testosterone, and growth hormone, are known to promote in vitro proliferation of erythroid cells. Therefore it is not surprising that mild or moderate normocytic anemia generally accompanies a number of endocrine deficiency states including hypothyroidism, Addison disease, hypogonadism, and panhypopituitarism. Of note, anemias secondary to endocrine failure are all readily corrected when adequate hormone replacement is given.

HYPOTHYROIDISM

In the anemia of hypothyroidism (myxedema), red cell life span is normal, and erythropoiesis is effective. A minority of patients have macrocytic red cells, usually due to either cobalamin or folate deficiency. Patients with autoimmune hypothyroidism (Hashimoto thyroiditis) have an increased incidence of other autoimmune disorders as well, including pernicious anemia. The plasma volume is often reduced along with the red cell mass, and thus the anemia in hypothyroid patients may be masked. Because the signs and symptoms of hypothyroidism are often subtle and elusive, this diagnosis should be considered in any patient with unexplained anemia.

ADDISON DISEASE

The anemia of Addison disease (glucocortical and mineralocortical hormone deficiency) is also masked by a decrease in plasma volume. Upon hormone replacement, the plasma volume is rapidly reconstituted, and the hemoglobin level falls to about 80% of the pretreatment level. With continued therapy, the red cell mass returns to normal.

HYPOGONADISM AND HYPOPITUITARISM

Testosterone has a physiologic influence on the red cell mass. As shown in Chapter 3, Figure 3-1, during adolescence the hemoglobin level of normal males increases from about 13 to 15 g/dL. Eunuchoid males generally have a hemoglobin level of about 13 g/dL. Pituitary dysfunction or ablation is also associated with mild, normocytic anemia.

SELF-ASSESSMENT STUDY QUESTIONS

1. What protein plays the most central role in the pathogenesis of the anemia associated with inflammation?
   A. Transferrin.
   B. Ferroportin.
   C. Ferritin.
   D. Hepcidin.
   E. Tumor necrosis factor.

2. What laboratory test findings are most indicative of the anemia of chronic inflammation?
   A. High serum iron level, high total transferrin level, high ferritin level.
   B. Low serum iron level, low total transferrin level, high ferritin level.
   C. Low serum iron level, low total transferrin level, low ferritin level.
   D. Low serum iron level, high total transferrin level, low ferritin level.
   E. High serum iron level, high total transferrin level, low ferritin level.

3. A patient with uremia and severe anemia failed to respond to treatment with recombinant human erythropoietin (rhEpo). What is the most common cause for this problem?
   A. Inadequate iron stores.
   B. Development of anti-rhEpo antibody.
   C. The presence of acute inflammation.
   D. Uremic waste products that suppress erythropoiesis.
   E. Hemolysis.

CHAPTER

8

Thalassemia

H. Franklin Bunn and David G. Nathan

LEARNING OBJECTIVES

After studying this chapter you should be able to:

- Outline the changes in globin gene expression that occur during fetal development.
- Explain the molecular genetics and inheritance of alpha and beta thalassemias.
- Grasp the cellular pathogenesis of alpha and beta thalassemias.
- Describe the clinical and laboratory features of beta thalassemia minor (trait) and beta thalassemia major and the different types of alpha thalassemia.
- Understand the pathophysiologic principles underlying treatment of beta thalassemia major.

The thalassemias are an inherited group of disorders in which mutations in genes expressing alpha globin or beta globin result in impaired hemoglobin synthesis and microcytic anemia of varying severity. The thalassemias are subdivided into alpha (α) or beta (β) according to which globin genes are defective. Heterozygotes are generally asymptomatic, whereas individuals who inherit thalassemia genes from each parent often have life-threatening clinical manifestations. The thalassemias have attracted worldwide interest and attention because of their high prevalence and clinical importance. Moreover, an ever-expanding body of information on the molecular pathogenesis of the thalassemias has provided critical insights into fundamental problems in biology, particularly tissue-specific and development-specific gene regulation.

THE GLOBIN GENES

A diagram of the layout of the human globin genes is shown in Figure 8-1. A tandem pair of α-globin genes is located on chromosome 16, downstream from two embryonic α-like genes called *zeta* (ζ). The high homology of the α-globin genes leads to frequent unequal meiotic crossover events, which are the basis for the deletions that cause the α-thalassemias, discussed at the end of this chapter.

The β-globin gene is a member of a family located on chromosome 11. As in the α-globin gene family, epsilon (ϵ), the most 5' (upstream) of these genes, is expressed only in early embryos. Downstream from this gene are two tandem gamma (γ) genes whose product is found in fetal hemoglobin (Hb F, $\alpha_2\gamma_2$), the

81

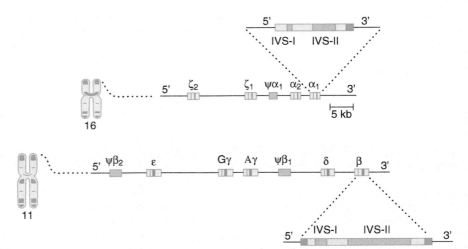

FIGURE 8-1 Organization of the α-globin family on chromosome 16 and the β-globin family on chromosome 11. IVS, intervening segments (also called introns); ψ, a non-expressing pseudogene. The three exons of the globin genes are shown in pale blue.

hemoglobin that predominates throughout most of gestation. The delta (δ) gene product forms a minor hemoglobin component, Hb A$_2$ (α$_2$δ$_2$), which has no functional importance but is useful in the diagnosis of the thalassemias (discussed later in this chapter.) The most 3′ (downstream) member of the family is the β gene whose product combines with α-globin to form Hb A (α$_2$β$_2$), the major hemoglobin component of adult red cells.

Figure 8-2 shows the expression of globin genes during development. Throughout gestation there is coordinate synthesis of globin products from the

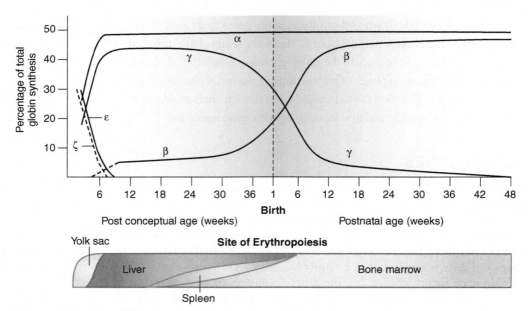

FIGURE 8-2 The sites of erythropoiesis and the pattern of globin synthesis during development.

two chromosomes, permitting the sequential and orderly production of functional tetrameric hemoglobins. In the transition from embryo to fetus to birth, the globin genes on both chromosomes are "read" sequentially from left to right (5′ to 3′). During the first month of gestation, embryonic hemoglobins ($\zeta_2\varepsilon_2$, $\alpha_2\varepsilon_2$, $\zeta_2\gamma_2$) are formed in erythroid cells located primarily in the yolk sac. During the remainder of fetal life, the sites of erythropoiesis gradually shift from the liver and spleen to the bone marrow. Fetal red cells contain predominantly Hb F ($\alpha_2\gamma_2$). Shortly before birth, there is a dramatic switch from γ-globin to β-globin expression, which is complete by the time an infant is 6 to 8 months old. From then on, over 95% of the hemoglobin in normal red cells is adult Hb A ($\alpha_2\beta_2$). The remaining hemoglobin consists of two minor components, Hb A_2 and Hb F. The molecular basis of the switch from γ- to β-globin synthesis remains one of the foremost problems in hematology research and, as discussed later, impacts importantly the pathogenesis and treatment of β-thalassemia as well as of sickle cell disease (Chapter 9).

During their maturation, erythroid cells become increasingly dedicated to the production of hemoglobin. Far upstream of the globin genes are regulatory elements called locus control regions at which erythroid-specific transcription factors bind cooperatively to response elements in the DNA to assure tissue-specific, high-level, and closely matched transcription of α and β (or γ) globin ribonucleic acids (RNAs). Like other precursor RNAs, globin RNA must be processed into messenger RNA (mRNA) and transported from the nucleus to cytoplasm for translation (protein synthesis) to occur. All globin genes have three exons and two introns. As shown in Figure 8-3, precursor RNA processing involves sequential splicing of the two introns followed by capping at the 5′ end of the RNA, which greatly enhances translation efficiency, along with cleavage and polyadenylation

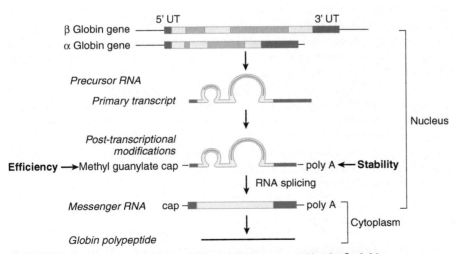

FIGURE 8-3 Processing of ribonucleic acid (RNA) expressed by the β-globin gene.
UT, untranslated. (Modified with permission from Chapter 21. MJ Cunningham, VG Sankaran, DG Nathan, SH Orkin. The Thalassemias, in: Orkin SH, Nathan DG, eds. *Nathan and Oski's Hematology of Infancy and Childhood.* 5th ed. Philadelphia, PA, Saunders; 2008: 1019.)

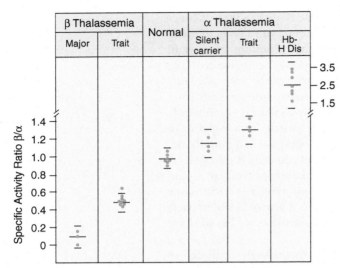

β Thalassemia		Normal	α Thalassemia		
Major	Trait		Silent carrier	Trait	Hb-H Dis

FIGURE 8-4 **The β/α globin biosynthetic ratio in different forms of thalassemia.** Peripheral blood was incubated with a radiolabeled amino acid, followed by separation of globin subunits. (Modified with permission from Nathan DG. Thalassemia. *N Engl J Med.* 1972;286:586. Copyright © 1972 Massachusetts Medical Society, all rights reserved.)

of the 3′ untranslated region, which enhances mRNA stability. Mutations at critical sites involved in splicing, capping, and polyadenylation can result in defective globin synthesis and therefore thalassemia.

As erythroid precursors reach full maturation, over 95% of protein synthesis is dedicated to globin production. This remarkable up-regulation is matched by markedly enhanced synthesis of heme. In erythroblasts and reticulocytes, globin released from the polyribosome combines with heme to form subunits capable of assembly into heterotetramers such as Hb A ($\alpha_2\beta_2$). This assembly depends on balanced synthesis of α and β subunits. As shown in Figure 8-4, globin chain synthesis is imbalanced in the thalassemias. The presence of excess free globin chains is an important contributor to the pathogenesis of these disorders.

β-THALASSEMIA

As shown in Figure 8-1, chromosome 11 contains a single β-globin gene. Individuals who inherit a β-thalassemia mutation from one parent and a normal β-globin gene from the other are heterozygotes, often designated as having β-thalassemia trait or β-thalassemia minor. Individuals who inherit the same β-thalassemia mutation from each parent are true homozygotes. Because multiple types of mutations can give rise to β-thalassemia, an individual often inherits a different mutation from each parent and is therefore a compound heterozygote. If homozygotes or compound heterozygotes have severe disease, they are designated as having β-thalassemia major or Cooley anemia, whereas if they have milder clinical manifestations, they have β-thalassemia intermedia.

Over 100 million people in the world are heterozygous carriers of a β-thalassemia mutation, nearly two-thirds from Asia and the rest divided between Africa, Europe, and the Americas. Affected individuals come primarily from tropical areas. Reasonably convincing evidence suggests that β-thalassemia heterozygotes are protected against infantile falciparum malaria, which is often fatal. Thus natural selection has enabled β-thalassemia genes to gradually rise to high levels in populations where malaria is endemic.

GENE DEFECTS CAUSING β-THALASSEMIA

The β-thalassemias are caused by diverse mutations involving the promoter, coding sequences, intron-exon boundaries, and the polyadenylation site of the β-globin gene. The mutant alleles are conveniently subdivided into two groups: β^0, in which no β-globin is detectable, and β^+, in which a small amount of normal β-globin protein is produced. Most β^0-thalassemia alleles involve single base substitutions in the coding region of the β polypeptide that introduce premature stop codons or small insertions or deletions that cause shifts in the reading frame of the mRNA. In either case, the resulting truncated polypeptide is dysfunctional and so unstable that it is undetectable in the patient's red cells. Other less common genetic mechanisms that result in β^0 alleles include deletions and mutations at splice junctions.

In β^+-thalassemia, the defective gene permits the production of normal β-globin, but the amount is markedly reduced. This type of β-thalassemia is usually due to a single base substitution that either creates a new (false) splice site or lowers the efficiency of a normal splice site. In both instances, some normal splicing occurs, and some normal β-globin is made, albeit in decreased amounts. When the alternate splice site is used, a nonsense mRNA is produced that cannot form a stable or useful protein product. Less often β^+-thalassemia is caused by mutations in the 5′ promoter or in a 3′ site in β-globin RNA where it is cleaved prior to polyadenylation.

CELLULAR PATHOGENESIS OF β-THALASSEMIA

Because inadequate amounts of β-globin are produced, there is a deficiency in the amount of hemoglobin per red cell. Therefore, the mean cell hemoglobin concentration and the mean cell volume (MCV) are decreased. Red cell production is impaired because of intramedullary destruction of erythroid precursors (ineffective erythropoiesis, Chapter 3). In addition, the survival of circulating red cells is somewhat decreased. These abnormalities are present to a slight degree in heterozygous carriers and to a marked degree in homozygotes or compound heterozygotes. In severely anemic patients, increased erythropoietin production markedly stimulates erythropoiesis in marrow cavities of all the bones as well as in extramedullary sites such as the liver and spleen, resulting in enlargement of these organs.

The markedly enhanced destruction of erythroid cells in these patients can be explained by *chain imbalance*. As shown in Figure 8-4, the β/α synthesis ratio is about 0.5 in heterozygotes and only 0.1 in homozygotes or compound heterozygotes. In the latter individuals, α-globin subunits are present in huge excess. Some, as depicted in Figure 8-5, partner with γ-globin to form Hb F, the dominant hemoglobin in red cells of patients with the severe types of β-thalassemia. The remaining free α-globin is poorly soluble and forms a precipitate in erythroid precursor cells. Its heme groups auto-oxidize, releasing toxic reactive oxygen species, that, as depicted in Figure 8-6, damage the erythroid cell membrane, leading to recognition and destruction by macrophages in the marrow, liver, and spleen. This severely ineffective erythropoiesis greatly impairs red cell production, and, when coupled with decreased survival of circulating red cells, results in severe anemia. As in other disorders characterized by ineffective erythropoiesis, β-thalassemia leads to inappropriately enhanced absorption of iron from the gut and progressive iron overload. As in most other types of severe anemia, erythropoietin production is markedly increased, resulting in the expansion of erythroid precursors not only in the bone marrow but also in extramedullary sites such as the liver and spleen. The enhanced proliferation of erythroid cells inside marrow cavities can lead to bony abnormalities described in the following section.

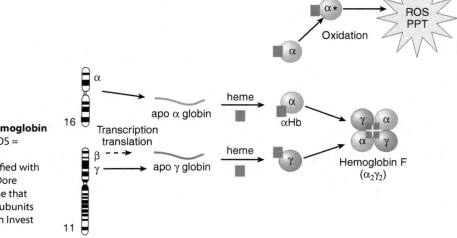

FIGURE 8-5 Assembly of hemoglobin subunits and hemoglobin tetramer in β-thalassemia. ROS = reactive oxygen species; PPT = hemoglobin precipitate. (Modified with permission from Yu Y, Kong Y, Dore LC et al, An erythroid chaperone that facilitates folding of α-globin subunits for hemoglobin synthesis, J Clin Invest 2007, 117: 1856-1865.)

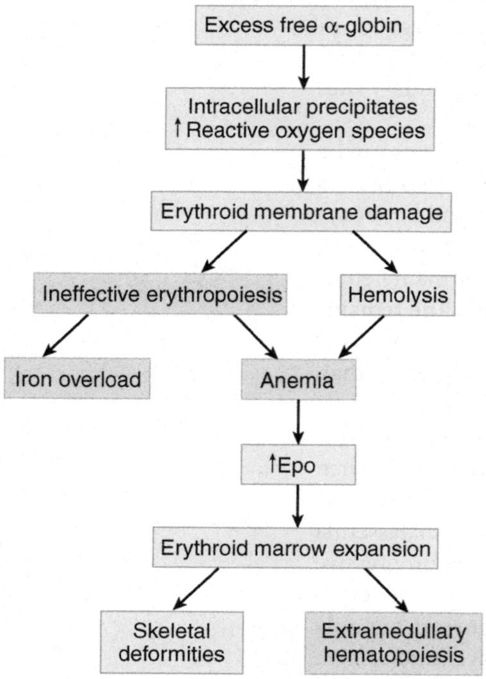

Excess free α-globin

↓

Intracellular precipitates
↑Reactive oxygen species

↓

Erythroid membrane damage

↓   ↓

Ineffective erythropoiesis   Hemolysis

↓   ↓   ↓

Iron overload   Anemia

↓

↑Epo

↓

Erythroid marrow expansion

↓   ↓

Skeletal deformities   Extramedullary hematopoiesis

FIGURE 8-6 Flow diagram summarizing the cellular pathogenesis of β-thalassemia.

CLINICAL MANIFESTATIONS

β-Thalassemia Heterozygotes

Individuals with β-thalassemia trait are asymptomatic and have a normal life expectancy. Although most have normal hemoglobin levels, many are slightly anemic. All individuals with β-thalassemia trait have microcytosis with MCVs in the range of 75 to 80 fL. Some have elevated non-conjugated bilirubin levels, reflecting enhanced erythroid cell destruction due to a modest degree of ineffective erythropoiesis. In a small minority of heterozygotes, the spleen is slightly enlarged. In addition to microcytosis, the blood smear reveals red cell stippling and target cells (Fig. 8-7). The diagnosis of β-thalassemia trait is usually made by first ruling out iron deficiency and then demonstrating an elevation of Hb A_2 levels by electrophoresis. A small fraction of individuals with the phenotype of β-thalassemia trait have an allele in which the δ and β genes are both deleted. They have low or normal Hb A_2 levels and a modest elevation in Hb F. Individuals with β-thalassemia trait require no treatment and need to be reassured that this condition is benign and does not pose a health problem. Potential parents should be counseled about the risk of having a severely affected child if both partners have β-thalassemia trait.

β-Thalassemia Major (Cooley Anemia)

Individuals at the severe end of the clinical spectrum (often designated as having *Cooley anemia*) have marked anemia

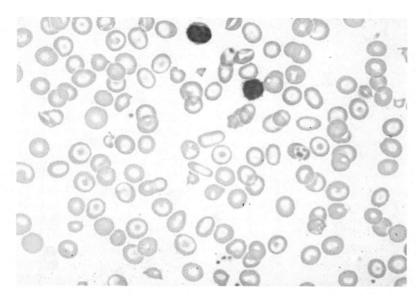

FIGURE 8-7 **Blood smear from an individual with β-thalassemia minor.**

and, unless given meticulous medical care, usually do not survive beyond childhood. As depicted in Figure 8-6, the marked, sustained erythropoietin-mediated stimulus to red cell production leads to extramedullary erythropoiesis and enlargement of the liver and spleen. Iron overload develops because of enhanced absorption of iron from the gastrointestinal tract coupled with accumulation of iron following blood transfusion. Fair-skinned patients often have a light bronze appearance, owing to a combination of pallor, icterus, and enhanced skin pigmentation. The extension of massive erythroid hyperplasia into bone marrow cavities in the skull causes deformities such as expansion of the frontal bones and/or maxillary bones ("chipmunk face"). Enlargement of the mandible can result in malocclusion of the jaw. Because of multiple-organ and multiple-system involvement, symptoms are varied and complex but are generally centered on the anemia and cardiac failure. In particular, sustained high cardiac output can lead to heart failure unless patients are adequately transfused. If iron overload is not treated, patients develop life-threatening cardiomyopathy, along with hepatic fibrosis and endocrine failure, particularly of the pituitary gland and gonads. The expansion of erythroid marrow into the peripheral skeleton leads to osteopenia and occasionally pathologic fractures of long bones (Fig. 8-8).

The diagnosis of β-thalassemia major is usually straightforward. Severe transfusion-dependent anemia

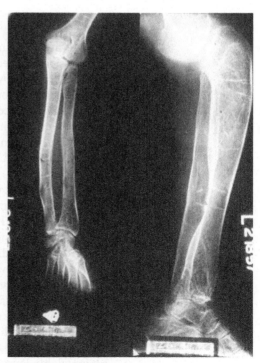

FIGURE 8-8 **Radiographs of the distal long bones in the arm and leg of a child with β-thalassemia major.**

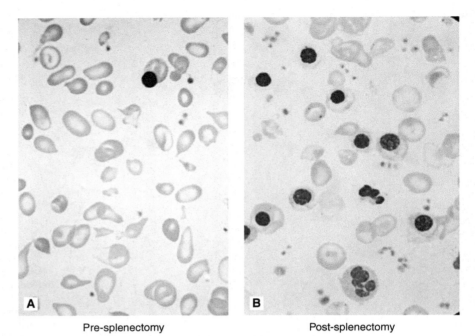

Pre-splenectomy   Post-splenectomy

FIGURE 8-9 **Blood smear from a patient with β-thalassemia major before (A) and after (B) splenectomy.**

begins at approximately age 6 months with the switch from γ-globin to β-globin expression. The red cells (shown in Fig. 8-9) are extremely microcytic (MCV about 55-70 fL) and show huge variations in size and shape. Normoblasts are present in the peripheral blood, and their numbers are markedly increased in patients who have had a splenectomy (Fig. 8-9 B). In patients with $β^0/β^0$ thalassemia, nearly all of the hemoglobin is Hb F. Patients who are $β^+/β^0$ or $β^+/β^+$ have a variable amount of Hb A that accompanies the Hb F. Because of both enhanced absorption from the gut and blood transfusions, serum iron, transferrin saturation, and ferritin are all elevated.

The antenatal diagnosis of homozygous or compound heterozygous β-thalassemia can be established from analysis of DNA obtained by chorionic villous biopsy. The marked heterogeneity of β-thalassemia genotypes makes antenatal diagnosis technically challenging. Moreover, even if a diagnosis is established, the unpredictable degree of clinical severity, religious and cultural considerations, and the development of new and better therapies may dissuade parents from interrupting the pregnancy. Despite these caveats, in selected areas and with well-organized surveillance, antenatal diagnosis has been remarkably effective in drastically lowering the number of babies born with severe β-thalassemia.

Patients with β-thalassemia major require meticulous multi-disciplinary care. The mainstay of treatment is red cell transfusion sufficient to maintain hemoglobin levels above 10 g/dL. Many patients benefit substantially from splenectomy, which improves survival of endogenous red cells and therefore reduces the transfusion requirement. An adequate transfusion program will prevent the

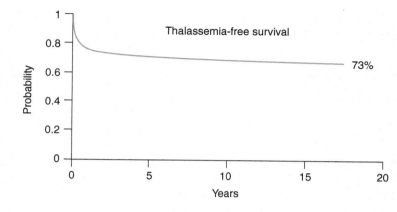

FIGURE 8-10 **Disease-free survival plot of 866 patients with β-thalassemia major following stem cell transplantation from HLA-identical donors.**

development of skeletal deformities, enhance growth and development, and obviate high output cardiac failure. However, transfusions pose a risk of infections such as HIV and hepatitis and development of antibodies (immunization) that may complicate matching of blood. Of even greater concern, transfusions inexorably increase the rate at which iron overload develops. Therefore all patients must be treated with iron chelators sufficient to put the patients into negative iron balance. Recent development of effective oral chelating agents may alleviate the need for daily subcutaneous administration.

Although chronic transfusion and chelation therapy are remarkably effective in preventing the morbid complications mentioned earlier, it is not only burdensome for the patient and his/her care providers but also imposes a huge economic burden. Stem cell transplantation, covered in detail in Chapter 26, offers a compelling alternative. Figure 8-10 shows a survival plot of a large number of patients with β-thalassemia major from Italy. About three-fourths of the patients were successfully transplanted without serious consequences over a period of up to 20 years. These patients can be considered cured. Moreover, despite the large initial financial outlay, stem cell transplantation is highly cost-effective over time. The chief limitation is that only about 25% of thalassemia patients have compatible stem cell donors. Alternative approaches to reverse the pathophysiology of β-thalassemia major include the development of pharmacologic agents that induce γ-globin expression and, further down the road, effective gene therapy.

β-Thalassemia Rx:

Splenectomy
RBC Transfusion
Iron chelation
Stem cell transplant
Induction of Hb F
Gene therapy

β-Thalassemia Intermedia

Some individuals who inherit a β-thalassemia gene from each parent have clinical manifestations and complications less severe than those seen in β-thalassemia major and are designated as having β-thalassemia intermedia. In some cases, the milder clinical phenotype can be explained by: β+-thalassemia genes that allow expression of Hb A; high expression of γ-globin genes; or co-inheritance of α-thalassemia, which ameliorates globin chain imbalance. Patients with β-thalassemia intermedia by definition are not transfusion dependent. However, they are generally somewhat symptomatic from anemia and nearly always develop clinically significant iron overload as well as bone changes. For unclear reasons, many of these patients develop progressive pulmonary hypertension leading to cor pulmonale.

Interaction of β-Thalassemia With Common Hemoglobin Variants

The two most common structural hemoglobin variants are Hb E ($\alpha_2\beta_2^{26glu\rightarrow lys}$) and Hb S ($\alpha_2\beta_2^{6glu\rightarrow val}$). Compound heterozygous individuals who inherit a β-thalassemia gene from one parent and one of these structural variants from the other are commonly encountered and generally have a severe clinical phenotype. The β^E mutation is a single base substitution at the boundary between exon 1 and intron 1, leading to impaired splicing and therefore lowered β-globin expression. Accordingly, Hb E produces a phenotype resembling a very mild form of β^+-thalassemia. Individuals who are either heterozygous or homozygous for Hb E have microcytosis but no significant clinical manifestations. In contrast, individuals who are β^E/β-thalassemia compound heterozygotes often have a severe phenotype indistinguishable from that of β-thalassemia major. Because the gene frequency of β^E is very high in populous southeastern Asia, β^E/β-thalassemia is commonly encountered and is a major cause of morbidity and early mortality.

The gene frequency of β^S is comparably high in central Africa, Arabia, and India. Accordingly, β^S/β-thalassemia compound heterozygotes are commonly encountered in these regions as well as in areas to which central Africans have migrated, such as Italy and Greece. Because the β-thalassemia allele expresses either no or very little β^A, the major hemoglobin component in β^S/β-thalassemia red cells is Hb S, and therefore the potential for sickling in these cells is greatly enhanced. As explained in Chapter 9, patients with the genotype β^S/β^0 have clinical manifestations as severe as those of sickle cell (β^S/β^S) patients, whereas those with the genotype β^S/β^+ have significantly milder manifestations.

α-THALASSEMIA

More than 10 million individuals around the world are heterozygote carriers of an α-thalassemia gene, a prevalence somewhat less than that of β-thalassemia. Affected individuals are predominantly from tropical areas in Asia and Africa. As in β-thalassemia, there is strong epidemiologic evidence that inheritance of a single α-thalassemia gene confers protection against falciparum malaria. Gene deletion accounts for the vast majority of α-thalassemia. As depicted in Figure 8-11, deletions have arisen because of unequal meiotic crossover between adjacent α-globin genes. Because individuals normally inherit two α-globin genes, one from each parent, there are four types of α-thalassemia, depending on how many genes have been deleted (Table 8-1). The most common abnormal haplotype is −α, in which there is only one functioning α gene. About 30% of black Africans are heterozygous for this genotype. Thus, they have a deletion of one of four α-globin genes. In the southern Mediterranean and in Southeast Asia, −α is also very common. The − − haplotype involves deletion of both of the tandem α-globin genes. This genotype is common in southeastern Asia but rare elsewhere (Fig. 8-11).

TABLE 8-1 Genotypes and Laboratory Test Values in A-Thalassemia

Condition	No. of α Genes Deleted	Genotype	MCV (fL)	Hb Electrophoresis	Smear
Normal	0	αα/αα	80-95	2.5% Hb A$_2$	Normal
Silent carrier	1	–α/αα	72-82	2.0% Hb A$_2$	Slight microcytosis
α-Thalassemia trait	2	–α/–α or	65-78	1.5% Hb A$_2$	Microcytosis, target cells
		αα/– –	65-78	1.5% Hb A$_2$	Microcytosis, target cells
Hb H disease	3	–α/– –	60-72	10% β$_4$ (Hb H)	Target cells, Heinz bodies
Hydrops fetalis	4	– –/– –	60-75	>90% γ$_4$ (Hb Bart)	Bizarre RBCs, circulating normoblasts

α, alpha; MCV, mean cell volume; Hb, hemoglobin; RBCs, red blood cells

The various genotypes in α-thalassemia (–α/αα, –α/–α, – –/αα, – –/–α, and – –/– –) correlate with the clinical phenotypes in accord with the number of α-globin genes deleted. Individuals with a single α-globin gene deletion (–α/αα) are called *silent carriers*. They have an entirely normal clinical and hematologic phenotype except for slight microcytosis. As shown in Figure 8-4, measurement of globin synthesis in reticulocytes shows a modest increase in the β/α ratio compared with normals. Individuals with two-deletion α-thalassemia may either be homozygous for the –α allele or heterozygous for the – – allele. The two types of two-deletion α-thalassemias have the same clinical phenotype: they are entirely asymptomatic and have normal or near-normal hemoglobin levels with significant microcytosis, occasional target cells, and an increased β/α synthesis ratio (Fig. 8-4). Two-deletion α-thalassemia should be suspected in African and Asian individuals with no or minimal anemia and moderate microcytosis, once iron deficiency and β-thalassemia trait have been ruled out by appropriate laboratory tests.

As shown in Table 8-1, the more serious forms of α-thalassemia require the inheritance of a – – allele with a –α allele (Hb H disease, – –/–α) or with another – – allele (hydrops fetalis, – –/– –) and are therefore seen almost exclusively in Southeast Asians. Although Hb H disease and hydrops fetalis are much less commonly encountered than the mild forms of α-thalassemia, awareness of these conditions in the United States has been heightened by the influx of large numbers of refugees following the Vietnam War. Individuals with Hb H disease have prominent microcytosis and target cells, shown in Figure 8-12, along with a marked increase in β/α synthesis

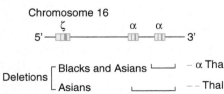

FIGURE 8-11 Molecular basis of α-thalassemia. Simplified layout of the α-globin gene family showing the single deletion responsible for the –α thalassemia allele and the more extended deletion responsible for the – – allele.

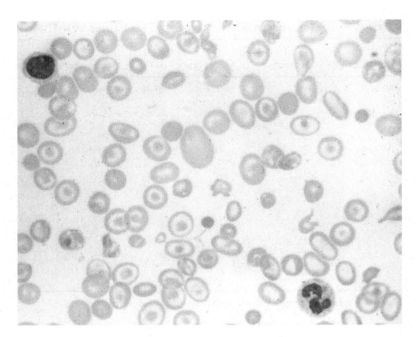

FIGURE 8-12 **Blood smear from a patient with hemoglobin H disease, three-gene deletion α-thalassemia (–α/– –).**

(Fig. 8-4). Because of the large decrement in α-globin production, excess γ-globin accumulates in red cells of the fetus, newborn, and infant and assembles to form an abnormal hemoglobin tetramer known as Hb Bart (γ_4). Following the switch in globin expression in later infancy (Fig. 8-2), the red cells contain an excess of β-globin, which self-associates to form another abnormal hemoglobin, Hb H (β_4). Hb H is relatively insoluble and forms intracellular precipitates called Heinz bodies, which impair red cell deformability and cause premature destruction by macrophages. Thus, individuals with Hb H disease have moderate (and occasionally severe) hemolytic anemia. The treatment for this condition is primarily supportive. If significant iron overload occurs, it should be treated with iron chelation. Splenectomy is of doubtful efficacy.

The inheritance of a – – allele from each parent results in the total absence of α-globin and thus a complete inability to produce Hb F and Hb A. As a result, during gestation nearly all of the hemoglobin is Hb Bart (γ_4). In order for hemoglobin to transport oxygen efficiently, it must be a heterotetramer composed of two pairs of structurally distinct subunits (e.g., α + γ or α + β). In contrast, homotetramers such as Hb Bart have a high affinity for oxygen and lack subunit cooperativity. Even though the blood of a fetus with – –/– – thalassemia is fully oxygenated, it does not release the oxygen to tissues, and therefore the baby suffers from severe tissue hypoxia. At term it is markedly edematous (Fig. 8-13) and moribund, and thus is either stillborn or dies a day or so after birth. The blood morphology reveals dramatic microcytosis, abnormalities in red cell shape, and a profusion of immature nucleated erythroid cells, as shown in Figure 8-14. The possibility of having a – –/– – fetus should be anticipated in Asian families where one or both parents

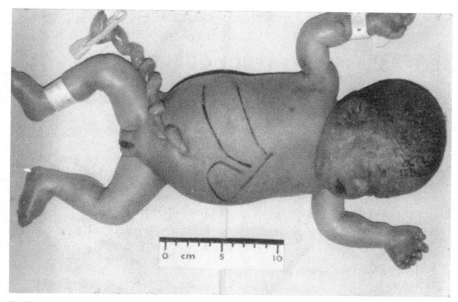

FIGURE 8-13 **Photograph of a stillborn baby with hydrops fetalis due to four-gene deletion α-thalassemia (– –/– –).** (Reproduced with permission, courtesy of Drs. Mary Tang and Elizabeth Lau, Boston Medical Center.)

have microcytosis and especially when there has been a previous baby with hydrops fetalis. Reliable antenatal diagnosis can be done by DNA analysis on a chorionic villus biopsy. If – –/– – α-thalassemia is established early in pregnancy, most parents will elect to terminate the pregnancy. If the diagnosis is not made until the second trimester or early in the third trimester, the fetus can be salvaged by intrauterine blood transfusions. Following birth, stem cell transplantation (Chapter 25), if successful, can be curative, but a compatible donor is found only

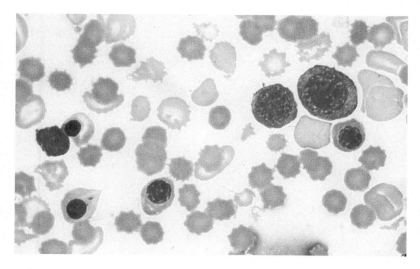

FIGURE 8-14 **Blood smear from a newborn baby with hydrops fetalis due to four-gene deletion α-thalassemia (– –/– –).**

in about 25% of cases.

SELF-ASSESSMENT STUDY QUESTIONS

1. Which of the following statements about β-thalassemia major is correct?
    A. Patients rely on hemoglobin A_2 ($\alpha_2\delta_2$) for oxygen-carrying capacity after birth because synthesis of β-globin is impaired.
    B. Adequate transfusion therapy suppresses ineffective erythropoiesis.
    C. Transferrin-bound iron causes heart disease.
    D. Although hematopoietic stem cell transplantation is effective therapy, it is much more costly than standard treatment with transfusions and iron chelation.
    E. Newborns are severely anemic.

2. The primary cause of death in $--$ / $--$ α-thalassemia is:
    A. Iron overload.
    B. Edema.
    C. Severe anemia.
    D. Liver failure.
    E. Hypoxia.

3. A hematologic evaluation of a 25-year-old man revealed a hemoglobin of 11 g/dL, a hematocrit of 37%, a mean cell volume of 73 fL, and a modestly enlarged spleen. What is the best course of action?
    A. Avoidance of food that contains excess iron.
    B. Hematologic evaluation of the patient's wife.
    C. Avoidance of body contact sports for fear of splenic rupture.
    D. Splenectomy.
    E. Folic acid, 1 mg/day.

Sickle Cell Disease

H. Franklin Bunn

LEARNING OBJECTIVES

After studying this chapter you should understand:

- The inheritance of sickle cell disease and the difference between hemoglobin SS homozygotes, hemoglobin AS heterozygotes, and compound heterozygotes (hemoglobin SC and hemoglobin S/β-thalassemia).
- The molecular basis for polymerization of deoxyhemoglobin S.
- The process of sickle vaso-occlusion.
- The clinical manifestations of sickle cell disease: acute pain crises and progressive organ damage.
- The treatment of sickle cell disease: supportive care and prevention of sickling.

In 1910, Dr. James Herrick, while teaching a course in laboratory medicine, noted that a student from the West Indies had blood with normal-appearing red cells along with a population of "thin sickle-shaped and crescent-shaped red cells" similar to what is shown in Figure 9-1. Dr. Herrick found that this student was anemic and had breathlessness, palpitations, and occasional bouts of icterus. During the ensuing decade, a number of similar cases were reported, nearly all of them individuals of African ancestry. Most of these patients complained of intermittent attacks of severe pain. In vitro studies demonstrated that when blood from these patients was deoxygenated, all of the red cells were transformed into irregular and elongated "sickle cells."

In the late 1940s, the era of molecular medicine was launched with the discovery by Linus Pauling that the hemoglobin from sickle cell anemia patients had an abnormal electrophoretic mobility, indicating that its structure was different from that of normal hemoglobin. Moreover, Pauling found that healthy relatives of these patients often had a 50:50 mixture of the normal and abnormal hemoglobins.

In 1957, Vernon Ingram showed that hemoglobin (Hb) S was identical to normal Hb A except for the replacement of glutamic acid, the sixth amino acid in beta (β)-globin, with valine. This was the first demonstration of a human disease arising from a single structural mutation.

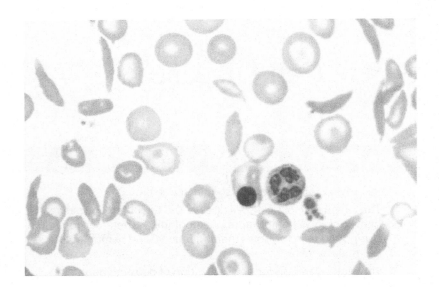

FIGURE 9-1 **Peripheral blood film of a patient with sickle cell anemia.**

GENETICS

Careful observations of families showed that sickle cell anemia is inherited in an autosomal recessive manner, as shown in Figure 9-2.

SICKLE TRAIT

About 10% of black Americans are heterozygotes, inheriting a sickle globin gene (βS) from one parent and a normal (βA) gene from the other parent. As shown in Table 9-1, these individuals with sickle cell trait (Hb AS or AS) have no significant clinical problems unless they are subjected to severe stress, such as marked dehydration or hypoxia. Rarely AS individuals sustain splenic infarction, stroke, or sudden death following strenuous military or athletic training, particularly at high altitude. As discussed later in this chapter, the renal medulla is particularly susceptible to sickling. Many AS individuals have impaired ability to form concentrated urine (hyposthenuria), and a few have recurrent episodes of painless

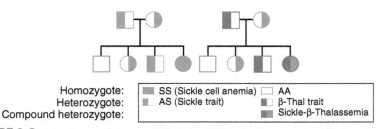

Homozygote:		SS (Sickle cell anemia)	□ AA
Heterozygote:		AS (Sickle trait)	β-Thal trait
Compound heterozygote:			Sickle-β-Thalassemia

FIGURE 9-2 **Inheritance of sickle cell disease.** A) When both parents have sickle cell trait (Hb AS) half of their offspring are expected to have sickle cell trait and one-fourth to have homozygous sickle cell anemia. B) When one parent has sickle cell trait, and the other has β-thalassemia trait, one-fourth of their offspring are expected to be compound heterozygotes (Hb S/β-thalassemia) with a symptomatic sickling disorder.

hematuria as a result of medullary infarction. However, damage to other organs is extremely uncommon in sickle trait individuals. They have normal life expectancy.

The gene frequency for Hb S is highest in Africa (Fig. 9-3), particularly in regions where malaria is endemic. Extensive analysis of polymorphisms adjacent to the β-globin gene has shown that the β6 valine mutation has arisen independently at four different times and places. This finding and the remarkably high frequency of the Hb S allele in central African populations (in which the prevalence of heterozygosity may be as high as 30%) indicate that the AS genotype confers a substantial selective advantage in this part of the world. There is strong epidemiologic evidence and somewhat less compelling experimental support for the notion that AS heterozygotes are less likely to succumb to falciparum malaria, particularly during infancy before immune defense becomes fully developed.

TABLE 9-1 Sickle Cell Disorders

Genotype	Prevalence	Clinical Severity
SS	~1/400	4+
S/β-thal⁰	Less	4+
S/β-thal⁺	Less	3+
SC	Less	3+
AS (S trait)	~1/10	0

SICKLE CELL DISEASE: Hb SS, Hb S/β-THALASSEMIA, Hb SC

According to simple Mendelian genetics, about one-fourth of the children of parents with sickle trait (about 1 in 400 babies born to African American parents) will be homozygotes and have red cells containing primarily Hb S and no Hb A. As discussed in detail in this chapter, these individuals have severe hemolytic anemia

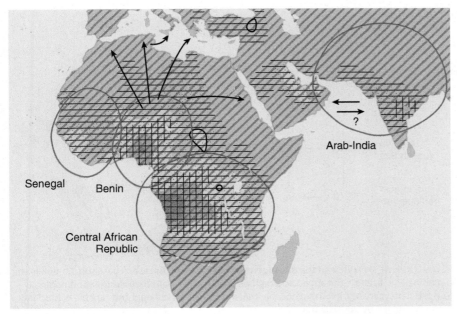

FIGURE 9-3 Map of Africa, the Middle East, and southern Europe, showing four independent origins of the sickle cell (β6 Glu→Val) mutation. The arrows show migration patterns.

and episodes of vaso-occlusion that cause acute bouts of pain and progressive organ damage. A similar clinical phenotype is encountered in individuals who are compound heterozygotes—inheriting the sickle gene from one parent and, from the other, either a β-thalassemia gene (Fig. 9-2B) or a gene that encodes Hb C, another β-globin structural mutant. Patients with S/β^0 thalassemia[1] are unable to make any Hb A and are as severely affected as those with Hb SS (or SS) disease. In contrast, patients with Hb S/β^+-thalassemia or with Hb SC disease have less morbidity and a longer life span (Table 9-1).

MOLECULAR PATHOGENESIS

An overview of the pathogenesis of sickle cell disease is presented in Figure 9-4. The overarching question, which continues to defy easy answers, is how replacement of one of the 146 amino acids in β-globin causes a disease that can wreak havoc on nearly every organ system and display a wide range of clinical phenotypes. A partial understanding has come from rigorous study of 1) the structure of the sickle hemoglobin polymer, 2) the kinetics of polymerization, 3) the impact of recurrent episodes of sickling on the red cell membrane, and 4) the influence of Hb F on disease severity.

STRUCTURE OF THE SICKLE CELL FIBER

Electron micrographs of deoxygenated SS red cells reveal the presence of elongated parallel fibers of about 20 nm diameter that are oriented parallel to the long axis of sickling. Each fiber consists of a helical polymer composed of seven double strands (Fig. 9-5), each containing deoxyhemoglobin S molecules that

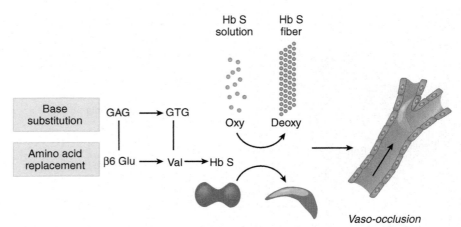

FIGURE 9-4 **Overview of the pathogenesis of sickle cell disease.** A base substitution in the β-globin gene results in the amino acid replacement β6 Glu→Val. When sickle cell hemoglobin $(\alpha_2\beta_2^S)$ is deoxygenated, it forms a polymer that makes the red cell rigid and capable of blocking blood flow in the microcirculation.

---

[1]See Chapter 8 for distinction between β^0 and β^+ thalassemia.

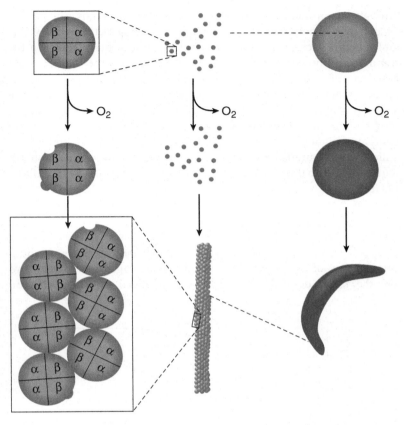

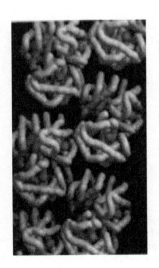
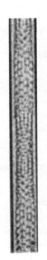
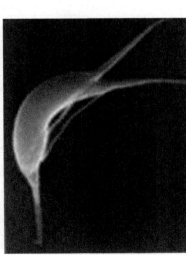

FIGURE 9-5 **Red cell sickling and formation of the sickle polymer.** Right: Deoxygenation of the red cell induces deformation into the sickle and other abnormal shapes. Left: Deoxygenation of Hb S leads to exposure of β6 Val (blue) and a complementary hydrophobic site elsewhere on the β-globin to which β6 Val binds, leading to the formation of a double strand of aggregated Hb S molecules. Middle: Seven double strands aggregate to form a 14-strand helical polymer. (Modified with permission from Bunn HF, Pathogenesis and treatment of sickle cell disease, *N Engl J Med.* 1997;762-769. Copyright © 1997 Massachusetts Medical Society, all rights reserved.)

interact through lateral and axial contacts (Fig. 9-5). Importantly, the double strand is stabilized by non-covalent hydrophobic bonding between β6 valine and a complementary "acceptor" site on another portion of the β-chain on the partner strand. In addition, the double strand is stabilized by other non-covalent contacts between molecules. When the hemoglobin is reoxygenated, conformational changes disrupt these contacts, and the polymer "melts" into individual molecules. The potential to form polymer is greatly affected by the presence of non-S hemoglobin in the red cell. Red cells of SS patients contain 2% to 20% Hb F ($\alpha_2\gamma_2$), compartmentalized in a subset of cells (F cells). Because of amino acid sequence differences in gamma (γ)-globin, it cannot provide a proper hydrophobic acceptor site for binding to the β6 valine site, and therefore Hb F inhibits the polymerization of Hb S.

KINETICS OF FIBER FORMATION

The rate at which polymerization and sickling occur depends primarily on intracellular concentration of Hb S and the extent of deoxygenation. These two variables are the major determinants of the time required for the formation

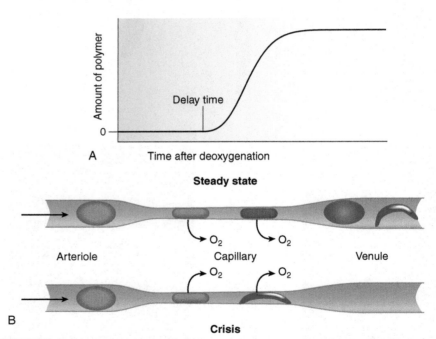

FIGURE 9-6 **Kinetics of sickling.** A) Time course for the emergence of the polymer and sickling of red cells following deoxygenation. The delay time is the time elapsed before the rapid and concerted formation of the polymer. B) Blood flow in the microcirculation. Under steady-state conditions, which pertain in the vast majority of times and sites, red cells are progressively deoxygenated during flow through the capillaries. However, the duration of flow is less than the delay time, and thus the cell does not sickle until it is in a venule that has a relatively wide lumen. Under rare circumstances of either excessive deoxygenation or relatively slow flow, the transit time for passage through the capillary exceeds the delay time, resulting in sickling and obstruction of blood flow. (With permission courtesy, Dr. William Eaton.)

of the polymer. During this "delay time," deoxygenated Hb S aggregates to form a critical nucleus of about 15 molecules. As depicted in Figure 9-6, once this occurs there is a rapid and explosive propagation of polymer extending throughout the cell, deforming it into irregular sickle or holly leaf shapes. If polymer formation occurs before the red cells exit the narrow lumen of the microcirculation, obstruction to flow may occur, resulting in local tissue hypoxia, deoxygenation of red cells perfusing neighboring tissue, and further sickling. Amplification of this vicious cycle may result in a larger area of ischemia and infarction.

PERTURBATIONS OF THE RED CELL MEMBRANE

Recurrent hypoxia-dependent sickling stretches and deforms the red cell membrane, leading to the accumulation of intracellular calcium and the loss of potassium and water. As SS red cells become progressively dehydrated, the increasing intracellular hemoglobin concentration greatly lowers the delay time, thereby enhancing sickling. The most dehydrated cells appear on blood films as dense, irreversibly sickled forms, as shown in Figure 9-1. Other acquired structural alterations in the stressed membranes of SS red cells increase their adherence to endothelial cells lining the vessels in the microcirculation. In addition, leukocytes, which roll on the surface of endothelial cells, can serve as docking sites for sickle cells (Fig. 9-7). Red cell–endothelial cell adhesion slows the transit time of the red cell in the microcirculation and therefore increases the probability that sickling will occur in narrow-lumen vessels. Acute inflammation causes up-regulation of adhesive molecules on the surface of endothelial cells and leukocytes. This response may contribute to the higher frequency of vaso-occlusive events among patients with acute bacterial or viral infections.

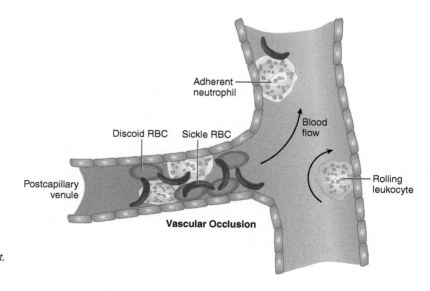

FIGURE 9-7 Sickle cell vaso-occlusion. Sickle red cells tend to adhere to endothelial cells lining the microcirculation, particularly within inflamed tissues. In addition, leukocytes, which roll along the surface of endothelial cells, can capture and bind to sickle red cells. (Modified, with permission, Frenette PS, Atweh GF. Sickle cell disease, old discoveries, new concepts and future promise, *J Clin Invest.* 2007;117:850.)

EFFECT OF Hb F

The most important variable affecting the clinical severity of sickle cell disease is the level of Hb F. As mentioned earlier, Hb F is distributed unevenly among SS red cells. Because Hb F is a potent inhibitor of polymerization, F cells are resistant to sickling and survive much longer in the circulation than non-F SS cells. The ability to produce Hb F varies considerably among different populations. Among American patients with SS disease, clinical severity is inversely proportional to Hb F levels. Among populations in the eastern region of the Arabian peninsula and India (Fig. 9-3), SS patients have high Hb F levels and relatively mild disease. These epidemiological observations have been a powerful incentive for development of pharmacological agents for induction of γ-globin expression and Hb F production. Currently, genome-wide scanning is being actively pursued in search of gene polymorphisms that may modulate sickle cell severity and complications.

DIAGNOSIS

A number of methods are available to test for sickle cell hemoglobin. Simple inexpensive screening tests take advantage of the low solubility of deoxyhemoglobin S and provides a sensitive and reasonably specific way of detecting Hb S. These tests are suitable for large field studies, as they require only a drop of blood and use stable reagents, but do not distinguish between homozygotes and heterozygotes. Newborn screening is mandatory in most states in the United States. It is generally done by transfer of a heel-stick blood specimen to a piece of filter paper, which is then mailed to a central laboratory. A positive result on one of these screening tests needs to be pursued with a follow-up blood specimen for determination of hemoglobin, hematocrit, and red cell indices as well as an electrophoresis of the patient's hemoglobin (Fig. 9-8). Individuals with Hb

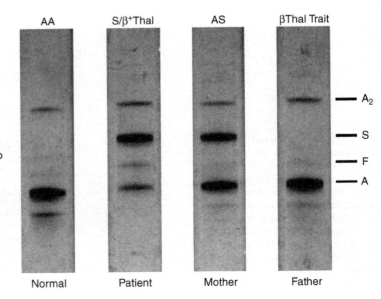

FIGURE 9-8 Diagnosis of Hb S/β⁺-thalassemia by electrophoresis. The normal Hb AA individual has predominantly Hb A and 2% Hb A$_2$. The father has an increased Hb A$_2$ level (3.5%), indicative of β-thalassemia trait. The mother has nearly equal amounts of Hb A and Hb S, indicative of sickle cell trait. The patient inherited the β-thalassemia gene from his father and the βS gene from his mother. He has predominantly Hb S. The presence of a small amount of Hb A indicates that he has Hb S/β⁺-thalassemia. Note that the patient also has a slightly increased Hb F level.

AS have Hb S and Hb A in nearly equal proportions. Hb SS homozygotes and individuals with S/β^0-thalassemia have predominantly Hb S along with a variable amount of Hb F. As shown in Figure 9-8, those with S/β^+-thalassemia also have a small amount of Hb A. Hb SC individuals have nearly equal proportions of Hb S and Hb C. Because of the high level of Hb F in newborns, those with Hb SS, Hb S/β-thalassemia, and Hb SC have no clinical or hematologic abnormalities. They do not become anemic or develop signs and symptoms of sickle cell disease until they are at least 6 months of age, around the time that the switch from γ-globin expression to β-globin expression is complete. Nevertheless, accurate diagnosis of neonates is important in identifying those who are homozygotes or compound heterozygotes, enabling them to benefit from parental counseling and enrollment in a health care network, in anticipation of the complex medical problems that lie ahead.

PRENATAL DIAGNOSIS

When both parents carry the β^S gene, they are understandably concerned about whether future children will have SS disease. This is especially true if they already have experienced the stresses and challenges of caring for a child with the disease. Prenatal diagnosis can be made safely and with nearly 100% accuracy on DNA from a chorionic villus biopsy, usually taken at the end of the first trimester of gestation. If the fetus is SS, the parents face the larger question of whether to interrupt the pregnancy, one that involves moral, religious, and economic issues that are well beyond the scope of this book.

CLINICAL MANIFESTATIONS

Patients with homozygous sickle cell disease as well as those with Hb S/β-thalassemia and Hb SC disease have a variety of clinical problems, outlined in Table 9-2. Among the constitutional manifestations are delayed growth and development. In addition, sickle cell patients are at increased risk of developing serious infections, due to pneumococcus as well as a broad range of other bacterial pathogens. Repeated splenic infarctions lead to loss of organ function and therefore defective clearance of circulating bacteria. Occasionally infarcts in the spleen or other sites of vaso-occlusion become infected, leading to abscess formation.

ANEMIA

Hb SS homozygotes have severe hemolytic anemia with hemoglobin values between 6 and 9 g/dL and elevated reticulocyte counts. The mean red cell lifespan is 10 to 15 days. As a result of accelerated red cell destruction, sickle cell patients have laboratory test findings characteristic of hemolysis, as described in Chapter 3. Patients with Hb S/β^+-thalassemia and Hb SC disease have less

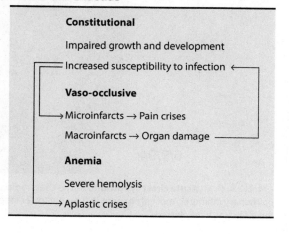

TABLE 9-2 Clinical Manifestations of Sickle Cell Disease

Constitutional

Impaired growth and development

Increased susceptibility to infection

Vaso-occlusive

Microinfarcts → Pain crises

Macroinfarcts → Organ damage

Anemia

Severe hemolysis

Aplastic crises

severe hemolysis. In Hb SS patients, infection will suppress erythropoiesis and cause a fall in hemoglobin level (Table 9-2). In particular, parvovirus B19 has a tropism for erythroid progenitors and therefore can trigger a drop in the hemoglobin levels of sickle cell patients to extremely low levels.

VASO-OCCLUSION

The morbidity and mortality of sickle cell disease are due primarily to recurrent vaso-occlusive phenomena. As outlined in Table 9-2, these can be divided into microinfarctions, which manifest as acute, episodic attacks of pain, and macroinfarctions, which cause progressive and usually irreversible damage to a wide range of organs.

Pain Crises

Throughout their lives, most sickle cell patients are plagued with recurrent attacks of acute pain caused by vaso-occlusion. These episodes account for most of the hospital admissions of sickle cell patients. Pain crises are sporadic and highly unpredictable. Usually, they appear suddenly and are localized to a limited area, particularly the abdomen, chest, back, or joints. As mentioned earlier and in Table 9-2, pain crises are often preceded by a viral or bacterial infection. Most patients are able to distinguish sickle cell pain from pain due to some other type of acute process such as biliary colic, a perforated viscus, or abscess.

The acute chest syndrome, a pulmonary vaso-occlusive crisis, is the most common cause of death in both children and adults with Hb SS disease. The diagnosis is based on the combination of acute chest pain, pulmonary infiltrate(s) and arterial hypoxemia. Because it is often difficult to distinguish between pulmonary vaso-occlusion and pneumonia, all patients should be treated with antibiotic therapy. If there is rapid expansion in the size of the infiltrate(s) or deterioration of

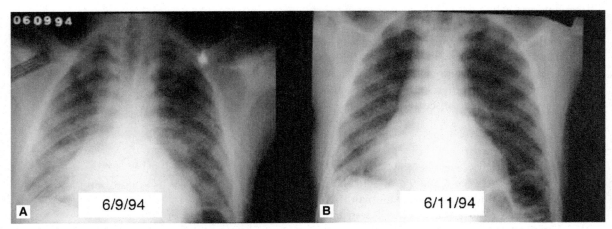

FIGURE 9-9   **Acute chest syndrome.** A) The chest radiograph on the left is from an acutely ill, hypoxemic patient with pulmonary infiltrates, most prominent in the right lower lobe. B) Forty-eight hours after treatment with exchange transfusion, the infiltrates have cleared.

pulmonary function, progressive vaso-occlusion is likely, and prompt intervention is necessary. As shown in Figure 9-9, replacing at least half of the patient's Hb SS red cells with normal (Hb AA) red cells (so-called exchange transfusion) can result in surprisingly rapid clinical improvement and resolution of pulmonary infiltrates. In some patients, acute chest syndrome is triggered by fat emboli shed into the circulation from infarcted bone marrow, a common site of painful vaso-occlusion.

Chronic Organ Damage

Over time, most sickle cell patients sustain damage to various organs due to the cumulative effect of recurrent vaso-occlusive episodes.

Neurologic   Roughly one-fourth of sickle cell patients develop a central neurologic complication at some point in their lifetimes. Noninvasive studies in children have revealed a surprising and sobering frequency of abnormalities of cerebral blood flow that are associated with subclinical impairment of cognition along with increased risk of vaso-occlusive stroke. As patients get older, hemorrhagic strokes may occur. A rigorous and sustained program of red cell transfusions has proven effective in preventing strokes during childhood. It is not known yet whether hydroxyurea therapy (discussed later in the prevention Sickling section) will be as effective.

Cardiopulmonary   Sickle cell patients commonly have impairment of pulmonary function. Resting arterial PO_2 is usually low, in part because of intrapulmonary arterial-venous shunting. Repetitive bouts of acute chest syndrome, described earlier, and chronic hypoxemia can lead to pulmonary hypertension and occasionally to cor pulmonale. In addition, many sickle cell patients have left ventricular dilatation and decompensation, probably due to a combination of chronic anemia, hypoxia, and iron overload.

Hepatobiliary   Like other patients with chronic hemolytic anemia, those with sickle cell disease are very likely to develop gallstones. Nearly all Hb SS patients and many with Hb S/β-thalassemia and Hb SC disease have abnormal liver function, owing to a combination of hepatic vaso-occlusion, hepatitis transmitted via blood transfusions, and iron overload.

Genitourinary   The hypertonic milieu of the renal medulla dehydrates red cells and increases the intracellular hemoglobin concentration, thereby promoting sickling. Therefore, all individuals with Hb S, even Hb AS heterozygotes, develop hyposthenuria (the inability to concentrate urine) and some have episodes of painless hematuria. Hyposthenuria has little deleterious effect on its own, but makes patients (and thus their red cells) prone to dehydration, which can increase the risk for vaso-occlusion. In addition, Hb SS patients develop progressive impairment of glomerular function. As they survive into the fifth and sixth decades of life, renal failure becomes an important contributor to morbidity and mortality. Males with sickle cell disease occasionally develop episodes of priapism,

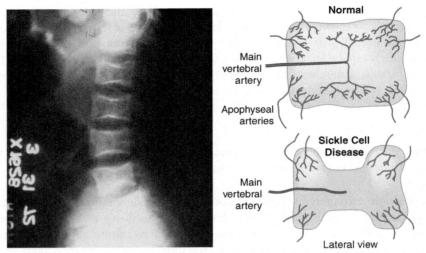

FIGURE 9-10 **A deformity of the lumbar vertebrae in a patient with sickle cell disease.**
Lateral radiographic view showing biconcave or "fish mouth" vertebrae. The collapse of the inner part of the vertebral body occurs because the corners are well-perfused with blood vessels, whereas the inner portion is at the mercy of a single blood vessel.

acute painful engorgement of the penis, due to vaso-occlusion in the sinuses of the corpus cavernosum.

Skeletal   Vaso-occlusion within a bony matrix leads to aseptic necrosis, particularly of the hips and shoulders, and may cause sufficient disability to require joint replacement. Figure 9-10 shows the characteristic deformity of the lumbar spine due to vaso-occlusion in the interior of the vertebral body.

Dermal   Many sickle cell patients are plagued by chronic ulceration of the skin overlying the ankle bones (Fig. 9-11). These lesions probably arise from a combination of minor trauma, local infection, and circulatory compromise by vaso-occlusion. These ulcers are often extremely refractory to treatment.

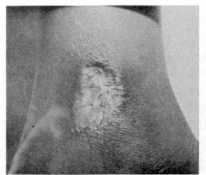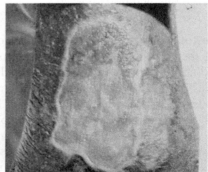

FIGURE 9-11 **Ankle ulcers in patients with sickle cell disease.**

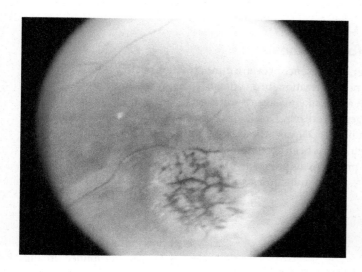

FIGURE 9-12 Sickle cell retinopathy. The "black sunburst" is essentially an accumulation of hemoglobin-laden macrophages in the aftermath of a retinal hemorrhage.

Ocular Sickle cell disease is the leading cause of monocular blindness among people of African ancestry. The retina can be damaged by a variety of events including arterial occlusion, hemorrhage, and proliferation of blood vessels in response to ischemia. Figure 9-12 shows the retina of a patient who sustained a localized hemorrhage, the resolution of which led to the accumulation of hemosiderin-laden macrophages. Proliferative retinopathy is the most commonly encountered ocular complication, surprisingly affecting patients with Hb SC disease and Hb S/β^+-thalassemia about twice as often as those with Hb SS and Hb S/β^0-thalassemia.

THERAPY

SUPPORTIVE

Pain Crises

The management of acute pain episodes remains a very challenging problem. The mainstays of treatment have changed very little in the last 50 years. Nearly all patients experiencing severe pain should receive nasal administration of oxygen to minimize hypoxia and deoxygenation-induced sickling. Close attention must be paid to fluid, electrolyte, and acid-base balances. Pain treatment requires considerable skill and experience, as it is important to give the patient the benefit of analgesia without depressing the central nervous system and suppressing ventilation. Avoidance of chronic narcotic dependency is another important objective.

Febrile Episodes

This must be evaluated and treated promptly and effectively because sickle cell patients are at increased risk of overwhelming sepsis. Nevertheless, with good judgment, at least half of febrile episodes can be managed on an outpatient basis. Because sickle cell patients are at higher risk of developing life-threatening bacterial infections, physicians should have a low threshold for the administration of antibiotics.

PREVENTION OF SICKLING

Induction of Hb F Synthesis

As mentioned earlier, the presence of even a minor fraction of Hb F in a Hb SS red cell greatly inhibits Hb polymerization. In an attempt to pharmacologically increase the production of Hb F, anti-leukemia agents were tested largely on an empirical basis. Although several agents were effective, hydroxyurea was shown to be the safest and most predictable. It blocks DNA synthesis by inhibiting the enzyme ribonucleotide reductase. Hydroxyurea has been given to thousands of patients with Hb SS disease. In most patients, it produces a significant, often marked, increase in the Hb F level. The mechanism of γ-globin induction is unclear. Patients treated with hydroxyurea develop increased hemoglobin levels, have less hemolysis, and show a marked reduction in irreversibly sickled cells in the peripheral blood (Fig. 9-1). As exemplified in Figure 9-13, hydroxyurea treatment reduces the frequency and severity of vaso-occlusive events.

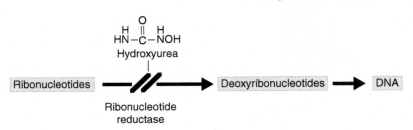

Reduction in Intracellular Hemoglobin Concentration

Based on the realization that Hb S polymerization is markedly concentration-dependent, clinical trials are investigating the safety and efficacy of drugs that inhibit sickling-induced K^+ efflux and Hb SS cell dehydration. The efficacy of one promising agent has been demonstrated in transgenic sickle cell mice and recently in a few patients.

Stem Cell Transplantation

Hematopoietic stem cell transplantation is the only curative therapy available for patients with sickle cell anemia. However, as explained in detail in Chapter 26, this

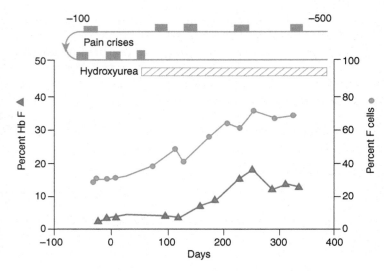

FIGURE 9-13   Response of a sickle cell patient to treatment with hydroxyurea. As shown in the blue rectangles in the wraparound plot at the top of the figure, the patient had numerous episodes of pain crisis during the 500 days prior to treatment. Following initiation of hydroxyurea therapy, there was a progressive rise in percent Hb F and in the fraction of red cells containing Hb F, accompanied by a dramatic reduction in the frequency of pain crises. (Modified with permission from Goldberg MA, Brugnara C, Dover GJ, et al. Treatment of sickle cell anemia with hydroxyurea and erythropoietin. N Engl J Med 1990; 323:366-372. Copyright © 1990 Massachusetts Medical Society, all rights reserved.)

formidable therapy poses serious risks of graft rejection, graft-versus-host disease, and life-threatening infections. A number of complex independent factors need to be carefully weighed in making a decision as to whether the patient is an appropriate candidate for stem cell transplantation. Thus far, stem cell transplantation has been restricted to young Hb SS adults with histories of stroke, acute chest syndrome, or frequent acute pain crises. It is anticipated that during the next decade advances in stem cell transplantation will result in a significant reduction in morbidity and mortality, thereby making this therapy more widely available to sickle cell patients.

Because of improvements in therapy, morbidity and mortality among sickle cell patients have decreased markedly in the last two decades. A major contributor has been the use of prophylactic penicillin, which has been effective in preventing pneumococcal and meningococcal sepsis. It is too early to know whether hydroxyurea therapy will have a positive impact on life expectancy. It is hoped that in the future safe and effective gene therapy can be developed, perhaps using recent technology that allows point mutations to be corrected more efficiently and precisely. This challenging goal is commanding a worldwide research effort.

SELF-ASSESSMENT STUDY QUESTIONS

1. What is the most common cause of death in both children and adults with homozygous sickle cell anemia (Hb SS)?
   A. Acute chest syndrome.
   B. Acute splenic infarction and splenic sequestration.
   C. Infarctive stroke.
   D. Hemorrhagic stroke.
   E. Acute pain crisis.

2. Hydroxyurea has proven to be both effective and safe in the therapy of sickle cell disease. What is the primary mechanism by which hydroxyurea benefits these patients?
   A. Induction of arteriolar vasodilation, resulting in prevention of acute vaso-occlusion.
   B. Enhancement of the ability of Hb S to unload oxygen to ischemic tissues.
   C. Inhibition of thrombosis at the sites of sickle vaso-occlusion.
   D. Maintenance of red cell hydration and prevention of sickle cell deformation.
   E. Induction of Hb F production, thereby decreasing Hb S polymerization.

3. A 17-year-old high-school senior has had recurrent episodes of acute pain in her back, knees, and elbows, which the school nurse attributed to arthritis. Because of progressive fatigue and shortness of breath, the patient was finally evaluated by a physician who found her to be anemic and referred her to a hematologist. Her physical examination results were unremarkable except for a resting heart rate of 90/minute and a soft systolic ejection murmur. Laboratory tests revealed a hemoglobin of 7.5 g/dL and a reticulocyte count of 12%, and a blood film showed many sickle-shaped red cells. Hemoglobin electrophoresis revealed 12% Hb A, 9% Hb F, 75% Hb S, and 4% Hb A_2. What is the most likely diagnosis?
   A. Homozygous sickle cell disease (Hb SS).
   B. Heterozygous sickle cell disease (Hb SA).
   C. Sickle cell β^0-thalassemia.
   D. Sickle cell β^+-thalassemia.
   E. Sickle cell Hb C disease.

10 Hemolytic Disorders of the Red Cell Membrane and Red Cell Metabolism

H. Franklin Bunn and Samuel E. Lux

LEARNING OBJECTIVES

After studying this chapter you should have a coherent understanding of:

- The organization and function of the major proteins of the red cell membrane and cytoskeleton.
- The pathogenesis and clinical features of hereditary spherocytosis.
- The genetics and pathogenesis of **glucose-6-phosphate dehydrogenase** deficiency.

DISORDERS OF THE RED CELL MEMBRANE

MOLECULAR ANATOMY OF THE RED CELL MEMBRANE

As mentioned in Chapter 1, the red cell has two relatively simple yet highly important responsibilities—the transport of oxygen from the lungs to respiring organs and tissues and the transport of carbon dioxide in the reverse direction. Because of its relatively long life span of 120 days, a single red cell makes about 170,000 circuits through the microcirculation and, in doing so, travels roughly 100 miles! The efficiency of both gas transport and flow through narrow channels in the capillary and splenic circulation is enhanced by the ability of the red cell to change shape. Thus, in order for a red cell to fulfill its functions, its membrane must have a high degree of durability and flexibility.

The basis for the remarkable mechanical properties of the red cell is a network of proteins that assemble to form a specialized membrane skeleton, depicted in Figure 10-1. The primary building blocks of the membrane skeleton are alpha (α)-spectrin and beta (β)-spectrin, which bind to each other to form long, stable dimers. Self-association of spectrin dimers and docking of spectrin to a complex of actin filaments, with the aid of protein 4.1, creates a flexible, branching, hexagonal network that covers the entire inner surface of the membrane. The membrane skeleton is tethered to the membrane's lipid bilayer by vertical interactions with a complex composed of the anion exchange channel (band 3), ankyrin, and protein 4.2. These horizontal and vertical interactions within the membrane skeleton and with the lipid bilayer are critical determinants of the pliability and tensile strength of the red cell membrane.

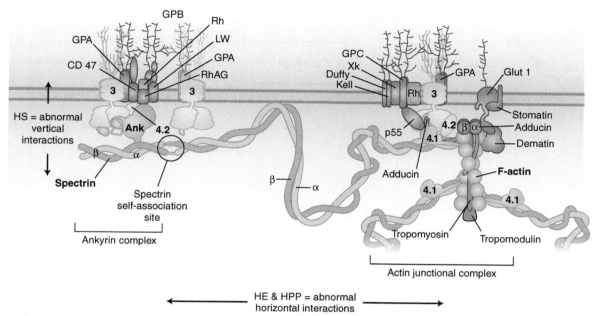

FIGURE 10-1 **Cross-section of the red cell membrane.** The membrane skeleton is composed principally of spectrin (*green*), which binds to itself at one end and attaches to short filaments of F-actin (*blue*) at the other end, aided by protein 4.1 (*orange*). Up to six spectrins can bind to one actin filament, making the skeleton a hexagonal array. The membrane skeleton is attached to band 3 (*pink*), the anion exchanger, via ankyrin near the spectrin self-association site, and to band 3 via proteins 4.1 and 4.2 (*yellow*) at the actin end of spectrin. Other proteins (*gray*) participate in large protein complexes at each of these sites. Defects in the "vertical" connections between the membrane skeleton and band 3 result in hereditary spherocytosis. Defects in the "horizontal" interactions that hold the membrane skeleton together cause hereditary elliptocytosis or its severe variant, hereditary pyropoikilocytosis. (Modified with permission from Grace RF and Lux SE, Disorders of the Red cell membrane. In: Orkin SH, Nathan DG, eds. *Nathan and Oski's Hematology of Infancy and Childhood.* 5th ed. Philadelphia, USA, Saunders; 2008: 671.)

As discussed in the following sections, molecular defects in vertical interactions cause hereditary spherocytosis, whereas defects in horizontal interactions result in the formation of elliptical red cells.

HEREDITARY SPHEROCYTOSIS

Under the microscope, normal red cells appear as biconcave discs. Adoption of this shape requires a significant amount of excess membrane surface area and gives the red cell considerable deformability, allowing it to traverse narrow strictures in the microcirculation, especially within the spleen. In contrast, a cell with a minimal ratio of surface area to volume would assume the shape of a sphere and be non-deformable. A relatively simple laboratory test called *osmotic fragility* can provide an accurate assessment of the surface area to volume ratio of red cells (Fig. 10-2). When exposed to solutions of decreasing salt (NaCl) concentration, the red cell swells progressively until it becomes a sphere. With further reduction in salt concentration, the non-distensible membrane ruptures, leading to release

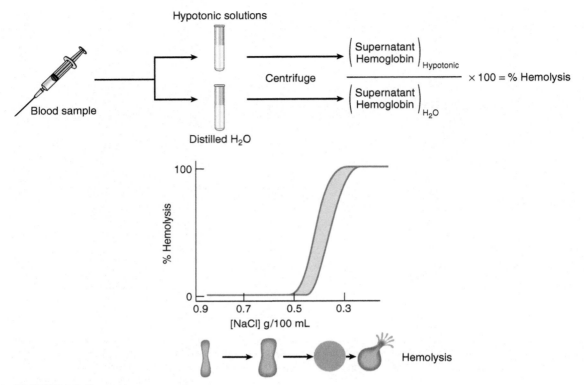

FIGURE 10-2 The osmotic fragility test.

of the cell's content of hemoglobin. Spherocytes have a low ratio of surface area to volume and undergo lysis at a higher salt concentration than that required for lysis of normal cells. In contrast, target cells, which have a higher surface area to volume ratio, undergo lysis at a lower salt concentration.

In patients with hereditary spherocytosis (HS), the presence of non-deformable spherocytes causes hemolysis of varying severity. It is one of the most commonly encountered inherited hemolytic anemias, with an incidence of about 1 in 5000. In the great majority of cases, an autosomal dominant inheritance pattern is apparent. In most of these patients, the causative mutations involve ankyrin, band 3, or β-spectrin. Those with recessive HS owing to biallelic mutations in α-spectrin have much more severe hemolysis. In contrast, individuals with biallelic mutations in protein 4.2 have mild HS. As shown in Figure 10-1, all of these proteins participate in the "vertical" assembly of a complex that stabilizes the interaction of the membrane skeleton with the lipid bilayer. Mutations that result in either impaired production or, less commonly, altered function of one of these proteins cause shedding of membrane microvesicles and thus a decrease in the ratio of surface area to volume. These rigid spherocytes are trapped in the spleen, where they are either destroyed or "conditioned" to become even more spherocytic.

The severity of HS varies considerably. Although all affected individuals have hemolysis with increased reticulocyte counts, those with mild anemia (compensated hemolysis) have minimal or no symptoms and often are not diagnosed until later in life. Most patients have a modestly enlarged, palpable spleen. Those with more marked hemolysis have symptoms of severe anemia and are often mildly icteric. Like other patients with chronic hemolysis, patients with HS, even adolescents or young adults, commonly develop gallstones caused by the precipitation of poorly soluble nonconjugated bilirubin, serum levels of which are elevated owing to the enhanced rate of red cell destruction, as explained in Chapter 3. Patients with HS may have sudden worsening of anemia because of either acute suppression of erythropoiesis, such as during parvovirus B19 infection, or enhanced hemolysis, such as during the transient splenic hyperplasia that accompanies infectious mononucleosis.

The diagnosis of HS should be suspected in any patient with life-long hemolytic anemia, especially when family members are also anemic. In moderate or severe cases, spherocytes are readily detected in the peripheral blood film, appearing as small, dark, red cells with no central pallor (Fig. 10-3). When the hemolysis is mild, the spherocytes are less apparent and are often overlooked. Consistent with the dark red color of spherocytes seen on the blood film, the mean cell hemoglobin concentration (MCHC) is increased in a portion of the red cells. Spherocytes are also the prime morphologic feature of an acquired disorder, immune hemolytic anemia (Chapter 11). The diagnosis of HS can be confirmed by the osmotic fragility test, as described in Figure 10-2. The presence of osmotically fragile cells, that is, those with a decreased surface area to volume ratio, can be enhanced by a 24-hour incubation period at 37°C before the test is performed.

Because spherocytes are trapped by and destroyed in the spleen, splenectomy always greatly decreases the rate of hemolysis and increases the hemoglobin level. Furthermore, the much lower degree of heme catabolism lessens the odds for

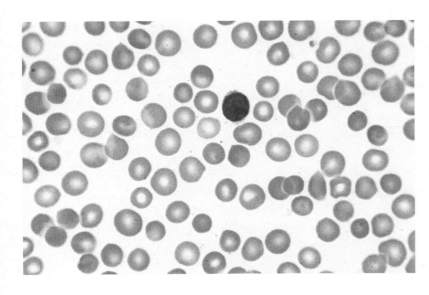

FIGURE 10-3   Blood film: hereditary spherocytosis.

developing bilirubin gallstones. Thus, splenectomy is recommended in all patients with severe HS. However, especially in very young children, splenectomy increases the risk of sepsis from encapsulated bacteria such as meningococcus and pneumococcus, which are normally opsonized and cleared by the spleen. Therefore, surgery should be avoided in very young children (<3 years) and often is not performed in patients at any age who have compensated hemolysis and little or no anemia. All patients should receive appropriate antimicrobial vaccinations prior to splenectomy, and most physicians treat patients with prophylactic penicillin for at least a few years after the operation. There is controversy as to whether patients with moderate hemolysis should have their spleens removed, because of the concern regarding postsplenectomy sepsis. Partial splenectomy is gaining favor in the treatment of moderately severe HS, because it is assumed that this procedure lessens the risk of sepsis.

HEREDITARY ELLIPTOCYTOSIS

Occasional families have mild hemolysis in association with elongated, elliptical red cells, as shown in Figure 10-4, a condition known as hereditary elliptocytosis (HE). These individuals have inherited, generally in an autosomal dominant manner, a molecular defect in proteins involved in the horizontal interactions depicted in Figure 10-1. As a result, *in vitro* studies have demonstrated that spectrin αβ-dimers in the HE membrane skeleton fail to assemble into stable hexagonal arrays. Most often HE is due to missense mutations in α-spectrin, especially in the domain through which αβ-spectrin dimers self-associate. Less often, HE is caused by mutations in the self-association domain of β-spectrin or by a deficiency of protein 4.1.

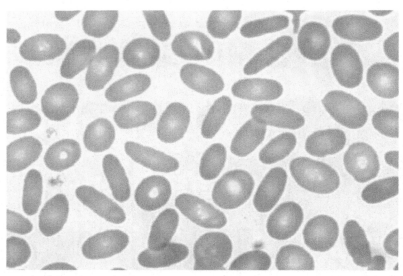

FIGURE 10-4 **Hereditary elliptocytosis.**

Most individuals with HE have modest hemolysis and either mild or no anemia, and therefore do not require treatment. However, at birth some individuals with HE have severe hemolysis and marked abnormalities of red cell shape (poikilocytosis). During the first year of life, these abnormalities evolve into mild HE. Some individuals whose parents have mild HE are born with even more bizarre deformities of red cell shape, designated hereditary pyropoikilocytosis, a severe, often transfusion-dependent hemolytic anemia that does not abate with time.

OTHER INHERITED RED CELL MEMBRANE DISORDERS

Severe hemolytic anemia can be caused by dominantly inherited defects in the control of red cell cation content. In hereditary xerocytosis, red cells are severely dehydrated, owing to excessive efflux of potassium that exceeds the influx of sodium from the plasma. As a consequence, the osmotic fragility test shows osmotic resistance, the opposite of that seen in HS. Red cell morphology is remarkably normal, with only a modest number of target cells. Xerocytes have a high MCHC and are therefore rigid and rapidly cleared by macrophages in the liver and spleen. The opposite pertains in the very rare hereditary stomatocytosis, in which red cells are overhydrated owing to excess influx of sodium and water. As shown in Figure 10-5, stomatocytes have a mouth-like slit rather than a circular area of central pallor. Patients with hereditary xerocytosis and stomatocytosis have a very high risk of thromboembolism after splenectomy, possibly because the asplenic state prolongs the circulation of damaged red cells that promote coagulation in some way. For this reason, splenectomy should be avoided in these patients whenever possible.

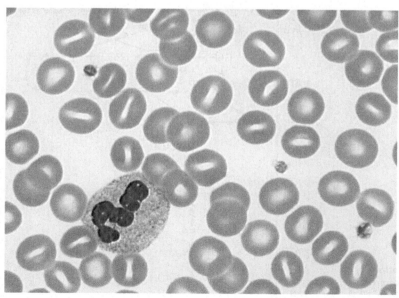

FIGURE 10-5 **Hereditary stomatocytosis.**

DISORDERS OF RED CELL METABOLISM

In keeping with the red cell's relatively simple structure and limited function, it has rather modest metabolic capabilities. Devoid of both nucleus and organelles, the red cell subsists on the glycolytic (Embden-Meyerhof) pathway (Fig. 10-6), which supplies only two moles of adenosine triphosphate (ATP) per mole of glucose metabolized. In contrast, cells containing mitochondria can reap 38 moles of ATP per mole of glucose. Nevertheless, this small supply of energy is sufficient for active transport of cations across the red cell membrane, the synthesis of 2,3-diphosphoglycerate (2,3-DPG) to modulate hemoglobin oxygen affinity (as explained in Chapter 3), and the reduction of heme iron from ferric to ferrous, so that hemoglobin can bind with oxygen.

Despite its simple metabolic requirements, the red cell is uniquely vulnerable to mutations that impair the stability of metabolic enzymes. In contrast to most other cell types, during its 120-day life span the red cell does not synthesize any new protein. As a result, mutations causing a modest decrease in enzyme stability can produce a pathogenic metabolic defect in red cells while leaving other cells in the body unaffected.

HEXOSE MONOPHOSPHATE SHUNT AND GLUCOSE-6-PHOSPHATE DEHYDROGENASE DEFICIENCY

Normally, a small proportion of glucose is metabolized through the hexose monophosphate shunt, which supplies reducing equivalents in the form of

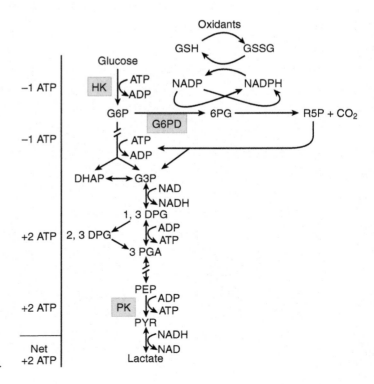

FIGURE 10-6 Red cell metabolic pathways.
HK = hexokinase; G6PD = glucose-6-phosphate dehydrogenase; GSH = reduced glutathione; 2,3-DPG = 2,3-diphosphoglycerate; PK = pyruvate kinase.

reduced glutathione. When the red cell is challenged by oxidant stress, a much higher fraction of glucose is metabolized through this pathway. As shown in Figure 10-6, glucose-6-phosphate enters the hexose monophosphate shunt and is oxidized to 6-phosphogluconate, transferring reducing electrons on to nicotinamide adenine dinucleotide phosphate (NADP) to form NADPH. This reaction is catalyzed by the enzyme glucose-6-phosphate dehydrogenase (G6PD). The production of NADPH permits the conversion of oxidized glutathione to reduced glutathione via the enzyme glutathione reductase. Enhanced production of reduced glutathione enables the red cell to detoxify oxidants such as hydrogen peroxide, superoxide, and other reactive oxygen species, which are produced by immune cells in response to infection and by the liver as part of the metabolism of certain drugs and chemicals. If the supply of reduced glutathione is overwhelmed, either by a very large oxidant stress or by enzymatic defects in the hexose monophosphate shunt, the red cell undergoes serious and irreversible damage. Both lipids and red cell membrane proteins become oxidized. Hemoglobin becomes denatured and falls out of solution into dense, intracellular precipitates called Heinz bodies, shown in Figure 10-7. Heinz bodies are also seen in α-thalassemia when three of the four α-globin genes are deleted (hemoglobin H disease, Chapter 8) and in individuals who have inherited mutant hemoglobins that result in improper protein folding and subunit assembly. The presence of these rigid inclusions causes the red cell to be trapped in the narrow interstices of the spleen. Sometimes splenic macrophages surgically excise the portion of the red cell that contains a Heinz body. In these

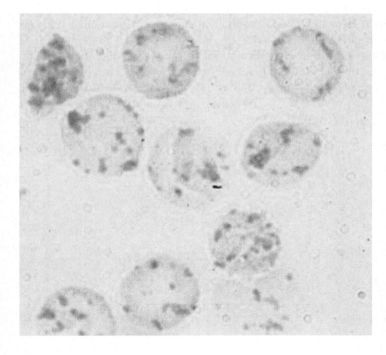

FIGURE 10-7 **Heinz bodies in a patient with oxidant hemolysis.** A special stain is required to reveal these intracellular precipitates of hemoglobin.

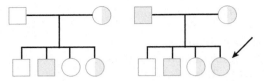

16% of black families   2% of black families

FIGURE 10-8 Inheritance of glucose-6-phosphate dehydrogenase deficiency in African and African American families. Half-filled circles: female heterozygotes; filled circles: female homozygotes (*arrow*); filled squares: male hemizygotes.

circumstances, the red cell may escape with a concave gap in its perimeter, appearing like a cookie after a large bite has been taken.

Deficiency of G6PD is common in parts of the world where malaria is endemic and accounts for nearly all of the inherited abnormalities of the hexose monophosphate shunt pathway. The gene encoding G6PD is located on the X chromosome, and hemizygous males carrying functionally defective G6PD mutants are accordingly more severely affected. Because of random inactivation of one of their X chromosomes, females who are heterozygous for a functionally defective G6PD mutant have, on average, half normal red cells and half G6PD-deficient red cells. Even when exposed to oxidant stress, these females are free of clinical consequences unless X chromosome inactivation is highly skewed toward the one bearing the deficient gene. Because males have a single X chromosome, half of the sons of a heterozygous mother will be G6PD deficient. Homozygous females are encountered much less frequently but have a clinical phenotype identical to that of affected (hemizygous) males. Figure 10-8 shows family trees that illustrate these points.

G6PD deficiency is probably the most prevalent genetic disorder worldwide, affecting many millions, particularly those living in tropical areas. The African (Gd^{A-}), Mediterranean (Gd^{Med}), and Southeast Asian (Gd^{Mahidol} or Gd^{Canton}) variants are so common in their respective locales that they can be regarded as polymorphisms. There is convincing epidemiologic evidence and suggestive experimental evidence that these variants confer protection against falciparum malaria and thus become fixed at a high level of gene frequency in susceptible populations. All of these common G6PD mutants are missense mutations that make the enzyme less stable. In addition, over 100 other structurally distinct G6PD mutants have been reported, most in single families.

As shown in Figure 10-9, even normal G6PD loses over half of its enzymatic activity during the red cell's 120-day life span. However "old" normal red cells have more than enough activity for protection against oxidant stress. In contrast, the

FIGURE 10-9 Decay in enzymatic activity of normal glucose-6-phosphate dehydrogenase (G6PD) and the African and Mediterranean variants during the red cell's life span. The dashed horizontal line shows the level of G6PD needed to protect red cells from oxidant stress.

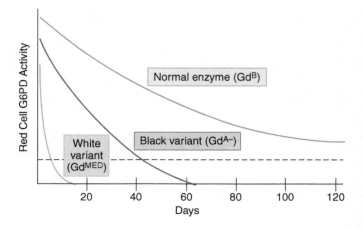

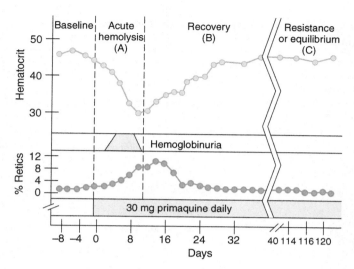

FIGURE 10-10   Effect of administration of the oxidant drug primaquine to a glucose-6-phosphate dehydrogenase-deficient soldier. Top: hematocrit; bottom: percentage of reticulocytes.

activity of the African Gd^{A-} variant decays more rapidly and is nearly absent in red cells older than 60 days. The Mediterranean variant (Gd^{Med}) is even more unstable; its activity disappears before red cells reach 20 days of age.

Individuals with the common forms of G6PD deficiency do not have hemolysis or any other clinical manifestations unless they are challenged with some type of oxidant stress. Figure 10-10 is a historical account from the 1950s of the clinical course of a Black soldier who participated in a study to evaluate the hematologic effects of primaquine, a drug used to treat malaria. The man had normal initial blood cell counts but, similar to about 10% of other African American soldiers in this study, when given primaquine, he developed acute intravascular hemolysis marked by a sudden drop in hemoglobin and hematocrit and the development of hemoglobinuria and reticulocytosis. Importantly, even with continuation of the drug at the same dose, the hemoglobin and hematocrit subsequently stabilized and then slowly recovered to pretreatment levels. All of these findings can be explained by the decay in G6PD activity as red cells circulate in vivo. As shown in Figure 10-9, exposure of red cells expressing the Gd^{A-} variant to an oxidant stress results in the abrupt lysis of all cells greater than 60 days old, that is, about half of the person's red cell mass. However, once these old cells are lysed, the remaining cohort of young cells is resistant to oxidants, except for the small fraction of cells that reach 60 days of age with each subsequent day. Thus, as the drug is continued, the red cell life span falls to 60 days, but otherwise healthy individuals easily compensate for this by increasing the production of red cells from the marrow. Once a new equilibration is reached, the person's reticulocyte count stabilizes at about 2%, and the hemoglobin and hematocrit levels are normal.

A variety of drugs can trigger acute hemolysis in G6PD-deficient individuals (Table 10-1). Individuals with the more severe Mediterranean variant are more likely to have drug-induced hemolysis than those with the African variant. In Black individuals with the common Gd^{A-} variant, bacterial or viral infection is at least as likely as drugs to cause hemolysis, presumably due to release of oxidants from activated macrophages and neutrophils.

TABLE 10-1 Drugs Commonly Associated with Hemolysis in G6PD-Deficient Individuals

Antimalarials	Analgesics
Primaquine	Acetylsalicylic Acid (Aspirin)*
Quinacrine (Atabrine)	Acetophenetidin (Phenacetin)*
Sulfonamides	**Sulfones**
Sulfanilamide	Diaminodiphenylsulfone (Dapsone)
Sulfasalazine (Azulfidine)	**Miscellaneous**
Sufisoxazole (Gantrisin)*	Dimercaprol (BAL)
Nitrofurans	Methylene Blue
Nitrofuradantoin	Naphthalene (Moth Balls)
Nitrofurazone	Vitamin K (Water-Soluble Analogues)*
	Ascorbic Acid (Vitamin C)*

*Hemolysis infrequent. Requires high drug concentrations in G6PD Mediterranean. Does not cause hemolysis in G6PD A.

GLYCOLYTIC PATHWAY

Because the red cell depends on glycolysis for its energy requirements, it is not surprising that mutations in enzymes in this pathway can cause hemolytic anemia. Most of these glycolytic enzyme defects are inherited in an autosomal recessive manner and generally stem from missense mutations that affect protein stability. All are extremely rare except for pyruvate kinase deficiency. As shown in Figure 10-6, pyruvate kinase catalyzes the conversion of phosphoenolpyruvate to pyruvate with the concomitant production of ATP. It is likely that the impaired survival of pyruvate kinase–deficient red cells is due to a fall in ATP to levels insufficient to meet the red cell's energy requirements. Like other red cell enzyme defects, abnormalities of red cell morphology in pyruvate kinase deficiency are nonspecific and unimpressive. Diagnosis requires specific enzyme assays. Severely affected patients may benefit modestly from splenectomy.

SELF-ASSESSMENT STUDY QUESTIONS

1. In what acquired anemia is the red cell morphology most similar to that of hereditary spherocytosis?
   A. Heart valve hemolysis.
   B. Immune hemolytic anemia.
   C. Paroxysmal nocturnal hemoglobinuria.
   D. Myelodysplasia.
   E. Aplastic anemia.

2. An African American soldier developed an acute hemolytic anemia shortly after taking the antimalarial drug Dapsone. By mistake, he continued to take the drug continuously for the next 6 months. What would be the most likely blood cell counts at that time?
   A. Hemoglobin 7 g/dL, reticulocytes 14%.
   B. Hemoglobin 7 g/dL, reticulocytes 2%.
   C. Hemoglobin 10 g/dL, reticulocytes 14%.
   D. Hemoglobin 10 g/dL, reticulocytes 2%.
   E. Hemoglobin 14 g/dL, reticulocytes 2%.

3. Six months after the soldier had continued to take dapsone, what would be the most likely life span of his red cells?
   A. 5 days.
   B. 15 days.
   C. 30 days.
   D. 60 days.
   E. 120 days.

11

Acquired Hemolytic Anemias

H. Franklin Bunn

LEARNING OBJECTIVES

After studying this chapter you should be able to:

- Explain the mechanisms underlying antibody-mediated autoimmune hemolysis.
- Understand the causes of immune hemolytic anemia as well as its diagnosis and treatment.
- Describe the pathogenesis and clinical features of disorders that cause traumatic hemolysis.

Hemolytic anemias are encountered less often than anemias due to decreased red cell production or blood loss. By far the most common hemolytic anemia in both pediatric and adult medicine is sickle cell disease (Chapter 9). Next in prevalence are acquired hemolytic anemias. Familiarity with the pathophysiology of this group of disorders is essential because these patients often pose formidable challenges in both diagnosis and management.

An overview of the hemolytic anemias is presented in Chapter 3 and summarized in Table 3-2. As indicated in Table 11-1, with the exception of the rare disorder *paroxysmal nocturnal hemoglobinuria*, all of the acquired hemolytic anemias are extracorpuscular. This means that red cells from a compatible donor are hemolyzed as readily as the patient's own red cells. Acquired hemolysis is most often caused by immune-mediated destruction or traumatic mechanical damage of red cells.

IMMUNE HEMOLYTIC ANEMIAS

Immune hemolysis can be triggered by:

- Autoantibodies binding to antigens on the patient's red cells.
- Alloantibodies binding to antigens on transfused red cells.

This chapter will deal with autoimmune hemolytic anemia. Alloimmune hemolysis will be covered in Chapter 25 (Transfusion Medicine).

Autoimmune hemolytic anemia is conveniently divided into two categories based on the temperature dependence of autoantibody binding to red cells, summarized in Table 11-2.

TABLE 11-1   Acquired Hemolytic Anemias

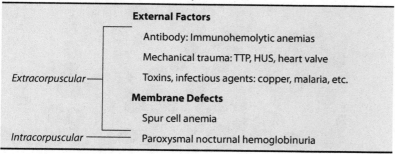

External Factors

Extracorpuscular
- Antibody: Immunohemolytic anemias
- Mechanical trauma: TTP, HUS, heart valve
- Toxins, infectious agents: copper, malaria, etc.

Membrane Defects
- Spur cell anemia

Intracorpuscular
- Paroxysmal nocturnal hemoglobinuria

WARM AUTOANTIBODIES

Warm autoantibodies bind avidly to the patient's red cells at body temperature. They are immunoglobulin G (IgG) antibodies with specificity for Rh group antigens found on red cells of nearly all individuals. IgG-coated red cells are cleared primarily in the spleen, where they are engulfed by resident macrophages that have receptors for the constant region (Fc) of the heavy (H) chain of IgG. Figure 11-1A shows a macrophage from a patient with warm antibody hemolytic anemia that has just ingested two red cells and is about to destroy them. Alternatively, the patient's IgG-coated red cells may bind to the surface of the macrophage but escape total engulfment. Under these circumstances, the macrophage nibbles at the red cell membrane and removes a small portion of it. As shown in Figure 11-1B, this depletion of the red cell surface area results in the formation of a spherocyte. Spherocytes are the predominant morphologic feature

TABLE 11-2   Hemolytic Autoantibodies

	Warm	**Cold**
Autoantibody	IgG	IgM
Specificity	Rh complex	I antigen
I° site of clearance	Spleen	Liver
Mode of recognition	Common IgG H chain	C3
Blood film	Spherocytes	Agglutination

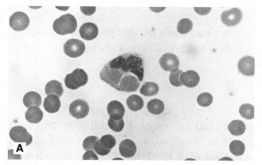

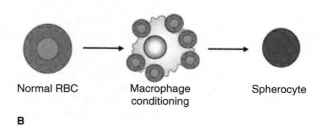

Normal RBC → Macrophage conditioning → Spherocyte

A

B

FIGURE 11-1   Conditioning of antibody-coated red cells by macrophages. A) Erythrophagocytosis of two red cells by a macrophage in a patient with immune hemolytic anemia. (Used with permission from Lichtman MA, Lichtman's Atlas of Hematology. www.accessmedicine.com. McGraw-Hill, New York.) B) Conversion of a normal, disk-shaped red cell into a spherocyte by macrophage conditioning.

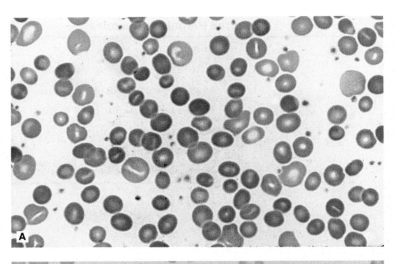

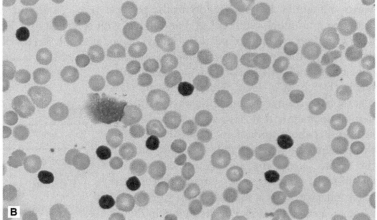

FIGURE 11-2 **Blood films from patients with autoimmune hemolytic anemia due to a warm antibody.** A) Idiopathic. B) Secondary to chronic lymphocytic leukemia. Note the presence of many spherocytes in both. (Used with permission from Lichtman MA, Lichtman's Atlas of Hematology. www.accessmedicine.com. McGraw-Hill, New York, New York.)

in two disorders: warm antibody autoimmune hemolytic anemia (Fig. 11-2A) and hereditary spherocytosis (Chapter 10). Even though these two types of anemia have very different pathogenic mechanisms, they produce identical morphologic alterations in red cells.

Patients with warm antibody immune hemolysis usually present with fatigue, shortness of breath, and general symptoms of anemia. Physical examination often reveals slight icterus and splenomegaly.

COLD AUTOANTIBODIES

Cold autoantibodies bind to the patient's red cells with much higher affinity at low temperature than at body temperature. As a result, binding of cold autoantibodies to red cells is restricted to cool areas of the body, such as the extremities and the ear lobes. In the vast majority of cases, they are IgM macroglobulins that have specificity for the I antigen, which (like the Rh complex) is found on nearly all adult red cells. The large pentameric IgM binds the C3 component of complement much more efficiently than does IgG. As red cells return from the periphery and the blood warms, the IgM falls off the surface, but complement remains attached. C3-coated red cells are prey to two modes of destruction. If complement components are fully assembled, the cell will lyse and release its cytosolic contents into the plasma. More often, however, full fixation of complement does not occur, but sufficient C3b is deposited on the red cell surface for it to be recognized by C3 receptors on macrophages in the liver and elsewhere, which clear the cells from the circulation.

The clinical presentation of patients with cold-type autoantibodies is fully in accord with the pathogenic events described earlier. Most patients have extravascular hemolysis and a clinical presentation similar to that of patients with warm autoantibody hemolysis. Others, however, have a more dramatic clinical picture, in which vascular sludging in parts of the body exposed to low temperature (toes, fingers, ear lobes) results in pain, cyanosis, and even gangrene. In another subset of patients with cold-type autoantibody, the full fixation of complement, particularly following cold exposure, results in acute intravascular hemolysis with hemoglobinuria and a sudden drop in hemoglobin level.

Table 11-3 classifies autoimmune hemolytic anemias according to etiology. In about half of cases, the cause is unknown (idiopathic). In a small fraction of patients the autoimmune process is incited by drugs, some of which act as haptens. More often, drugs, particularly the cephalosporins, trigger autoantibody formation by an unknown mechanism. Patients with idiopathic or drug-induced disease usually have warm IgG autoantibodies. In the remainder of patients, an underlying disease is responsible for the development of autoimmune hemolysis. Lymphoproliferative disorders, particularly chronic lymphocytic leukemia and non-Hodgkin lymphoma (Chapter 22), account for most of these cases. Figure 11-2B shows a blood film of a patient with chronic lymphocytic leukemia who has developed autoimmune hemolysis. Patients with systemic lupus erythematosus are also at risk of developing immune hemolysis. In both lymphomas and systemic lupus erythematosus, the hemolysis is often due to a combination of warm and cold autoantibodies. Patients with either lymphoma or systemic lupus erythematosus are also at high risk of developing autoimmune thrombocytopenia (Chapter 14). Those with mycoplasma pneumonia and infectious mononucleosis occasionally develop transient acute hemolysis secondary to cold autoantibodies.

TABLE 11-3 Causes of Autoimmune Hemolysis
Idiopathic
Drug induced
Cephalosporins
α-Methyldopa
Penicillin
Quinidine
Secondary to underlying disease
Lymphoproliferative: CLL, NHL
Connective tissue: SLE, etc.
Infections: *Mycoplasma*, etc.

LABORATORY DIAGNOSIS

Patients with autoimmune hemolytic anemia generally have straightforward hemolysis with elevation of the reticulocyte count as well as of unconjugated bilirubin

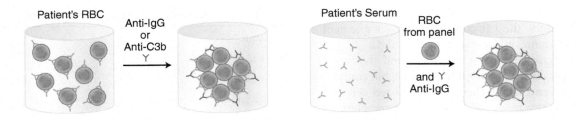

FIGURE 11-3 **The antiglobulin (Coombs) test.** A) Direct antiglobulin test: antiserum against IgG or C3 is added to the patient's red cells (RBC). If they are coated with antibody or complement, agglutination occurs. B) Indirect antiglobulin test: the patient's serum is added to a sample of red cells expressing a known set of blood group antigens, followed by addition of anti-human immunoglobulin (Ig). Agglutination signifies that the patient's serum contains antibodies that recognize antigenic determinants on the test sample. (Courtesy of Dr. Peter Marks.)

and lactate dehydrogenase in the serum. Serum haptoglobin is usually undetectable. As mentioned earlier, the peripheral blood film often reveals spherocytes.

The diagnosis is definitively established by the direct antiglobulin or Coombs test, which is depicted in Figure 11-3A. Following the addition of an animal anti-human IgG antibody, red cells will form visible clumps if they are coated with IgG immunoglobulin. The direct antiglobulin test can also utilize anti-C3 to detect complement on the surface of red cells of patients with a cold autoantibody. If cold autoantibodies are present, clumps of red cells may be seen in the blood film (agglutination) due to the fall in temperature between the time the blood is drawn and when the film is prepared. Usually, cold agglutinins are of no clinical significance, but some are associated with the cold-induced symptoms and signs described earlier.

The indirect antiglobulin test, shown in Figure 11-3B, detects antibody that can bind to a cognate red cell antigen. Patients with warm-type hemolysis usually have a high titer of autoantibody in the serum, which, as mentioned earlier, has specificity for the Rh group of red cell antigens. However, as explained in Chapter 25, the primary application of the indirect antiglobulin test is in blood banking, where it is used to identify and characterize the specificity of alloantibodies in serum of patients who are about to receive transfused red cells.

TREATMENT

Similar to that of other autoimmune disorders, the mainstay of therapy is immunosuppression. Initial treatment usually entails the administration of high-dose corticosteroids, with gradual tapering once the hemolysis abates. Patients with warm autoantibodies who fail to respond or require a high dose of steroids to remain in remission are treated either with splenectomy or with rituximab, a monoclonal antibody directed against CD20 on B lymphocytes. This treatment is virtually identical to that used for the treatment of immune thrombocytopenia (Chapter 14). Patients with cold-type immune hemolysis are usually more difficult to treat. A simple but critically important measure is avoidance of exposure to cold, including the warming of blood prior to transfusion. Occasionally, a patient needs to move to a warmer climate before the hemolysis is controlled. Steroids and splenectomy are much less effective in cold antibody disease. However, some impressive remissions have been achieved with rituximab therapy.

TRAUMATIC HEMOLYTIC DISORDERS

Although the red cell is remarkably sturdy and can tolerate considerable stretching and deformation during 120 days of travel through the microcirculation, extreme turbulence or other mechanical stresses can cause red cells to fracture into small fragments called schistocytes or become irreversibly deformed into shapes resembling a triangle or a helmet, as illustrated in Figure 11-4.

The most prevalent and challenging types of traumatic hemolysis are thrombotic thrombocytopenic purpura and hemolytic uremic syndrome. The formation of platelet microthrombi is critical in the pathogenesis of these disorders, which are covered in detail in Chapter 14. In addition, similar red cell morphology is observed in a sizable minority of patients with an important acquired bleeding disorder, disseminated intravascular coagulation, which is covered in Chapter 16. However, hemolysis is seldom a dominant feature of disseminated intravascular coagulation. Severe thrombocytopenia is a critical feature in all of these disorders.

Grossly turbulent blood flow can also cause traumatic damage to red cells without affecting platelet function or number. The primary example is traumatic hemolysis owing to a malfunctioning artificial heart valve. As shown in Figure 11-4, the blood film reveals striking abnormalities in red cell shape, but, in contrast to the low platelet counts in other disorders mentioned above, the platelet count is normal.

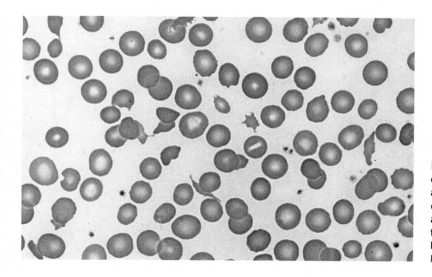

FIGURE 11-4 Traumatic hemolysis due to turbulent flow across an artificial heart valve. Red cells with different types of abnormal shapes are present. (Used with permission from Lichtman MA, Lichtman's Atlas of Hematology, www.accessmedicine.com McGraw-Hill, New York.)

OTHER EXTERNAL CAUSES OF HEMOLYSIS

Infectious pathogens and toxins can cause severe intravascular hemolysis. By far the most important of these worldwide is malaria. This protozoal infection is transmitted by *Anopheles* mosquitoes. Sporozoites injected into the dermis travel to the liver, where they develop into schizonts, which release multiple merozoites into the bloodstream. After infecting red cells (Fig. 11-5A), the parasite undergoes further multiplication. Falciparum is the most severe form of malaria because it elicits the formation of knobs on the red cell surface that promote adherence to receptors on venule and capillary endothelium, resulting in sequestration of the parasite in certain venous beds and the spleen. Along with the constitutional symptoms of fever and malaise, patients infected with falciparum malaria can have life-threatening complications such as encephalopathy due to sequestration of parasites in cerebral vessels, lactic acidosis, and loss of renal function. The pathogenesis of anemia in

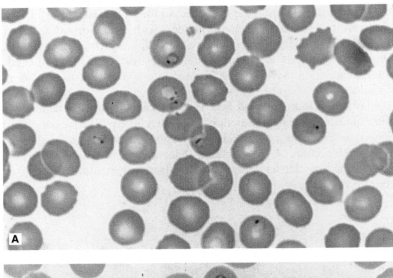

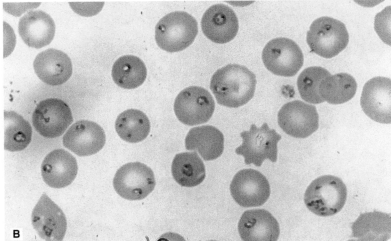

FIGURE 11-5 **Blood films from patients with hemolysis due to parasitic infestations.** A) Falciparum malaria. B) Babesiosis (*Babesia microti*). (Used with permission from Lichtman MA, Lichtman's Atlas of Hematology. www.accessmedicine.com. McGraw-Hill, New York.)

malaria is complex, but premature destruction of infected red cells in the spleen plays a major role. Some patients have severe intravascular hemolysis and hemoglobinuria (blackwater fever).

Babesiosis is a protozoan infection with a reservoir in animals and transmission to humans by tick bite. Most cases in the United States are localized to the northeast coastline, particularly the islands off of Cape Cod. Like malarial organisms, *Babesia* enters red blood cells (Fig. 11-5B) and causes a debilitating illness with fever, chills, malaise, and mild hemolytic anemia. Asplenic individuals are at particularly high risk of developing severe and potentially fatal infections. A skilled observer can distinguish *Babesia* parasites within infected red cells from malaria organisms by subtle differences in morphologic appearance.

ACQUIRED MEMBRANE DISORDERS

Most disorders of the red cell membrane are inherited, and these topics are covered in the preceding chapter. There are two rare but illuminating acquired membrane abnormalities that cause hemolytic anemia: spur cell anemia and paroxysmal nocturnal hemoglobinuria.

SPUR CELL ANEMIA

Patients with liver disease, particularly those with biliary obstruction, have red cells that appear on the blood film as targets, with a puddle of red hemoglobin in the center of the cell rather than an area of relative pallor (see Fig. 3-7 and Fig. 11-6). These cells have an increased ratio of surface area to volume, owing to the passive accumulation of extra cholesterol and phospholipid in the lipid bilayer of the red cell membrane. Target cells have normal pliability and a normal life span in the circulation. In contrast, an occasional patient, usually with severe alcoholic liver disease, will develop more marked increases of lipid on red cell membranes, resulting in bizarre red cells with spikes and thorny projections on

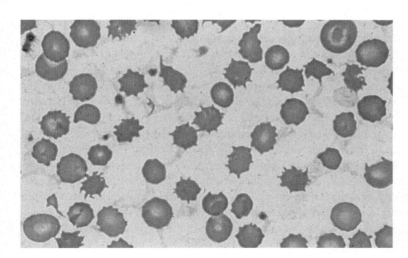

FIGURE 11-6 **A blood film from a patient with spur cell anemia.** (From Lichtman MA, Lichtman's Atlas of Hematology, www.accessmedicine.com. McGraw-Hill, New York.)

the cell surface. In contrast to target cells, these so-called spur cells are rigid and are rapidly destroyed in the circulation. This is an extracorpuscular abnormality. If normal red cells are transfused into a patient with spur cell anemia, they too become spiculated and assume the same abnormal morphology.

PAROXYSMAL NOCTURNAL HEMOGLOBINURIA

Paroxysmal nocturnal hemoglobinuria (PNH) is one of a small and distinguished group of disorders in which the investigators who study it may outnumber the patients who are afflicted. Teachers are appropriately chary about foisting very rare diseases upon overloaded students. However, PNH is a disorder of sufficient scientific and medical interest that an understanding of its pathogenesis, clinical features, and treatment is well worth pursuing.

During the last 100 years, occasional previously healthy patients have been reported to develop severe anemia accompanied by passage of red-brown urine following bed rest. Clinical investigation over the ensuing decades established that these patients had intravascular hemolysis and that the pigment in their urine was free hemoglobin. One astute early investigator wondered if the nocturnal hemoglobinuria could be due to the slight drop in pH resulting from hypoventilation during sleep. This hypothesis was tested by asking a patient to sleep through the night with mechanical ventilatory assistance from a crude, external vacuum-driven respirator (iron lung). This maneuver proved to be fully effective in preventing night-time hemolysis. The significance of this finding was clarified by the demonstration that the fixation of complement on red cells is enhanced by a small drop in pH and that PNH red cells are much more sensitive to the lytic action of complement than are normal cells. A diagnostic blood test was developed, based on the enhanced lysis of PNH red cells at low pH.

As these laboratory studies were underway, hematologists began to appreciate a broader clinical spectrum of PNH. Many patients with hemolytic anemia had a positive acid lysis test without any history of hemoglobinuria, nocturnal or otherwise. In some, the anemia was due to impaired red cell production rather than hemolysis. Most of these patients also had leukopenia and thrombocytopenia, and a few had bone marrow aplasia. Finally, it was appreciated that a dominant clinical feature of the disease was a high risk of developing thromboembolic complications, often life-threatening.

These confusing revelations came into focus through the discovery that PNH is an acquired clonal disorder of the hematopoietic pluripotent stem cell. A variable fraction of a PNH patient's red cells, white cells, and platelets were shown to be hypersensitive to complement and to have arisen from the same abnormal clone. More recently, the gene PIG-A was found to be mutated in the hematopoietic cells, but not in the other cells, of patients with PNH. PIG-A is located on the X chromosome, meaning that any cell in a male or female that acquires a somatic inactivating mutation in the single active PIG-A gene will be unable to express the normal PIG-A protein. PIG-A catalyzes the transfer of a glycosyl phosphatidyl inositol group to certain proteins, a modification that is necessary for their expression on the plasma membrane of cells. Thus, the surface of cells derived from PIG-A defective hematopoietic clone is deficient in glycosyl phosphatidyl inositol-linked proteins. Among these

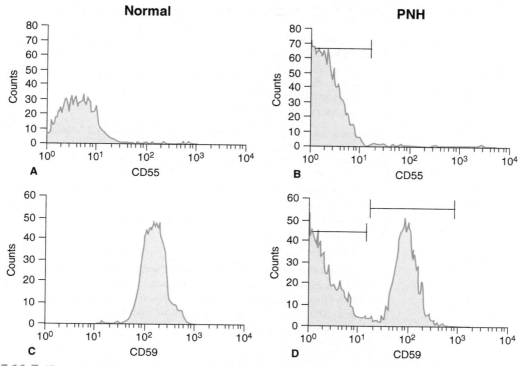

FIGURE 11-7 **Flow cytometric staining patterns of red cells from a normal individual and one with paroxysmal nocturnal hemoglobinuria (PNH).** About half of the red cells in the PNH patient are deficient in CD55 and in CD59.

are CD55 and CD59, two proteins that play a key role in down-regulating activated complement. Figure 11-7 shows flow cytometry results demonstrating uniform expression of CD55 and CD59 on the red cells of a normal individual, whereas the red cells from a patient with PNH include a substantial fraction that is deficient in these two surface proteins.

The remarkable advances in the molecular pathogenesis of PNH have led to a partial understanding of the clinical features of the disease, particularly the enhanced sensitivity of the clonal hematopoietic progeny to complement. The mechanisms underlying the development of marrow aplasia and thrombosis are less clear. However, recent experience with a novel therapy has provided additional clues to pathogenesis. The administration of a monoclonal antibody directed against the terminal portion of the complement cascade has been shown to be remarkably effective not only in reducing, and in many cases eliminating, hemolysis but also in preventing thrombotic complications.[1]

---

[1]This therapeutic advance comes with a price, however. Individuals with inherited deficiencies of complement are known to be at high risk for severe and frequently fatal infections due to *Neisseria* meningococcus, and (predictably) cases of meningococcemia have occurred in those treated with the inhibitory antibody. It is hoped that vaccination and prophylactic antibiotics will obviate this limitation.

SELF-ASSESSMENT STUDY QUESTIONS

1. What diagnostic test is most indicative of autoimmune hemolysis?
   A. Red blood cell morphology.
   B. Direct antiglobulin test.
   C. Indirect antiglobulin test.
   D. Cold agglutinin test.
   E. Elevated serum globulin level.

2. A previously healthy, 50-year-old diplomat recently developed fatigue, weight loss, and mild jaundice. He had a hemoglobin of 7 g/dL, a reticulocyte count of 14%, spherocytes on a peripheral blood film, and a serum bilirubin level of 4 mg/dL total, of which 0.2 mg/dL was conjugated. What underlying illnesses is of most concern?
   A. HIV infection.
   B. Tuberculosis.
   C. Babesiosis.
   D. Malaria.
   E. Lymphoma.

3. A 40-year-old violinist had a 2-year history of hemoglobinuria detected in early morning urine specimens. She was severely anemic (hemoglobin 6.4 g/dL, reticulocyte count 5%). Flow cytometry of her peripheral blood leukocytes revealed a deficiency of CD55 and CD59. What complication is of most concern?
   A. Life-threatening thrombosis.
   B. Renal failure.
   C. Transition to acute leukemia.
   D. Sepsis.
   E. Cardiac failure and/or arrhythmia.

Erythrocytosis

H. Franklin Bunn

Some patients come to medical attention because of an increase in red cell mass, manifested by hematocrit and hemoglobin levels that exceed the upper limit of normal for age and sex. The terms *"erythrocytosis"* and *"polycythemia"* are often used interchangeably. The former is preferred because it covers all conditions in which the red cell mass is increased. *"Polycythemia"* is a more restrictive term, implying not only increased hemoglobin and hematocrit levels but also leukocytosis and thrombocytosis.

In the initial evaluation of the patient, it is important to consider whether the hematocrit and hemoglobin levels might be falsely elevated because of a reduction in plasma volume. False or "pseudo" erythrocytosis may be due to dehydration or loss of gastrointestinal fluid from vomiting or diarrhea. In addition to these acute conditions, modest elevations of hemoglobin (Hb) and hematocrit (Hct) levels may be caused by chronic contraction in plasma volume, most often encountered in hypertensive, overweight, middle-aged males, a condition known as stress erythrocytosis or Gaisböck syndrome. However, when levels exceed two standard deviations above normal (Hb >17.5 g/dL, Hct >54% in males; Hb >16.0 g/dL, Hct >46% in females), it is likely that the patient has true erythrocytosis.

Many individuals with erythrocytosis are asymptomatic. However, as the red cell mass increases, they develop a ruddy or florid facial complexion. With further increases, the patient may develop central nervous system symptoms, such as forgetfulness, lethargy, or headache, and may have signs of excess cardiac preload, such as distended neck veins and hepatic congestion. More often, the clinical presentation is dominated by symptoms and signs related to the underlying cause rather than the erythrocytosis per se.

Establishing the cause of erythrocytosis can be a diagnostic challenge that requires the application of sound pathophysiologic principles. Table 12-1 presents an etiologic framework based on different mechanisms responsible for the expansion of the red cell mass. In primary erythrocytosis, the increase is due to autonomous proliferation of erythroid progenitors in the marrow, independent

TABLE 12-1 Causes of Erythrocytosis

Primary (autonomous) erythrocytosis → Low plasma Epo

  Acquired: Polycythemia vera

  Inherited:

    Familial PV

    EPO receptor mutants

Secondary erythrocytosis

  Hypoxia → Appropriately high plasma Epo

    High altitude

    Cardiac right to left shunt

    Pulmonary disease

    Abnormal hemoglobin function

  Abnormal HIF signaling → Inappropriately high plasma Epo

    Tumors

    von Hippel-Lindau syndrome

    Inherited defects of HIF pathway

of external cues. In these patients, the abundant oxygen supply from the elevated hemoglobin concentration dampens expression of the erythropoietin (*Epo*) gene, and, as a result, plasma Epo levels are low. In contrast, secondary erythrocytosis is caused by an increased plasma erythropoietin level, which is either an appropriate physiologic response to hypoxia or a result of inappropriate autonomous up-regulation of Epo expression.

PRIMARY ERYTHROCYTOSIS

The most commonly encountered form of primary erythrocytosis is an acquired myeloproliferative disorder called *polycythemia vera*. These patients have a marked expansion of the red cell mass, owing to acquisition of a mutation in the tyrosine kinase JAK2, a signaling enzyme that plays a crucial role in hematopoietic cell differentiation. The remarkable ability of this mutation to trigger autonomous erythroid proliferation is depicted in Figure 12-1B. In addition to elevations

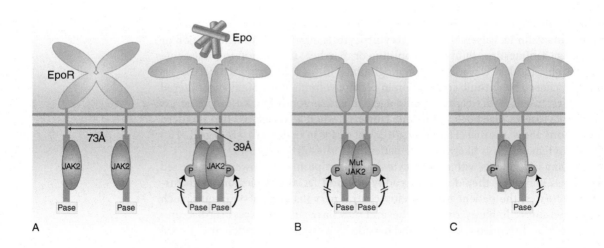

FIGURE 12-1 Erythropoietin (Epo)-dependent signaling. A) Normal erythropoiesis. When Epo binds to its dimeric receptor on erythroid progenitor cells, the two intracellular tails are pulled together, allowing phosphorylation of JAK2 kinase, which initiates the signal transduction cascade. A phosphatase (Pase), that binds to the C-terminal portion of the cytosolic domain of the Epo receptor, acts as a negative regulator, limiting the extent of signal transduction. B) Patients with polycythemia vera have acquired a mutant JAK2 kinase, which has enhanced activity sufficient to initiate and maintain signal transduction in the absence of Epo. C) Some individuals have familial erythrocytosis owing to the dominant inheritance of a C-terminal deletion of the Epo receptor. This truncated receptor cannot bind to the phosphatase and thus gives rise to autonomous, high-level signal transduction, signified by P*.

in hemoglobin and hematocrit levels, patients with polycythemia vera usually have leukocytosis, thrombocytosis, and modest splenomegaly. For more information on the molecular pathogenesis, clinical presentation, course, diagnosis, and treatment of this disorder, see Chapter 20.

Rare families have been reported in which the polycythemia vera clinical phenotype is inherited in an autosomal dominant manner. The mutation(s) responsible for the familial disease are not yet known. Other families have autosomal dominant inheritance of autonomous erythrocytosis with normal white cell and platelet counts. One affected individual was an elite cross-country skier who won several world championships. He and a large number of relatives had hemoglobin levels as high as 19 g/dL, despite low plasma erythropoietin levels. DNA sequencing revealed that those having erythrocytosis were heterozygous for a stop codon mutation that caused the truncation of the intracellular tail of the Epo receptor. As depicted in Figure 12-1C, in the normal Epo receptor, a phosphatase, binds to this site and functions as a brake, limiting the potency of signaling by the JAK2 kinase. In the absence of this negative control, receptor-mediated signaling and erythropoiesis are markedly enhanced. Subsequently, a number of other families have been identified around the world with erythrocytosis due to several other mutations causing similar truncations in the Epo receptor.

SECONDARY ERYTHROCYTOSIS

The major physiologic regulator of Epo expression is hypoxia. When low oxygen tension is sensed in the Epo-producing cells of the kidney, hypoxia-inducible transcription factor (HIF) is induced, triggering a marked induction in *Epo* transcription and increased levels of Epo protein in the plasma. A number of diverse inherited and acquired disorders can cause increased red cell mass owing to elevated levels of plasma erythropoietin. As shown in Table 12-1, it makes pathogenetic sense to group these disorders into those in which the elevated plasma Epo level is an appropriate response to some type of hypoxic stress and those in which the enhanced Epo production is autonomous and therefore inappropriate.

ERYTHROCYTOSIS DUE TO APPROPRIATE ENHANCEMENT OF EPO PRODUCTION

There are many different ways in which hypoxia elicits clinical symptoms, signs, and laboratory abnormalities. Perhaps the most commonly encountered situation involves conditions such as angina pectoris, in which compromised blood flow to an organ or tissue results in focal ischemia. However, secondary erythrocytosis is encountered only when the Epo-producing cells of the kidney sense hypoxia. The most common settings in which hypoxia leads to erythrocytosis are described in the following sections.

High Altitude

The purest form of secondary erythrocytosis is that seen in populations living at altitudes greater than 5000 feet above sea level. The pulmonary, cardiovascular, and hematologic adaptations to high altitude are complex. However, there is convincing evidence that increased red cell mass improves exercise tolerance, lessens fatigue, and enhances well-being in individuals living at high altitude. Erythrocytosis is more marked, and adverse consequences emerge, in high-altitude dwellers who are heavy smokers with obstructive lung disease and in miners who develop inhalational restrictive lung disease (pneumoconiosis).

Cardiac Hypoxemia

Patients with congenital heart disease may develop severe, prolonged hypoxemia because of shunting of blood from the right side to the left side of the heart. These patients have cyanosis owing to low oxygen saturation and therefore an increase in deoxyhemoglobin in arterial blood. The highest hemoglobin and hematocrit levels observed in clinical medicine are in patients with cyanotic heart disease. A modest increase in the red cell mass is beneficial for these patients, enabling enhanced delivery of oxygen to tissues. However, when hemoglobin levels exceed 18 g/dL, the viscosity of the blood rises sharply and is likely to compromise peripheral blood flow. Therefore, patients with cyanotic heart disease and extreme erythrocytosis are treated with phlebotomy. Congestive heart failure is a much more common problem in cardiac patients. With the development of pulmonary edema from left ventricular failure, there is a fall in arterial oxygen tension. However, the degree of hypoxemia is seldom severe enough or of sufficient duration to cause secondary erythrocytosis.

Pulmonary Hypoxemia

Although patients with chronic lung disease often have long periods of sustained hypoxemia, the erythropoietic response is less predictable and less robust. In some of these patients, low-grade pulmonary infection or inflammation may suppress red cell production. However, other patients, particularly those with chronic emphysema, develop sufficiently high hemoglobin levels that they require periodic phlebotomy. Some individuals, especially those who are obese or have upper airway obstruction, have intermittent apnea and alveolar hypoventilation during sleep. A small fraction of these individuals have sufficient periods of hypoxemia to cause mild erythrocytosis.

Increased Affinity of Hemoglobin for Oxygen

As pointed out in Chapter 3 and shown in Figure 3-3, the position of the oxygen dissociation curve is a critical determinant of oxygen delivery to tissues. An increase in oxygen affinity will result in a decrease in hemoglobin's ability to release oxygen during flow through the microcirculation. Unlike individuals at high altitude or patients with cardiac or pulmonary hypoxemia, those having hemoglobin with high oxygen affinity have normal arterial oxygen tension. Therefore, they are not hypoxemic. However, the reduction in unloading of oxygen to tissues results in cellular hypoxia. Thus the cells in the kidney that produce Epo sense hypoxia and up-regulate *Epo* gene expression, leading to expansion of the red cell mass. Three uncommon but highly instructive abnormalities can cause a life-long increase in hemoglobin oxygen affinity associated with erythrocytosis:

- Structural mutations of globin.
- Congenital methemoglobinemia.
- Defects in production of red cell 2,3-diphosphoglycerate (DPG).

About 25 different amino acid substitution mutations of hemoglobin have been described that cause an increase in oxygen affinity and secondary erythrocytosis. Figure 12-2A shows a pedigree in which erythrocytosis is inherited in an autosomal dominant manner. About half of the hemoglobin in red cells of affected individuals was Hb Bethesda, in which an amino acid substitution at the C-terminus of the β-globin increases oxygen affinity (Fig. 12-2B). Erythrocytosis is the only well-documented clinical finding in affected individuals with this and other high-affinity mutant hemoglobins.

Methemoglobin is incapable of binding to oxygen because the heme iron has been oxidized to the ferric form. In partially oxidized hemoglobin, the oxygen affinity of the remaining normal (ferrous) hemes is increased. Accordingly, individuals with congenital methemoglobinemia, due to a deficiency in the enzyme that catalyzes the reduction of heme iron, often have a modest increase in hemoglobin and hematocrit levels.

Secondary erythrocytosis is also seen in rare families with low levels of red cell 2,3-DPG owing to a deficiency of 2,3-DPG mutase, the red cell enzyme required for the synthesis of this glycolytic intermediate. As shown in Chapter 3, Figure 3-3, 2,3-DPG is an important regulator of the oxygen affinity of hemoglobin in red cells.

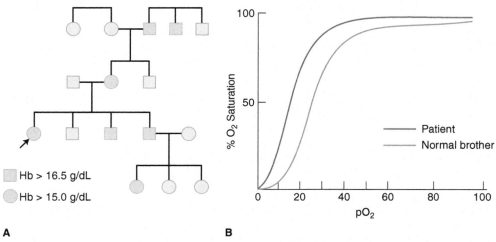

A   **B**

FIGURE 12-2 Familial erythrocytosis due to a high-affinity hemoglobin, Hb Bethesda. A) A pedigree of a family in which affected members have erythrocytosis owing to the autosomal dominant inheritance of a mutant hemoglobin (Hb Bethesda). The arrow denotes the individual in whom the mutant hemoglobin was initially identified. B) Oxygen binding curves of blood from a daughter with Hb Bethesda (designated by the arrow in Figure 12-2A) and from her unaffected brother.

ERYTHROCYTOSIS DUE TO INAPPROPRIATE EPO PRODUCTION

In other settings, erythrocytosis is a consequence of hypoxia-independent over-production of Epo. These forms of erythrocytosis are usually caused by tumors but also occasionally by genetic defects in the oxygen-sensing mechanism that regulates Epo production.

Erythrocytosis-Associated Tumors

Although most tumors are associated with mild to moderate normocytic anemia (Chapter 7), occasionally erythrocytosis appears as a paraneoplastic phenomenon. Interestingly, the tumors that most often cause erythrocytosis are carcinomas of the kidney and liver, the two organs in which Epo is expressed. Other tumors associated with secondary erythrocytosis are cerebellar hemangioblastoma, pheochromocytoma (adrenal medulla), Cushing adenoma (adrenal cortex), and uterine myomata (fibroid tumors). Many of these tumors are highly vascular, and several occur at increased frequency in patients with von Hippel-Lindau syndrome (described in the next paragraph), which is caused by inherited mutations in the *VHL* gene. Epo secretion by tumor cells is believed to be the cause of paraneoplastic erythrocytosis, although this has been proven in only a few cases.

Some families have an increased risk of developing cancer due to the autosomal dominant inheritance of a mutated tumor suppressor gene, one of a large class of genes that normally protect cells from malignant transformation. In such patients, if a cell anywhere in the body suffers a somatic inactivating mutation in the single normal allele, tumor suppressor function is completely lost. One prominent and widely studied tumor suppressor gene is VHL, which encodes a protein that plays a crucial role in oxygen sensing and the regulation of the HIF transcription factor, mentioned earlier in this chapter. As shown in Figure 12-3, in well-oxygenated cells, the alpha (α) subunit of HIF undergoes oxygen-dependent hydroxylation of specific proline residues. This prolyl hydroxylase functions as the oxygen sensor for HIF regulation. Proline hydroxylation of HIF-α results in specific binding of HIF-α to a protein complex containing the VHL protein enabling the polyubiquitination and proteasomal degradation of HIF-α. Thanks to this elegant regulatory mechanism, HIF-dependent transcription is turned on only in hypoxic cells, in which HIF fulfills a critical role by up-regulating genes whose products facilitate adaptation to hypoxia.

The tumors that occur in von Hippel-Lindau syndrome arise from cells that have completely lost VHL function. As a result, the tumor cells exhibit constitutive or ongoing HIF activity, irrespective of oxygen tension. The resultant overexpression of HIF-dependent genes is probably the primary

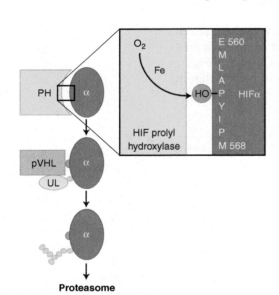

FIGURE 12-3 **The pathway by which the hypoxia-inducible transcription factor HIF is up-regulated by low intracellular oxygen tension.** In normally oxygenated cells, the alpha subunit (HIF-α) undergoes hydroxylation of two proline residues, one of which is shown here. This oxygen-dependent, posttranslational modification is catalyzed by a HIF-α-specific prolyl hydroxylase. The von Hippel-Lindau protein binds to hydroxylated HIF-α, enabling it to be polyubiquinated and rapidly degraded by the proteasome.

mechanism underlying the malignant transformation and, indeed, helps to explain the characteristic vascularity of von Hippel-Lindau syndrome–associated tumors, which secrete HIF-dependent proangiogenic factors such as vascular endothelial growth factor in large amounts.

Tumors most frequently encountered in von Hippel-Lindau syndrome are renal cell carcinoma, retinoblastoma, cerebellar hemangioblastoma, and tumors of the adrenal medulla and pancreas. About 15% of tumors occurring in those with von Hippel-Lindau syndrome are associated with secondary erythrocytosis. Of note, most sporadic renal cell carcinomas are also associated with somatic loss-of-function mutations in both copies of the *VHL* gene.

Inherited Defects of the Oxygen Sensing HIF Pathway

In an isolated enclave in central Russia, there is a high frequency of a particular mutation in the *VHL* gene that is not associated with development of tumors. However, although heterozygotes have no apparent clinical phenotype, homozygotes develop severe erythrocytosis due to elevated levels of Epo. Despite the absence of increased cancer risk, life expectancy is shortened due to complications of erythrocytosis. In other locales, rare families have been reported with erythrocytosis and high plasma Epo levels linked to mutations in the *HIF2-α* gene or a prolyl hydroxylase gene, which, as shown in Figure 12-3, regulates HIF-α. Thus, genetic defects in the system for oxygen sensing and HIF regulation can cause secondary erythrocytosis.

SELF-ASSESSMENT STUDY QUESTIONS

1. A 2-year-old girl had cyanosis and severe erythrocytosis. Which of the following disorders is most likely?
   A. Congenital heart disease.
   B. An Epo-secreting tumor.
   C. Mutant hemoglobin with low oxygen affinity.
   D. Mutant hemoglobin with high oxygen affinity.
   E. Congenital methemoglobinemia.

2. Affected members of a family with erythrocytosis all had very low levels of plasma Epo. What is the most likely cause of this inherited disorder?
   A. A mutant hemoglobin having high oxygen affinity.
   B. Low levels of red cell 2,3-DPG due to an inactivating mutation of 2,3-DPG mutase.
   C. Constitutive signaling caused by a mutation of Epo receptor.
   D. An activating mutation of the alpha subunit of HIF.
   E. An inactivating mutation of the gene encoding the von Hippel-Lindau protein.

PART II Hemostasis and Thrombosis

Hemostasis commands special attention among physicians and investigators. The importance and appeal of this discipline rests on exciting scientific advances as well as its obvious clinical relevance. The mechanisms underlying the initiation and control of blood coagulation constitute a complex but beautifully integrated system of cellular and molecular interactions that fulfill a biological function of crucial importance. As summarized in Chapter 1, the circulation of blood cells and plasma through the vascular tree is essential for providing the body's organs and tissues with nutrients and oxygen and for defense against infection and inflammation. Platelets, endothelial cells, and coagulation proteins cooperate in a complex and dynamic way to repair leaks in the vasculature and protect against hemorrhage in a high-pressure circulatory system.

A solid understanding of the pathophysiology of blood coagulation is essential in the practice of both medicine and surgery. Thrombosis is the leading cause of death in developed countries, impacting a broad range of common medical problems including diabetes, obesity, myocardial infarction, stroke, and pulmonary embolization.

Clinical and laboratory investigation of congenital bleeding disorders have been crucial in working out the structure and function of the blood clotting proteins. The two most famous patients with hemophilia are descendants of Queen Victoria. They are shown in the photographs on the right, convalescing from acute bleeding episodes. On the upper right, the queen's son, Prince Leopold of Albany, is attended by the celebrated British physician Sir William Jenner. Below, Prince Alexei, czarevitch of all the Russias and great-grandson of the queen, is attended by his mother, Czarina Alexandra.

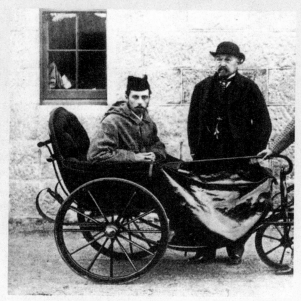

From the Hulton Getty Collection
Prince Leopold (left) and Sir William Jenner (right)

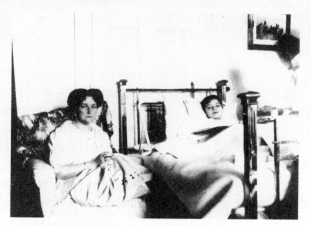

From the state archives of the Russian Federation, Moscow
Prince Alexei and his mother

13 Overview of Hemostasis

H. Franklin Bunn and Bruce Furie

Hemostatic system latent but poised for immediate participation

Blood coagulation limited to region of vessel injury

Hemostasis is a vital host defense system that has evolved in man and other vertebrates to maintain the integrity of a high-pressure closed circulatory system. Following a break in the vasculature, the formation of a blood clot either prevents hemorrhage or lessens its extent. An exquisitely modulated orchestration of cells and plasma proteins enables clot formation to be rapid, self-limited, and reversible. The classic paradigm of blood coagulation begins with the formation of a platelet thrombus at the site of vessel injury. Initially, platelets adhere to collagen exposed on the denuded surface of the injured vessel. This adhesion event then triggers activation of platelets by collagen, thrombin generated by tissue factor, or both, allowing them to aggregate and form a tight platelet plug that stanches the further egress of blood from the injured vessel. The clot is then reinforced and strengthened by the activation of the coagulation cascade, which results in the deposition of insoluble polymers composed of fibrin. The recruitment of specific inhibitors prevents unwanted extension of the clot beyond the site of injury. The final step, fibrinolysis, enables the vessel to be recanalized, thereby restoring blood flow. Recent studies have shown that these phases are less clearly demarcated in vivo than this idealized scenario would suggest. Indeed, the use of specific fluorescent molecular markers clearly shows that fibrin deposition occurs as the platelet plug is being formed.

This chapter will first present the dynamic sequence of events involved in formation of the platelet thrombus and the initiation, propagation, limitation, and lysis of the fibrin clot. This conceptual framework will guide the discussion of the pathophysiology, diagnosis, and treatment of bleeding and thrombotic disorders in this and the following chapters.

PLATELET ADHESION AND ACTIVATION

Plasma contains a large, elongated protein called *von Willebrand factor* (vWF) that forms multimeric polymers with molecular weights as high as 15 million Daltons. As discussed later in this chapter, vWF binds to and transports factor VIII, the protein deficient in patients with classic hemophilia. In addition, vWF fulfills a vital role in the formation of the primary platelet plug. It has binding sites for collagen as well as for a glycoprotein complex on the surface of platelets, GPIb-IX-V (hereafter referred to simply as *the GPIb complex*). Under high shear stresses, such as occur within flowing blood, vWF "unwinds" to an extended conformation in which it can bind to both platelet GPIb complexes and to collagen exposed by damage to the blood vessel. Thus, vWF is a kind of molecular "glue" that allows platelets to adhere to injured vessel walls.

The platelet is activated by adhesion as well as by thrombin generated by tissue factor. Thrombin activates platelets by cleaving the platelet thrombin "receptor" in its extracellular domain, causing a conformational change that transduces an activating signal. As depicted in Figure 13-1A, activation entails a sudden and irreversible change in platelet shape from a smooth disc to a spiky "sea urchin" with multiple pseudopods, markedly increasing the surface area of the platelet. Activation also leads to a conformational change in another platelet membrane glycoprotein, GPIIb/IIIa, which allows it to bind fibrinogen. Fibrinogen is bivalent and can therefore form bridges between GPIIb/IIIa receptors on two different platelets. This cross-linking event is the crucial step in platelet aggregation and the propagation of the primary platelet plug.

In addition to adhesion and thrombin, platelet activation can be triggered by other physiologically relevant stimuli, such as adenosine diphosphate (ADP). ADP is one of a number of molecules released from the dense granules of activated platelets. In the local milieu of the platelet plug, ADP binds to receptors on nearby unstimulated platelets and causes their activation. This is one of several amplification loops that ramp-up the hemostatic process in the immediate vicinity of a vascular injury, enabling rapid clot formation.

Activation of platelets also results in the release of arachidonic acid, a long-chain polyunsaturated fatty acid, from phospholipids on the plasma membrane. Arachidonic acid is converted to thromboxane A_2, a potent inducer of platelet aggregation, by a series of enzymes including cyclooxygenase. Inhibition of platelet cyclooxygenase explains the ability of aspirin to suppress platelet activation.

When platelets are activated, another morphologically distinct organelle, the alpha granule, releases proteins that contribute to hemostasis, including platelet factor 4, thrombospondin, fibrinogen, and factor V. In addition, P-selectin in the alpha granule membrane is translocated to the surface plasma membrane of the activated platelet where it plays an important role in the interaction of platelets with other cells, including leukocytes and the vascular endothelium. These processes provide an important link to the soluble coagulation system.

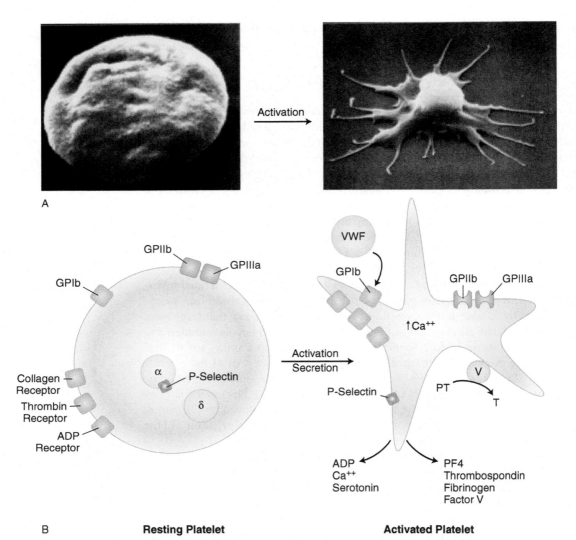

FIGURE 13-1 **Platelet activation.** A) Dramatic change in platelet morphology following activation. (Courtesy of Dr. James White.) B) Molecules on the surface of platelets that are either turned on or exposed upon activation and the substances released from activated platelets.

The factor Xa receptor, defined by phospholipid on the surface of the activated platelet, cooperates with factor V in the generation of thrombin, as shown in Figure 13-1B and discussed in more detail in the following section.

THE BLOOD COAGULATION CASCADE

Just as the formation of the platelet plug is a highly cooperative process, so is the concomitant formation of the fibrin clot. Amplification of a small signal (vascular injury) is transduced by a series of molecular interactions into a fibrin clot. The protagonists in this dramatic process are a set of plasma proteins that normally circulate as inactive zymogens. Figure 13-2 depicts a prototypical or consensus pathway. When the coagulation cascade is activated, either in vivo or in the test tube, a zymogen is converted into an active proteolytic enzyme capable of specifically cleaving the next zymogen in the set, and so on. This highly controlled limited proteolysis leads to the eventual formation of thrombin and generation of the fibrin clot.

During the last century, biochemical studies of in vitro clot formation have gradually led to the identification of the specific proteins that participate in the coagulation cascade, along with in-depth understanding of how they interact in a precisely controlled and orchestrated fashion. A substantial portion of this cumulative knowledge has come from rigorous investigation of families with inherited defects of specific coagulation proteins (see Chapter 15).

Figure 13-3 depicts the coagulation proteins involved in clot formation prior to the formation of fibrin. The zymogens, shown in image A (prothrombin and factors VII, IX, X, and XI), are synthesized in the liver. As this figure demonstrates, they have some striking structural similarities. All have a signal peptide at the N-terminus, and except for factor XI, a propeptide is immediately adjacent. These N-terminal portions are cleaved within the hepatocyte prior to the release of the mature zymogen into the circulation. All five zymogens have a large catalytic domain at the C-terminus that, when activated, functions as a serine protease that specifically cleaves and activates the next protein in the coagulation cascade. Four of these zymogens, factors VII, IX, X, and prothrombin, undergo a crucial post-translational modification in the Golgi body prior to secretion into the plasma.

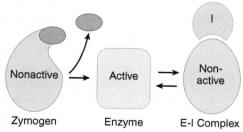

FIGURE 13-2 Consensus pathway responsible for the rapid and controlled formation of the fibrin clot. Zymogen activation by limited proteolysis from inactive to active enzyme (left) and inhibition of the enzyme (E) by a specific inhibitor (I).

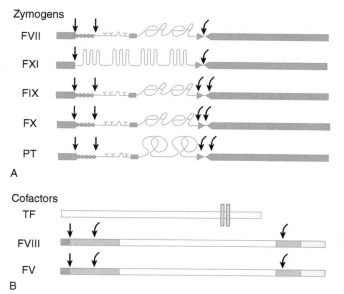

FIGURE 13-3 Proteins in the proximal coagulation cascade. A) Zymogens are converted to active enzymes by proteolytic cleavage. Blue rectangles at left = signal peptides; ●●●●● = propeptide; Y = specific sites of glutamic acid carboxylation. The curved arrows to the right show sites of cleavage releasing the C-terminal catalytic domain (*long blue rectangle on right*), which now functions as an active serine protease. B) Cofactors serve as docking sites for zymogens. Tissue factor is a transmembrane protein. (The lipid bilayer is shown as a pair of vertical rectangles.) Factors VIII and V are activated by proteolytic cleavage at sites shown by the curved arrows. (Modified with permission from Furie B and Furie BC. The molecular basis of blood coagulation. Cell. 1988. 53: 505-518.)

Specific glutamic acid residues in the region adjacent to the propeptide undergo vitamin K–dependent carboxylation. This additional negative charge facilitates the binding of calcium ions, an essential cofactor for optimal function.

Protein cofactors play an equally important role in the regulation of the coagulation cascade. They bind to platelet and endothelial cell membranes, serving as docking sites for the zymogens and contributing importantly to the amplification that is essential for the rapid formation of the fibrin clot. As shown in Figure 13-3B, tissue factor is a transmembrane protein on the surface of extravascular cells, cells within the vessel wall, and circulating microparticles. Like the zymogens mentioned earlier, factors VIII and V are actually pro-cofactors—soluble plasma proteins that require proteolytic cleavage for activation.

In the test tube, the formation of the fibrin clot proceeds by the intrinsic pathway depicted in Figure 13-4. Exposure of the plasma to the glass surface of the tube triggers the activation of factor XII to XIIa (the *a* stands for activated), which in turn, with the participation of high molecular weight kininogen, activates factor XI to factor XIa. Factor XIa, in the presence of calcium ions, catalyzes the activation of factor IX to factor IXa. Factor IXa forms a complex with activated factor VIII (factor VIIIa) on membrane surfaces in the presence of calcium ions to trigger the activation of factor X to factor Xa.

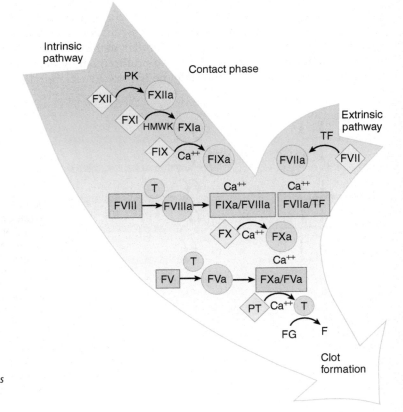

FIGURE 13-4 The blood coagulation cascade in vitro. A fibrin clot can be formed by activation of either the intrinsic or extrinsic pathway. In the test tube, surface contacts trigger the intrinsic pathway. Key: diamonds = zymogens; circles = active enzymes and cofactors; pink rectangles = pro-cofactors; green rectangles = bimolecular complexes; HMWK = high molecular weight kininogen; TF = tissue factor; PT = prothrombin; T in small circle = thrombin; FG = fibrinogen; F = fibrin. (Modified with permission from Furie B and Furie BC. The molecular basis of blood coagulation. In Hoffman R, Benz EJ, Shattil SJ, et al, eds. *Hematology, Basic Principles and Practice,* 3rd Edition, New York USA, Churchill Livingstone, 2001:1784.)

According to conventional wisdom, the extrinsic pathway depicted in Figure 13-4 is responsible for the initiation of the coagulation cascade in vivo. Tissue factor is constitutively expressed on cells within blood vessels. Upon vessel injury, tissue factor is exposed and binds to minute amounts of activated factor VII (factor VIIa) that are normally present in plasma. The procoagulant complex factor VIIa/tissue factor then initiates the coagulation cascade by converting factor X to factor Xa. As Figure 13-4 shows, this is the point at which the extrinsic and intrinsic pathways converge.

However, in vivo coagulation is more complicated. Low concentrations of tissue factor may be concentrated in the thrombus early in its development. The model that best reflects in vivo coagulation in humans is depicted in Figure 13-5.

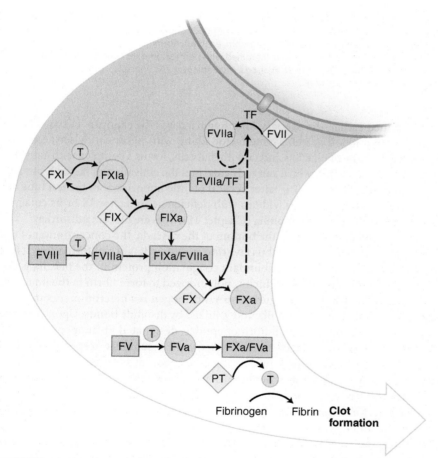

FIGURE 13-5   The blood coagulation cascade in vivo. The primary initiating event is the exposure of tissue factor (TF) on the injured blood vessel. Tissue factor forms a complex with activated factor VII (FVIIa), which not only catalyzes the activation of factor X but also the activation of factor IX. This dual role of the FVIIa/tissue factor complex contributes to the dramatic amplification of blood coagulation in vivo. Activated coagulation factors are shown as circles. (Modified with permission from Furie B and Furie BC. The molecular basis of blood coagulation. In Hoffman R, Benz EJ, Shattil SJ, et al, eds. *Hematology, Basic Principles and Practice,* 3rd Edition, New York USA, Churchill Livingstone, 2001:1785.)

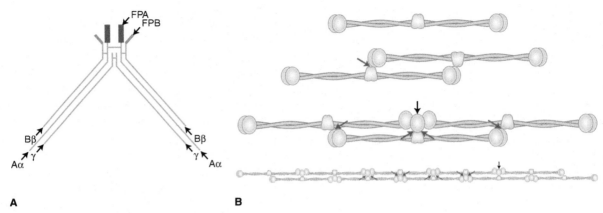

FIGURE 13-6 Fibrinogen and fibrin. A) Diagram of the dimeric structure of fibrinogen showing its three subunits connected by disulfide bonds. Fibrinopeptides A and B (FPA and FPB) are cleaved by thrombin, enabling fibrinogen to polymerize into fibrin by forming end-to-end as well as side-to-side contacts, as shown in panel B. (Modified with permission from Furie B and Furie BC. The molecular basis of blood coagulation. In Hoffman R, Benz EJ, Shattil SJ, et al, eds. *Hematology*, Basic Principles and Practice, 3rd Edition, New York USA, Churchill Livingstone: 2001: 1797, 1798.)

As mentioned earlier, the primary initiating trigger is the exposure of tissue factor on the injured blood vessel. Tissue factor, along with phosphatidylserine on the plasma membrane of platelets and endothelial cells, forms a complex with activated factor VII (factor VIIa), which not only catalyzes the activation of factor X but also the activation of factor IX. The latter event is of little importance in the test tube but is critical in vivo, because individuals with deficiencies of factor IX or its cofactor, factor VIII, suffer from hemophilia (Chapter 15), a severe bleeding disorder.

At each successive step in the bottom of the cascade, the concentration of the respective zymogen increases, thus favoring amplification of clot formation. It follows then that by far the most abundant coagulation protein in the plasma is the structural protein fibrinogen, which is polymerized to form fibrin in the final step in the cascade. As shown in Figure 13-6A, fibrinogen is a heterodimer composed of a pair of three subunits, Aα, Bβ, and γ, linked by disulfide bonds. Upon cleavage by thrombin (factor IIa), small fibrinopeptides, designated fibrinopeptide A and fibrinopeptide B, are released from the Aα and Bβ subunits, respectively. Measurement of fibrinopeptide A reflects the conversion of fibrinogen to fibrin and can be useful in monitoring patients with disseminated intravascular coagulation (Chapter 16). Upon cleavage, fibrinogen undergoes a conformational change that enables it to form noncovalent polymers via end-to-end interactions as well as side-to-side interactions between the linear strands. The strength and durability of the fibrin polymer is then greatly enhanced by the action of factor XIIIa, which catalyzes the formation of covalent crosslinks between the fibrin strands.

LIMITATION OF CLOT FORMATION

Thus far, this chapter has emphasized the importance of rapid clot formation and propagation in the cessation of bleeding. However, it is equally important that coagulation be limited to the site of injury, because its continued extension to

TABLE 13-1   Mechanisms Limiting Extension of Blood Clots

Inhibitor	Target	Effect
TFPI	Factor VIIa-TF complex	Inhibition of extrinsic pathway
Antithrombin	Heparin and endogenous glycoconjugates	Inhibition of factors VIIa, IXa, XIa, and thrombin
Activated protein C	Factors V and VIII	Inhibition of formation of factor Xa and thrombin
Plasmin	Fibrin	Fibrinolysis

TFPI, tissue factor pathway inhibitor; TF, tissue factor.

adjacent normal vessels could occlude blood flow, with possibly disastrous consequences. Thus, during evolution, molecules and pathways have emerged that limit the extent of clot formation (summarized in Table 13-1).

- Tissue factor pathway inhibitor (TFPI) is synthesized in endothelial cells and is present in plasma and platelets. It blocks the extrinsic coagulation pathway after its initial activation by binding first to factor Xa. This binary factor Xa/TFPI complex then docks onto and inactivates factor VIIa/tissue factor complexes, shutting down the extrinsic pathway after a small amount of factor Xa, and subsequently thrombin, has been generated. The intrinsic pathway provides a burst of procoagulant activity once factor VIIIa and factor Va are generated by the action of thrombin.

- Antithrombin (also referred to as *antithrombin III*) is the most important of a number of plasma protease inhibitors in regulating hemostasis. Antithrombin is also known as *heparin cofactor*. Upon binding to endogenous glycoconjugates on the surface of endothelial cells or the anticoagulant heparin, antithrombin changes its conformation and becomes a serine protease inhibitor (serpin) that inactivates not only thrombin but also factors VIIa, IXa, Xa, and XIa. Antithrombin is a scavenger that inactivates coagulation factors as they are carried in the blood away from the developing thrombus.

- Protein C, in the presence of protein S, is activated by thrombin bound to thrombomodulin on the surface of normal endothelial cells. Protein C and protein S undergo vitamin K-dependent carboxylation and share other structural features with factors VII, IX, X, and prothrombin (see Fig. 13-3). Activated protein C attenuates the coagulation cascade by specifically inactivating factors Va and VIIIa.

- The fibrinolytic pathway promotes dissolution of unwanted clot in adjacent non-injured tissues as well as eventual removal of clot during and following healing of injured tissues, thereby restoring blood flow. Fibrinolysis is triggered by tissue plasminogen activator and urokinase-type plasminogen activator, enzymes that convert the zymogen plasminogen into plasmin, a proteolytic enzyme that degrades fibrin.

These mechanisms for limiting blood coagulation often go awry in heredi-tary thrombotic disorders, discussed in detail in Chapter 17, and are the targets of several important anticoagulant therapies described later in this chapter.

LABORATORY EVALUATION OF PLATELET NUMBER AND FUNCTION

The platelet count (number of platelets per mm^3) is a routine part of a complete blood count. Purpura (superficial bleeding beneath the skin), mucosal bleeding, and other types of hemorrhage can occur if the platelet count is too low. In addi-tion, bleeding can be caused by congenital or acquired defects in platelet function. This topic is covered in the next chapter (Chapter 14).

Occasionally, laboratory assessment of platelet function provides useful information. The bleeding time is determined by making a controlled super-ficial incision on the forearm and monitoring the time that elapses before the bleeding stops. As shown in Figure 13-7, if the platelets are functionally nor-mal, the bleeding time becomes progressively prolonged as the platelet count falls below 100,000/mm^3. In contrast, in individuals with abnormal platelet function, such as those with uremia, von Willebrand disease (Chapter 15), or in those who have taken aspirin, the bleeding time is prolonged even though the platelet count is normal. Although the bleeding time has a sound pathophysiologic rationale, the test is cumbersome to set up and is subject to considerable variability and poor reproducibility. For these reasons, it is seldom used.

In contrast, in vitro assessment of platelet aggregation offers highly reliable, albeit lim-ited, information about platelet function and is therefore widely used in the evaluation of patients with bleeding disorders. Platelet-rich plasma is prepared from freshly drawn blood. Following the addition of an agonist, platelet GPIIb/IIIa receptors become competent to bind fibrinogen, which, in turn, promotes platelet aggregation. As platelets clump, the turbidity of the plasma decreases, allowing the process to be followed by increases in light transmission. The time course of normal platelet aggregation in response to agonists (ADP, epinephrine, collagen, and ristocetin) is shown in Figure 13-8. When used at the proper concentration, the first two of these agents trigger release of endogenous ADP from platelet-dense granules in a small

FIGURE 13-7 **Individuals' bleeding time measurements (in minutes) plotted against their respective platelet counts.** As the straight vertical and diagonal lines show, in those with normal platelet function, the bleeding time is not prolonged unless the platelet count is less than 100,000/mm^3. Individuals with ITP (solid blue circles) often have normal bleeding times despite very low platelet counts. Individuals with qualitative platelet defects, due to aspirin, uremia, or von Willebrand disease, have normal platelet counts but prolonged bleeding times.

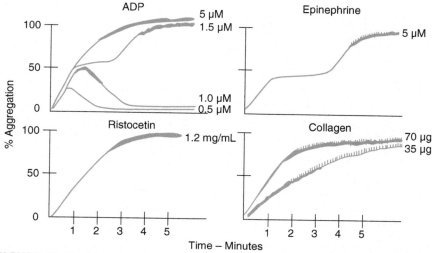

FIGURE 13-8 **Normal patterns of platelet aggregation following addition to platelet-rich plasma of four agonists: adenosine diphosphate, epinephrine, ristocetin, and collagen.**

subset of platelets; this ADP then activates the remaining platelets, inducing a second wave of platelet aggregation. In the presence of the antibiotic ristocetin, vWF in plasma binds to normal platelets and induces platelet agglutination. Aggregation requires calcium mobilization and the activation of the fibrinogen receptor, whereas agglutination merely depends on passive cross-linking of platelets mediated by bivalent binding of vWF to GPIb complexes and therefore occurs even with platelets that have been fixed with formalin. Ristocetin-induced agglutination is absent or attenuated in individuals with either von Willebrand disease or a deficiency of GPIb complexes, the binding site on platelets for vWF.

LABORATORY EVALUATION OF THE COAGULATION CASCADE

In contrast to the earlier-mentioned platelet function tests that are used only in special circumstances, laboratory assessment of the coagulation cascade is crucial in the diagnosis and monitoring of a broad range of medical, surgical, and obstetric patients with a variety of common and sometimes life-threatening disorders. The standard initial assessment includes the platelet count (discussed earlier), prothrombin time (PT), and partial thromboplastin time (PTT).

As shown in Figure 13-9, the PT is performed by the addition of recombinant tissue factor to plasma. Thus, the PT assesses the extrinsic pathway of coagulation. Normally, the plasma suddenly clots after about 12 seconds. A prolongation in the PT means that the patient has a functional deficiency of one or more of the clotting factors in the extrinsic pathway, specifically factors VII, X, V, prothrombin, or

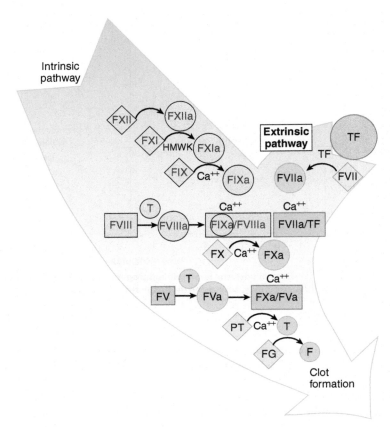

FIGURE 13-9 **The prothrombin time (PT) is used to monitor the extrinsic pathway of coagulation.** The addition of exogenous tissue factor (TF) to plasma activates factor VII, initiating the extrinsic cascade. The coagulation factors that participate in this pathway are shown in light blue diamonds (zymogens and fibrinogen), orange circles (activated enzymes, factor V cofactor, and Fibrin), and light green rectangles (protein complexes). (Modified with permission from Furie B and Furie BC. The molecular basis of blood coagulation. In Hoffman R, Benz EJ, Shattil SJ, et al, eds. Hematology, Basic Principles and Practice, 3rd Edition, New York USA, Churchill Livingstone, 2001: 1784.)

fibrinogen. In many laboratories and clinics, the report includes the international normalized ratio (INR), a standardization of the PT that takes into account the potency of the tissue factor employed.

In contrast, the PTT assesses the intrinsic pathway of coagulation. Kaolin, a porous diatomaceous earth, is added to plasma, providing an abundant artificial contact surface that initiates the cascade by activating factor XII. Figure 13-10 shows the clotting factors that participate in the clot formed in the PTT: factors XII, XI, IX, VIII, X, V, prothrombin, and fibrinogen.

The thrombin time (TT) is the time required for a clot to form after the addition of thrombin to plasma. Thus, it assesses the amount and functionality of fibrinogen as well as the presence of thrombin inhibitors such as the anticoagulant heparin (see page 155) or breakdown products of fibrinogen and fibrin, called *fibrin degradation products,* that interfere with fibrin formation.

The interpretation of the results of the PT, PTT, and TT can be viewed as a matrix, shown in Table 13-2. The combination of the PT, PTT, and TT is very useful in narrowing down what factor or factors are defective or deficient. Armed with this information, the laboratory can then perform specific factor assays, often by

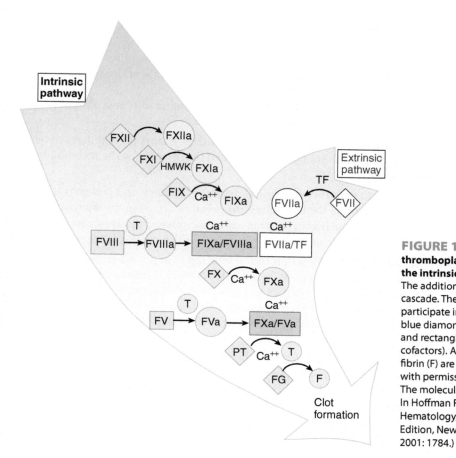

FIGURE 13-10 The partial thromboplastin time is used to monitor the intrinsic pathway of coagulation. The addition of kaolin initiates the intrinsic cascade. The coagulation factors that participate in this pathway are shown in light blue diamonds (zymogens and fibrinogen) and rectangles (factor V and factor VIII cofactors). Activated coagulation factors and fibrin (F) are shown as pink circles. (Modified with permission from Furie B and Furie BC. The molecular basis of blood coagulation. In Hoffman R, Benz EJ, Shattil SJ, et al, eds. Hematology, Basic Principles and Practice, 3rd Edition, New York USA, Churchill Livingstone, 2001: 1784.)

TABLE 13-2 Interpretation of Initial Laboratory Assessment of Hemostasis

Prothrombin Time	Partial Thromboplastin Time	Thrombin Time	Single Defects in the Coagulation Cascade
Prolonged	Prolonged	Normal	Factor V, factor X, prothrombin
Prolonged	Normal	Normal	Factor VII
Normal	Prolonged	Normal	Factors XII, XI, IX, or VIII
Normal or prolonged	Normal or prolonged	Prolonged	Fibrinogen or thrombin inhibitor

mixing the patient's plasma with plasma that is known to be deficient in a single clotting factor. In almost all of the inherited bleeding disorders (Chapter 15), only a single deficiency will be found.[1] In contrast, patients with acquired bleeding problems (Chapter 16) due to liver disease, vitamin K deficiency, or disseminated intravascular coagulation will have multiple deficiencies.

In addition to single factor assays, a number of other tests are commonly used to determine the cause of bleeding disorders.

- Assessment of *fibrinogen*, a normally abundant plasma protein that can be quantified by immunologic assay or tested functionally by the thrombin time.

- Measurement of *fibrinogen/fibrin degradation products* and *D-dimers* is useful in documenting the fibrinolytic process that occurs in the aftermath of clotting in vivo, such as in patients with disseminated intravascular coagulation (discussed in Chapter 16) or deep venous thrombosis (Chapter 17).

- Assessment of *vWF* function (often referred to as a vWF panel). These include: 1) measurement of factor VIII activity; 2) immunologic quantification of vWF, which carries factor VIII in the blood; and 3) ristocetin-induced platelet agglutination assays, which assess vWF function. This panel is particularly useful in the diagnosis of von Willebrand disease (Chapter 15).

- *Mixing studies* are used to detect the presence of inhibitors to blood clotting factors. For example, to evaluate a patient with a prolonged PTT, the patient's plasma is mixed with an equal volume of normal plasma, and the PTT test is repeated. Clotting factor levels that are >25% of normal are sufficient to give a normal PTT; therefore, if the patient has a simple deficiency in a clotting factor, the PTT of the mixture will be normal. In contrast, the PTT will be prolonged if the patient's plasma contains an inhibitor, such as an antibody, capable of inactivating a clotting factor in both the patient's plasma and the admixed normal plasma.

The application and interpretation of these tests in different clinical settings will be covered in Chapters 14 through 17.

ANTICOAGULANT AND FIBRINOLYTIC DRUGS

Patients with bleeding and thrombotic disorders are effectively treated with a variety of modalities including specific factor replacement, transfusions of red cells, platelets and plasma, and a wide range of drugs. These applications will be covered in the four chapters that follow. However, it is fitting that this chapter conclude with a consideration of anticoagulant and antifibrinolytic drugs because they are widely used in a number of commonly encountered disorders, and the mechanisms underlying their efficacy are based on the coagulation pathways described earlier.

---

[1]An important exception is von Willebrand disease, in which the plasma is deficient in both vWF and factor VIII.

- Vitamin K antagonists. Because carboxylation of factors VII, IX, X, and pro-thrombin is required for hemostatic effectiveness, blocking of this vitamin K-dependent post-translational modification has proven to be an effective way to retard blood clotting in vivo. The most commonly used vitamin K antagonist is warfarin, which is administered daily by mouth. Patients treated with warfarin must be monitored closely with regular measurements of the PT to ensure that warfarin levels are in a therapeutic range, because insufficient anticoagulation is ineffective in preventing thrombosis, whereas excessive anticoagulation increases the risk of serious bleeding.

- Heparin and heparin-like drugs. As explained in the previous section, polysaccharides, particularly heparin, activate the serine protease inhibitor antithrombin thereby inhibiting several steps in the coagulation cascade both in vivo and in vitro. Heparin must be administered parenterally, but patients do not need to be monitored as closely as those on warfarin. Unfractionated hepa-rin occasionally causes a potentially serious complication, heparin-induced thrombocytopenia, owing to an autoantibody against a complex of the drug and platelet factor 4 released from alpha granules. This immune response activates platelets, commonly causing thrombocytopenia and, in some patients, life-threatening venous and/or arterial thrombosis (see Chapter 17).

- Direct thrombin inhibitors. Knowledge of the three-dimensional structure of thrombin and the domain responsible for its proteolytic activity has led to the design and development of drugs such as argatroban that bind with high affinity and specificity to thrombin's active site. Argatroban is particularly useful in patients who cannot be anticoagulated with heparin because of the development of heparin-induced thrombocytopenia.

- Fibrinolytic drugs. Agents that activate the fibrinolytic pathway are often remarkably effective in opening vessel lumens occluded by thrombus and re-establishing blood flow. Initially, the proteolytic enzymes streptokinase and urokinase were used. More recently, recombinant tissue plasminogen activator has been shown to have superior efficacy. These therapies carry with them the risk of hemorrhage.

SELF-ASSESSMENT STUDY QUESTIONS

1. What is the primary molecular event underlying platelet aggregation and propagation of the platelet plug?
   A. Binding of vWF to platelet GPIb complex.
   B. Binding of vWF to platelet GPIIb/IIIa.
   C. Binding of fibrin to platelet GPIb complex.
   D. Binding of fibrinogen to platelet GPIb complex.
   E. Binding of fibrinogen to platelet GPIIb/IIIa.

2. What is the primary role of tissue factor?
   A. Activation of prothrombin.
   B. Activation of factor VII.
   C. Activation of factor X.
   D. Activation of thrombin.
   E. All of the above.

3. Which of the following proteins strengthens the fibrin clot by mediating covalent cross-linking?
   A. Thrombin.
   B. Fibrinogen.
   C. Factor Va.
   D. Factor VIIa.
   E. Factor XIIIa.

4. A 4-year-old boy has had recurrent bleeding episodes in his joints (hemarthroses). His maternal uncle has a similar history. Laboratory evaluation of both the boy and his uncle reveals normal platelet counts, prolonged partial thromboplastin times, prolonged prothrombin times, and normal thrombin times.

   Among the possibilities listed below, these two patients are most likely to be deficient in:
   A. Fibrinogen.
   B. Factor V.
   C. Factor VIII.
   D. Factor IX.
   E. Factor VII.

Platelet Disorders

H. Franklin Bunn and Bruce Furie

LEARNING OBJECTIVES

After studying this chapter you should be able to:

- Distinguish among the different causes of thrombocytopenia.
- Understand the pathogenesis of immune thrombocytopenic purpura and the principles of treatment.
- Understand the pathogenesis of thrombotic thrombocytopenic purpura and the principles of treatment.
- Define mechanisms that lead to qualitative platelet defects.

Platelets assume an important role in a wide variety of disease states. Morbidity related to platelet dysfunction is generally due to bleeding, but occasionally thrombosis is dominant. As summarized in Table 14-1, bleeding can occur if the platelet count is too low or if there is a qualitative defect in platelet function. In patients with platelet disorders, bleeding is usually superficial and localized to skin and mucous membranes, a phenomenon known as *purpura*. Petechiae are small, 2-to-5 mm, red or purple macules (spots) that appear most often in the distal lower extremities (Fig. 14-1A) but also on the conjunctiva and palate. Small petechiae often merge to form larger lesions. Very large, purpuric lesions are called ecchymoses (Fig. 14-1B). In contrast to telangiectasia, petechiae and ecchymoses do not blanch under pressure. Mucosal purpura is generally associated with severe thrombocytopenia and may be a harbinger of complications such as gastrointestinal bleeding or even brain hemorrhage. In contrast to the superficial bleeding seen in patients with thrombocytopenia and qualitative platelet disorders, defects in the soluble coagulation factors, such as hemophilia (Table 14-1), typically present with deep bleeding, such as hemarthroses.

Platelet defects:
Superficial bleeding
Petechiae, ecchymoses
Coagulation factor defects:
Deep bleeding
Hemarthrosis, etc

THROMBOCYTOPENIA

In a clear and informative parallel to anemia, thrombocytopenia can be due either to decreased platelet production or enhanced platelet destruction. The life span of normal platelets in the circulation is about 7 to 9 days. Therefore, if the bone marrow stops producing platelets, it takes nearly a week before severe thrombocytopenia develops. In contrast, an acute immune or consumptive process that suddenly and drastically curtails platelet survival can produce severe thrombocytopenia within hours.

TABLE 14-1 Overview of Platelet Disorders

Disorder	Etiology	Occurrence	Examples
Bleeding			
Thrombocytopenia	Acquired	Common	ITP, DIC, marrow aplasia or malignancy
Qualitative defect	Acquired	Common	Drugs, uremia, bone marrow disorders
	Hereditary	Rare	Bernard-Soulier syndrome, Glanzmann thrombasthenia
Thrombosis			
Thrombocytosis	Acquired	Uncommon	Myeloproliferative disorders

ITP, immune thrombocytopenic purpura; DIC, disseminated intravascular coagulation.

DECREASED PRODUCTION

Damage or suppression of pluripotent hematopoietic stem cells may result in not only thrombocytopenia but also anemia and leukopenia (pancytopenia) accompanied by marrow aplasia. Aplastic anemia and other causes of pancytopenia are covered in Chapter 4. Transient thrombocytopenia due to marrow aplasia and decreased platelet production predictably follows certain forms of chemotherapy or radiation therapy for cancer. Other drugs selectively inhibit platelet production. Occasionally, patients with severe alcoholism will present with thrombocytopenia that appears to be due to a toxic effect of ethanol on megakaryocytes. In most cases, the platelets gradually return to baseline levels following cessation of therapy or drinking. Somewhat less often, decreased platelet production is due to a primary bone marrow disorder such as acute leukemia or a myelodysplastic

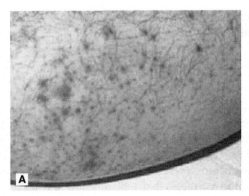
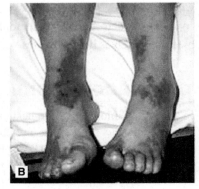

FIGURE 14-1 Purpura. A) Petechiae on distal lower extremity. B) Ecchymoses.

syndrome. Less severe thrombocytopenia can be due to megaloblastic anemia or to invasion of the bone marrow by tumors such as lymphoma or carcinoma.

The administration of thrombopoietin (Tpo) or Tpo-mimetic agents is seldom effective in the treatment of severe thrombocytopenia due to impaired platelet production. This may be due to the fact that endogenous plasma Tpo levels are already markedly elevated in these patients, owing to very low numbers of megakaryocytes in the bone marrow as well as platelets in the periphery. (See Chapter 2 for information on the regulation of platelet production by endogenous Tpo.) Because the platelet life span is usually normal in these patients, platelet transfusions produce a significant and beneficial rise in the platelet count unless or until the patient develops alloimmunization. In contrast, platelet transfusions are much less effective in patients in whom thrombocytopenia is due to enhanced destruction.

SEQUESTRATION

As explained in Chapter 1, the spleen in normal individuals contains (sequesters) about a third of the body's platelets. Patients who have splenomegaly due to a wide range of disorders (Chapter 1, Table 1-4) have a higher proportion of their platelets entrapped along with white and red blood cells. A significant reduction in one or more of the peripheral blood counts by splenic sequestration is called *hypersplenism*.

Patients with hypersplenism generally have platelet counts of 50,000 to 120,000/mm³. Thus, the degree of thrombocytopenia is almost never low enough to pose a risk of hemorrhage. Accordingly, splenectomy is not indicated for correction of the platelet count. However, some patients may have neutropenia that is sufficiently severe to warrant splenectomy.

INCREASED CONSUMPTION/DESTRUCTION

Severe thrombocytopenia is commonly caused by rapid destruction of platelets, most often due either to immune clearance or to consumption in conditions associated with intravascular thrombosis. In either case, the bone marrow produces increased numbers of platelets that have a short survival in the circulation. Because platelets normally become smaller as they age in vivo, the few platelets that are seen in blood films of patients with thrombocytopenia due to increased destruction tend to be larger than average.

IMMUNE THROMBOCYTOPENIA

Immunologic recognition followed by destruction of platelets is a relatively common cause of severe thrombocytopenia in individuals of all age groups. Most of these individuals come to medical attention because they develop purpura—hence the designation *immune thrombocytopenic purpura* (ITP). In children, the peak incidence is about 5 years of age. These previously healthy children typically develop a sudden onset of petechiae or ecchymoses within a few days or weeks following an infectious illness, usually viral. In the majority of these patients, the thrombocytopenia and purpura resolve within 6 months regardless of whether they have received therapy. Adults with ITP have a strikingly different clinical presentation and course. In these patients, the onset is insidious and seldom accompanied by a viral prodrome. The illness is chronic and, when severe, requires meticulous and often complex management. In both children and adults, if ITP is the primary diagnosis, patients normally have no symptoms or physical findings except for purpura. The spleen and lymph nodes are not enlarged. Some women also experience menorrhagia. Gastrointestinal bleeding is much less common. Rarely patients with ITP sustain cerebral hemorrhage.

PATHOGENESIS

There is overwhelming circumstantial evidence that in ITP platelets are destroyed by autoantibodies directed against platelet antigens. In early (less regulated) days of clinical research, it was noted that the intravenous administration of plasma from a patient with ITP to a normal volunteer resulted in the development of acute and severe thrombocytopenia and purpura. These studies led to the hypothesis that ITP patients had circulating autoantibodies directed against "public" antigens displayed on the surface of platelets in all individuals. These antibody-coated platelets are rapidly cleared by the interaction of the Fcγ receptor on tissue macrophages with the Fc (constant) portion of the immunoglobulin.

The primary public antigen targeted for immune attack in ITP is GPIIb/IIIa, which, as explained in Chapter 13, undergoes a conformational change during platelet activation and is the site of fibrinogen cross-linking. As shown in Figure 14-2, once the antibody-coated platelet is recognized and engulfed by the macrophage, GPIIb/IIIa as well as other platelet membrane proteins are degraded. These peptide antigens are then coupled with HLA class 2 molecules and displayed on the macrophage cell surface. This antigen-presenting complex interacts with the T-cell receptor on CD4 helper lymphocytes, inducing proliferation and recruitment of antigen-specific B-cell clones, which also proliferate and produce high levels of antibody against not only GPIIb/IIIa but also GPIb/IX and other platelet antigens.

The rapid destruction of platelets by resident macrophages results in Tpo-mediated stimulation of megakaryocyte production in the bone marrow. Thus, patients with ITP usually have increased numbers of marrow megakaryocytes (Fig. 14-3). Indeed, as a general rule, the level of platelet production parallels the number of megakaryocytes in the bone marrow. In this respect, the pathophysiology of ITP closely parallels that of immune hemolytic anemia (Chapter 11). In both disorders, the enhanced destruction of the blood cell in the peripheral circulation is accompanied by a compensatory hyperplasia of the respective precursors in the bone marrow. However, the plasma levels of the critical cytokines differ in the two disorders. In immune hemolytic anemia, as in nearly all other types of anemia, plasma erythropoietin levels are markedly elevated, in response to hypoxic stress (Chapter 1). In contrast, in ITP, plasma Tpo levels are generally normal or modestly elevated, owing to the clearance of this cytokine by hyperplastic marrow megakaryocytes.

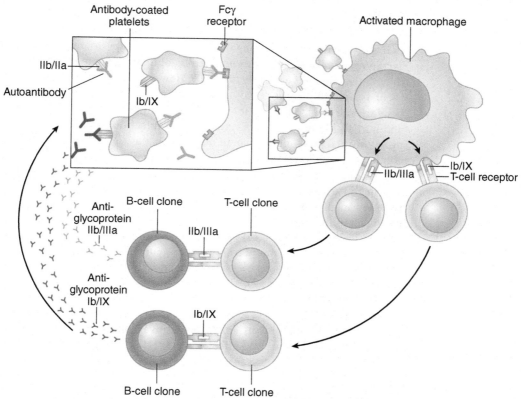

FIGURE 14-2 Amplification of the immune response in immune thrombocytopenic purpura. Phagocytosis of antibody-coated platelets by macrophages results in the presentation of platelet peptide neoantigens to CD4 helper T cells, which then trigger proliferation of B-cell clones, producing high levels of antiplatelet antibodies. (Modified with permission from Cines DB and Blanchette VS. Immune thrombocytopenic purpura. *New Engl J Med.* 2002; 346:995-1008. Copyright © 1972 Massachusetts Medical Society, all rights reserved.)

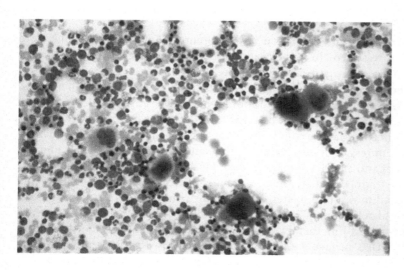

FIGURE 14-3 Bone marrow of a patient with immune thrombocytopenic purpura, showing increased numbers of megakaryocytes. Erythroid and myeloid lineages are normal.

DIAGNOSIS

Most often, immune thrombocytopenia arises spontaneously in otherwise healthy individuals with no underlying illness. The sudden development of purpura in an asymptomatic patient with normal hemoglobin level, white blood cell count, and differential count is very likely to be ITP. However, even in this setting the possibility of associated disorders should be investigated and ruled out. Immune thrombocytopenia is encountered in a substantial minority of patients with lymphoma and human immunodeficiency virus (HIV) infection, sometimes when these illnesses are at a preclinical stage. In other cases, the association with an underlying condition is obvious, such as immune thrombocytopenia seen in patients with acute mononucleosis, in those who have undergone bone marrow transplantation, and in those with systemic lupus erythematosus. Occasionally, drugs can cause immune-mediated destruction of platelets. The classic example is the antiarrhythmic agent quinidine, a drug that is now seldom used. Much more often the anticoagulant heparin (Chapter 13) is associated with immune thrombocytopenia. The drop in platelet count caused by heparin is generally modest, but affected patients are paradoxically at high risk of developing life-threatening venous and arterial thrombosis (see Chapter 17).

Other than a complete blood count, no other laboratory test is essential in making the diagnosis of ITP. However, it is prudent to check a baseline coagulation profile to rule out disseminated intravascular coagulation and to obtain screening tests for lupus and infection with HIV and Epstein-Barr virus. Unfortunately, no serological test for detecting antibody coating of platelets is nearly as reliable as the Coombs test for detecting antibody-coated red cells. As mentioned earlier, the presence of large platelets in the peripheral blood smear suggests that the thrombocytopenia is due to a decrease in platelet life span. If doubt persists, a bone marrow examination will provide more definitive evidence as to whether the thrombocytopenia is due to impaired production or increased destruction.

TREATMENT

Treatment of ITP

Steroids
Rituximab
Splenectomy
IV immunoglobulin

As mentioned earlier, most children with ITP remit spontaneously and therefore do not require treatment. In contrast, adult patients require treatment if the thrombocytopenia poses a significant risk of bleeding (platelet count <50,000/mm³). The treatment strategy for ITP closely parallels that of immune hemolytic anemia (Chapter 11). Administration of high doses of corticosteroids reliably results in a boost in the platelet count within the first week, and with continued treatment, the platelet count often reaches normal levels. Steroid therapy appears to suppress both the clearance of the antibody-coated platelets and the production of anti-platelet autoantibodies. Most patients relapse during or following the withdrawal of steroids. Alternative therapy is required in patients who either fail to respond to steroids or require prolonged treatment in order to maintain platelet counts in a safe range (>50,000/mm³). Currently, the recommended second-line therapy is rituximab, a monoclonal antibody directed against the CD20 surface antigen on B lymphocytes. If this treatment is not effective, splenectomy offers a good chance of prolonged remission. It should be noted that this is true even though splenomegaly is not a feature of ITP. Recent clinical trials have shown that Tpo-mimetic drugs are effective in patients with refractory ITP, but it is too early to know whether this treatment will become part of standard care. Patients with extremely low platelet counts and those being prepared for surgery generally respond promptly, albeit transiently, to the intravenous (IV) administration of high doses of immunoglobulin; the mechanism of this response is not known.

DISSEMINATED INTRAVASCULAR COAGULATION

Disseminated intravascular coagulation is a relatively common cause of thrombocytopenia due to enhanced platelet destruction. This often catastrophic complication is encountered in patients with a wide range of severe illnesses including sepsis, obstetrical emergencies, trauma, and cancer. In contrast to ITP, the coagulation profile is markedly abnormal. Rapid platelet consumption is secondary to inappropriate triggering of the coagulation cascade. This topic is covered in detail in Chapter 16.

THROMBOTIC THROMBOCYTOPENIC PURPURA

In thrombotic thrombocytopenic purpura (TTP), a relatively uncommon but sometimes life-threatening disorder, patients present with acute onset of hemolytic anemia and thrombocytopenia, sometimes preceded by viral-infection-like symptoms of fatigue, malaise, and fever. A substantial fraction of patients have central nervous system manifestations, such as seizures, coma, hemiplegia, and dementia. These findings may progress, but more often are transient or recurrent. A smaller number of patients have modest or moderate impairment of renal function. The anemia is often severe and accompanied by laboratory abnormalities stemming from acute hemolysis, including increased reticulocyte counts and elevated levels of serum lactate dehydrogenase and nonconjugated bilirubin. Occasionally, the intravascular hemolysis results in hemoglobinuria. The blood film (Fig. 14-5) reveals striking abnormalities of red cell shape, such as small fragments (schistocytes), helmet cells, and triangular cells, along with occasional nucleated red cells and marked thrombocytopenia. Importantly, the coagulation profile, assessed by partial thromboplastin time and prothrombin times, is normal, thereby distinguishing TTP from disseminated intravascular coagulation (Chapter 16). Thus TTP is a pentad of five features, summarized in the sidebar. The first two, thrombocytopenia and microangiopathic hemolysis, are major criteria required for diagnosis.

> **TTP**
> (THROMBOTIC THROMBOCYTOPENIC PURPURA)
>
> • Thrombocytopenia
> • Microangiopathic hemolysis
> • Neurologic dysfunction
> • Renal functional impairment
> • Fever

PATHOGENESIS

Pathologic examination of tissues from patients with TTP has revealed the presence of small platelet thrombi studding the endothelium of arterioles and capillaries. These thrombi contain abundant von Willebrand factor (vWF) and relatively little fibrin. The only plasma abnormality is the presence of unusually high molecular weight multimers of vWF in the plasma, shown in Chapter 15, Figure 15-3. Taken

vWF and Platelet Adhesion

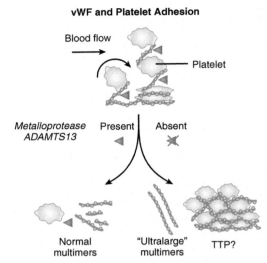

FIGURE 14-4 **Role of high molecular weight von Willebrand multimer and ADAMTS13 in the pathogenesis of thrombotic thrombocytopenic purpura.** (Modified from Sadler E, cover of journal *Blood* 98[6], 2001.)

together, these observations suggest that these abnormally large vWF multimers act like extra-sticky molecular glue, tethering platelets to the endothelial surface (Fig. 14-4). Very rare families have been encountered with chronic relapsing TTP. These individuals have an inherited deficiency of the protease ADAMTS13, which cleaves extra-large vWF into normal size multimers. In those with sporadic acquired TTP, a large majority of patients have inhibitory antibodies directed against ADAMTS13. These convergent insights have elucidated the molecular pathogenesis of this complex and formerly puzzling disease.

TREATMENT

Until 20 years ago, TTP was usually fatal. However, a decade prior to uncovering the role of ADAMTS13 in TTP, clinicians empirically discovered that plasma exchange is a remarkably effective therapy that can dramatically reverse the neurologic manifestations and reduce mortality in TTP. Elucidation of the importance of antibody inhibition of ADAMTS13 now provides a satisfying rationale for plasma exchange, which serves to both decrease the inhibitory antibody titer and to supply normal-sized vWF multimers.

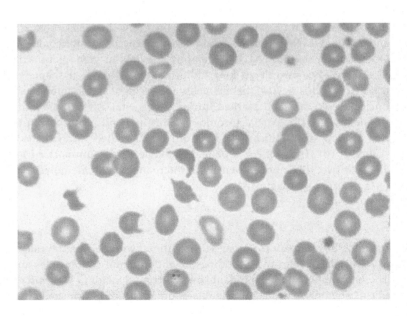

FIGURE 14-5 **Blood smear: thrombotic thrombocytopenic purpura.**

HEMOLYTIC UREMIC SYNDROME

Young children can develop acute microangiopathic hemolysis and thrombocytopenia accompanied by oliguria, proteinuria, and uremia, often following a diarrheal illness. In contrast to complications of TTP, neurologic complications are rarely encountered. This constellation of findings is designated *hemolytic uremic syndrome* (HUS). The anemia and thrombocytopenia are less severe than those seen in TTP, but the renal impairment is more severe. HUS is the most common cause of acute renal failure in young children. About 50% of cases are caused by an enteropathic strain of *Escherichia coli* (O157:H7), which releases a Shiga-like toxin. It is not understood how this toxin induces hemolysis and thrombocytopenia; damage to endothelial cells is suspected to incite the process. Supportive care is the mainstay of therapy. Children with enteropathic HUS have normal plasma levels of ADAMTS13 protease and do not benefit from plasma exchange.

Children with atypical (non-diarrheal) HUS commonly have a mutation in one of three proteins involved in the regulation of the complement cascade: factor H, membrane cofactor protein, or factor I. These patients have a more severe clinical course. About half require chronic dialysis therapy for renal failure.

In adults, there is a continuous spectrum between HUS and TTP. Measurement of plasma ADAMTS13 protease levels has not proven useful in predicting which patients respond to plasma exchange. Patients who have undergone bone marrow transplantation sometimes develop thrombotic microangiopathy with features overlapping those of TTP and HUS.

QUALITATIVE PLATELET DISORDERS

If platelet function is abnormal, bleeding may occur despite a normal or even high platelet count. Acquired qualitative platelet defects are very common; well-defined inherited defects are very rare, although uncharacterized hereditary thrombocytopathies are not uncommon.

ACQUIRED

Drugs may interfere with the biosynthesis of prostaglandins not only in platelets but also in endothelial cells. By far the most common offender is aspirin. As shown in Figure 14-6, aspirin inhibits cyclooxygenase, an enzyme that catalyzes the conversion of arachidonic acid to prostaglandins PGG2 and PGH2. Platelets and endothelial cells are affected differently by this inhibition. In the platelet, aspirin suppresses the level of thromboxane A$_2$. Thromboxane A$_2$ is released

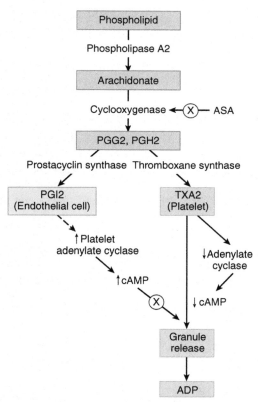

FIGURE 14-6 Pathway of arachidonate metabolism in the platelet and endothelial cell. Aspirin inhibits cyclooxygenase, thereby blocking production of thromboxane A$_2$ (TXA2) in the platelet and prostaglandin I$_2$ (PGI2) in the endothelial cell. Prostaglandin G$_2$ = PGG2; prostaglandin H$_2$ = PGH2. The circle with an X denotes inhibition. The dashed arrow in the lower left (—) represents the paracrine stimulation of platelet adenylate cyclase by PGI2 released from endothelial cells.

from platelets during activation, thus leading to activation of other platelets, and aspirin interferes with this process. In the endothelial cell, aspirin suppresses the formation of prostaglandin I_2, which is a vasodilator and protects the vessel from thrombus formation. Patients who take conventional doses of aspirin for relief from pain and/or inflammation are at risk of bleeding by virtue of impairment of platelet activation. Aspirin also has been shown to be effective in the prevention of arterial thrombosis (see Chapter 17). There is evidence that low doses (baby aspirin) lessen the risk of bleeding but are sufficient to have an anti-platelet effect. Furthermore, with low doses of aspirin, endothelial cells maintain production of anti-thrombotic prostaglandin I_2.

In addition to aspirin, a wide range of other non-steroidal anti-inflammatory drugs (NSAIDs) also lower platelet levels of thromboxane A_2 and therefore enhance the risk of bleeding. For this reason, patients are warned not to take these drugs prior to elective surgery. Moreover, aspirin and NSAIDs pose a much higher risk of significant hemorrhage in patients with underlying bleeding disorders such as hemophilia or von Willebrand disease and are thus contraindicated.

Patients with uremia also have impaired platelet function that can lead to serious bleeding, particularly in the gastrointestinal tract. The mechanism underlying this defect is unknown. Platelet function improves after uremic patients undergo dialysis therapy.

Patients with primary bone marrow disorders commonly have qualitative platelet defects superimposed on abnormalities in the platelet count. Those with myelodysplastic syndromes (Chapter 20) often have thrombocytopenia. Even when their platelet counts are normal, their bleeding times are often prolonged, and they are at an increased risk of clinical bleeding. In contrast, patients with myeloproliferative disorders (Chapter 20) usually have elevated platelet counts but, nevertheless, often have prolonged bleeding times. These patients are highly prone to developing either bleeding or thrombosis. Platelet aggregation studies are frequently abnormal in these patients, but the results have not been helpful in predicting either bleeding or thrombosis.

INHERITED

Rare families have been encountered with bleeding disorders owing to defective platelet receptor function. Molecular genetic studies have revealed the precise defect in several of these familial platelet disorders. This information, although not useful to the practicing physician, has provided invaluable insights into key proteins involved in platelet function as well as a clearer understanding of platelet aggregation tests.

Figure 14-7 shows platelet aggregation profiles that are particularly informative. As mentioned in Chapter 13, the binding of GPIIb/IIIa to divalent fibrinogen is required for the formation of crosslinks that lead to the aggregation of platelets in plasma. Patients with Glanzmann thrombasthenia have a bleeding syndrome owing to the inheritance of a defect in either the gene for GPIIb or GPIIIa. As a result, their platelets lack docking sites for fibrinogen binding. Even though agonists such as adenosine diphosphate, arachidonic acid, epinephrine,

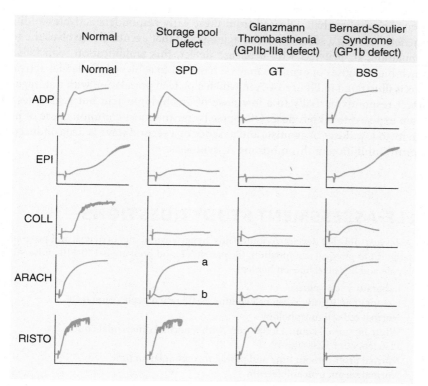

	Normal	Storage pool Defect	Glanzmann Thrombasthenia (GPIIb-IIIa defect)	Bernard-Soulier Syndrome (GP1b defect)
	Normal	SPD	GT	BSS
ADP				
EPI				
COLL				
ARACH		a b		
RISTO				

FIGURE 14-7 **Platelet aggregation studies in patients with qualitative platelet disorders.** a) High dose of arachidonic acid. b) Normal low dose. (Modified from White CC, Marder VJ, Colman RW, et al. Approach to the bleeding patient. In: Colman RW, Hirsh J, Marder VJ, et al, eds, *Hemostasis and Thrombosis—Basic Principles and Clinical Practice, 2nd Ed*, Philadelphia, USA, Lippincott, 1987, p. 1048.)

and collagen can activate their platelets, aggregation fails to occur due to the absence of fibrinogen cross-linking. The only agonist that triggers crosslinking of Glanzmann platelets is ristocetin, which "conditions" vWF to bind to platelet GPIb/IX, thereby providing an alternative, nonphysiologic mechanism for platelet agglutination.

Note that the opposite pertains in patients with Bernard-Soulier syndrome. These individuals have defective GPIb/IX, due to mutations in the gene encoding this receptor. Therefore, their platelets aggregate normally in response to adenosine diphosphate, arachidonic acid, epinephrine, and collagen but do not aggregate or agglutinate in the presence of ristocetin.

Abnormal platelet aggregation due to a storage pool defect is also shown in Figure 14-7. Families have been described with abnormalities either in the structure of the dense or alpha granules or in the ability to release granule contents during activation. Both types of defects lead to impairment of the "second wave" of aggregation that normally arises from the release of adenosine diphosphate from platelet granules. When a population of platelets is exposed to low concentrations of agonists, only a minor fraction is activated initially (the first wave). However, adenosine diphosphate released from these early responders activates additional platelets, starting a second wave of aggregation that eventually involves the whole population. In platelets with a release defect, this amplification loop fails, and much higher doses of agonists may be required to achieve full platelet activation. This is illustrated in Figure 14-7, in which a platelet population with a storage pool defect responds partially to a low dose of arachidonic acid but aggregates fully when exposed to a high dose. Of course by far the most common cause of insensitivity to low doses of agonists and absence of a second wave is drug-induced (eg, aspirin) inhibition of thromboxane A_2 synthesis.

SELF-ASSESSMENT STUDY QUESTIONS

1. A 24-year-old chef developed joint pains, hypertension, menorrhagia, and progressive fatigue. On physical examination, the patient's blood pressure is 170/110, pulse 90. She is pale and has petechiae on her legs.

   Laboratory test values:
   Hemoglobin 9 g/dL; mean cell volume 84 fL; reticulocyte count 0.5%
   Normal red cell morphology
   White blood cell count 11,000/mm³ with a normal differential count
   Platelet count 12,000/mm³
   Normal prothrombin time and partial thromboplastin time
   Normal serum iron and ferritin
   Large amounts of protein in urine
   Serum blood urea nitrogen 120 mg/dL; serum creatinine 5 mg/dL
   Anti-nuclear antibody positive, indicating systemic lupus erythematosus

   Which of the following tests is the most likely to have a positive or abnormal result?
   A. Platelet aggregation.
   B. Platelet agglutination.
   C. Bleeding time.
   D. Megakaryocyte morphology (seen on bone marrow examination).
   E. vWF screen.

2. What treatment is the best means to correct the patient's thrombocytopenia?
   A. Hemodialysis.
   B. Transfusion of platelets.
   C. Administration of iron, folate, and vitamin B_{12}.
   D. Administration of corticosteroids.
   E. Antihypertensive drugs.

3. Treatment with aspirin impairs the platelets' ability to produce which of the following?
   A. Adenosine diphosphate.
   B. Adenosine triphosphate.
   C. Arachidonic acid.
   D. Thromboxane A_2.
   E. Prostaglandin I_2.

4. A 36-year-old electrician had a mild viral illness last week. Over the last 3 days, he has noted a rash on his arms and legs, a fever (101°F), marked and progressive lethargy, and fatigue. On physical examination, the patient was semi-stuporous and had weakness on the right side of his body. The arms, legs, and mucous membranes were studded with petechiae.

    Laboratory test values:

    Hemoglobin 7 g/dL, mean cell volume 100 fL, reticulocyte count 12%; a peripheral blood smear revealed schistocytes and occasional nucleated red blood cells

    White blood cell count 15,000/mm³ with a slight shift to the left (increased number of neutrophils and band cells)

    Platelet count 7,000/mm³

    Blood urea nitrogen 40 mg/dL, creatinine 3 mg/dL

    Normal baseline coagulation study results

What is the most likely diagnosis?

A. Thrombotic thrombocytopenic purpura.

B. Immune thrombocytopenia.

C. Immune hemolytic anemia.

D. Immune hemolytic anemia and thrombocytopenia (Evans syndrome).

E. Sepsis.

5. How should this patient (Question 4) be treated?

A. High-dose steroids.

B. Broad-spectrum antibiotics.

C. Plasma exchange.

D. Splenectomy.

E. Hemodialysis.

CHAPTER

15

Inherited Coagulation Disorders

H. Franklin Bunn and Bruce Furie

> ### LEARNING OBJECTIVES
>
> After studying this chapter you should:
> - Understand the genetics, clinical features, diagnosis, and treatment of hemophilias A and B.
> - Understand the genetics, clinical features, diagnosis, and treatment of von Willebrand disease.

No hematologic disorder has more historical import and portent than hemophilia. Figure 15-1 shows the descendants of Queen Victoria and Prince Albert. One of their three sons, Leopold, Duke of Albany, suffered from a life-long bleeding disorder, as did nine grandsons and great grandsons, including members of the Russian, Prussian, and Spanish royal families. Particularly foreboding was the affliction of young Prince Alexie, the only son of Czar Nicholas and Czarina Alexandra. His illness was but one of many travails that beset the Russian royal family and led to their dethronement and execution during the Bolshevik revolution.

HEMOPHILIA A (FACTOR VIII DEFICIENCY)

Hemophilia A is the inherited bleeding disorder most often associated with severe morbidity, frequently requiring hospitalization. It is due to deficiency of factor VIII. When activated, factor VIII forms a complex with activated factor IX, enabling the efficient proteolytic activation of factor X (see bottom of sidebar and Chapter 13 for more information about factor VIII). Hemophilia A occurs in about 1 in 5000 male births. The gene encoding factor VIII is located near the tip of the long arm of the X chromosome. Thus, hemophilia A is inherited in an X-linked manner, with female heterozygous carriers passing the disease on to half of their sons. The royal families depicted in Figure 15-1 comprise a typical kindred demonstrating X-linked transmission. About 30% of patients have no family history of abnormal bleeding. Most of these cases are due to spontaneous mutations. Although hemophilia A can occur in homozygous females, often owing to consanguinity, most females who bleed abnormally are heterozygous carriers of the hemophilia gene. Although the mechanism for their low factor VIII levels is not known, skewed X-inactivation (lyonization) has been hypothesized.

Hemophilia

Hemophilia A (Factor VIII Deficiency)
Hemophilia B (Factor IX Deficiency)

Phenotypically Identical:
  Hemarthroses
  Hematoma
  GI and GU Bleeding

Severe	<1% factor
Moderate	1-4% " "
Mild	>4% " "

Screening Assays: ↑ PTT, NI PT

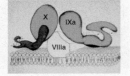

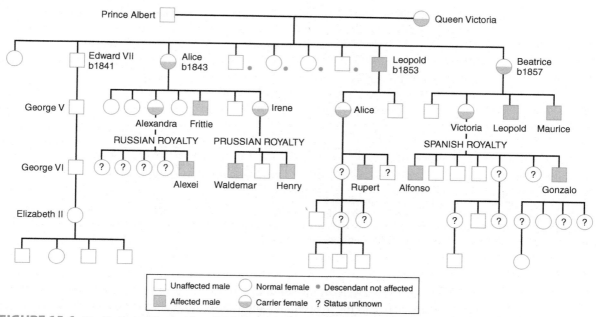

FIGURE 15-1   Family tree of Queen Victoria of England, Prince Albert, and their descendants. The frontispiece preceding Chapter 13 shows photographs of Prince Leopold, Duke of Albany, son of Queen Victoria, and Czarevich Alexei, son of Czar Nicholas and Czarina Alexandra of Russia.

CLINICAL PRESENTATION

Patients with hemophilia A tend to have deep bleeding into joints (hemarthroses) or muscle beds, rather than bleeding from mucosal surfaces. Patients with repeated joint hemorrhage develop chronic disability due to swelling, deformity, severe pain, limitation of motion, and contractures that can be corrected only by joint replacement. Less often patients have bouts of gastrointestinal or genitourinary bleeding and, rarely, intracerebral hemorrhage—a catastrophic event. Patients are assigned to one of three levels of severity according to plasma levels of factor VIII. These levels generally predict the phenotype of the patient. Those with 1% or less factor VIII (severe hemophilia) have an average of 20 to 30 episodes per year of either spontaneous bleeding or excessive bleeding after minor trauma. Patients with 1% to 4% factor VIII levels have moderate hemophilia, whereas individuals with greater than 4% factor VIII levels generally have bleeding episodes only after trauma or surgery.

GENETICS

As might be surmised from the range of phenotypes, hemophilia A is a genetically heterogeneous disease. A wide variety of mutations of the factor VIII gene have been identified in hemophilia patients, including missense mutations, nonsense mutations leading to premature termination of translation, frame shifts, deletions, and rearrangements. The most commonly encountered mutation, depicted

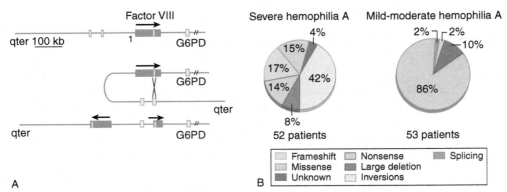

FIGURE 15-2 Mutations of factor VIII gene in hemophilia A. A) Inversion responsible for most cases of severe hemophilia A. B) Distribution of mutations in severe versus mild to moderate hemophilia A. (Modified with permission from Kaufman RJ and Antonarakis SE. Structure, biology and genetics of factor VIII. In Hoffman R, Benz EJ, Shattil SJ, et al, eds. *Hematology: Basic Principles and Practice,* 3rd Edition. New York, USA, Churchill Livingstone, 2001: 1858-1859.)

in Figure 15-2A, is an inversion that reverses the orientation of the 3' end of the gene relative to the 5' promoter and transcriptional start site. Alleles bearing this rearrangement, observed in about 50% of severe hemophilia A patients, make no factor VIII. As shown in Figure 15-2B, the great majority of mutations in patients with severe hemophilia A have either inversions, large deletions, nonsense mutations, or frame shifts, all of which preclude synthesis of full-length factor VIII. In contrast, those with moderate or mild hemophilia A usually have missense mutations in which full-length protein is produced but has impaired stability or function.

DIAGNOSIS

Because factor VIII is part of the intrinsic pathway of coagulation, the partial thromboplastin time in a patient with hemophilia A is prolonged, whereas the prothrombin time is normal. Moreover, there are no abnormalities in the platelet count or in tests of platelet function such as the bleeding time. Assay of factor VIII coagulant activity is used not only in establishing the diagnosis but also in monitoring patients with hemophilia A and assessing their need for therapy. This test entails measurement of the clotting time after the patient's plasma is mixed with factor VIII–deficient plasma. Molecular genetic testing is now available to diagnose hemophilia A during early fetal life for purposes of genetic counseling.

THERAPY

Currently, patients with hemophilia A are treated with infusions of either recombinant factor VIII or highly purified plasma-derived factor VIII prepared from human donor plasma. Both are equally effective and free of viral pathogens. The recombinant product costs 2 to 3 times as much as the plasma concentrates. Factor VIII has a plasma half-life of 8 to 12 hours. Thus, twice daily infusions are required to maintain levels adequate for hemostasis in patients with serious active bleeding (eg, intracranial, intraperitoneal, and gastrointestinal bleeds) or facing major surgery. Isolated joint hemorrhage is usually successfully treated with a single infusion sufficient to raise the plasma level of factor VIII to over 30%. Many children in the United States and in other developed countries are treated with prophylactic self-infusions of factor VIII three times a week in order to prevent damage to joints. Raising the factor VIII level from a baseline of 1% or less to 3% to 4% alters the phenotype of the patient dramatically. In the absence of human immunodeficiency virus (HIV) infection, patients with severe hemophilia treated with factor replacement have a life expectancy of about 65 years, whereas life expectancy in those with mild or moderate disease is near normal. The limiting factor is cost. Prophylactic treatment of children with factor VIII deficiency costs over $100,000 per year. In less developed countries, the high cost of factor VIII precludes most patients from being adequately treated, and many suffer a life of severe pain and disability. In patients with mild or moderate hemophilia A who produce some factor VIII, treatment with desmopressin releases von Willebrand factor (vWF) from stores in endothelial cells and results in a significant increase in plasma levels of factor VIII, due to the ability of vWF to bind and stabilize factor VIII. As a general rule, desmopressin infusion raises factor VIII levels 3-fold to 4-fold when given daily for up to 3 days.

Patients with hemophilia A are ideal candidates for gene therapy. Hemophilia A is a monogenetic disease that, in contrast to sickle cell disease, is not significantly confounded by concurrent genetic modifiers. Moreover, tight regulation of factor VIII gene expression is not necessary for safe and effective treatment of hemophilia A, because factor VIII levels from 10% to 150% of normal are adequate to achieve hemostasis and carry no apparent risk of thrombosis on the high end of the range. Contrast this with the situation in sickle cell anemia and thalassemia, in which erythroid-specific, precisely balanced and controlled globin gene expression is critical. Despite these inherent advantages, progress in this endeavor has been disappointing to date.

COMPLICATIONS

In addition to the consequences of repetitive hemarthroses mentioned earlier, two other major problems threaten the well-being and life expectancy of patients with hemophilia A. Prior to 1990, patients were treated with concentrates of pooled plasma that were contaminated with pathogenic viruses—in particular, hepatitis B and C as well as HIV. As a result, nearly all patients with hemophilia A severe enough to require infusions became infected with hepatitis B or C, and of these, nearly 20% developed hepatic cirrhosis. About two-thirds of these patients were also infected with HIV. The development of AIDS in hemophilia patients enormously complicates their management and for the last two decades has been the leading cause of death among adult patients with severe disease.

A second major complication is the development of antibodies that neutralize factor VIII. These inhibitors arise primarily in about 10% to 15% of severe hemophiliacs who lack the ability to produce even small amounts of endogenous factor VIII. The immune system in these patients sees the exogenously administered protein as "foreign" and mounts an antibody response. In some patients, inhibitor titers remain low enough to be overridden by infusion of large amounts of factor VIII. Moreover, the titer of low-level inhibitors generally does not rise with factor VIII infusions (non-inducible). Unfortunately, in others the titer of anti-factor VIII antibodies builds up to extremely high levels—enough to neutralize the total amount of factor VIII normally present in the circulation and all of the exogenous factor VIII that can reasonably be infused. Moreover, infusions of factor VIII in such patients usually result in an anamnestic antibody response. These patients are at very high risk of catastrophic bleeding. If there is minimal cross-reactivity between the anti-factor VIII antibody and porcine factor VIII, an effective therapeutic option is to switch to porcine factor VIII infusions. Alternatively, patients with high-titer inhibitors that neutralize porcine factor VIII can be treated with recombinant activated factor VII or by preparations that bypass the intrinsic pathway and directly trigger the activation of factor X to factor Xa.

HEMOPHILIA B (FACTOR IX DEFICIENCY)

The description in the beginning of this chapter of hemophilia among progeny of Queen Victoria makes no mention of whether afflicted family members suffered from factor VIII deficiency (hemophilia A) or factor IX deficiency (hemophilia B). It might have been anticipated that this family suffered from hemophilia A because its incidence is about 6-fold higher than that of hemophilia B. However, recent sequencing evidence has demonstrated that the mutation in this family involves the factor IX gene and produces severe hemophilia B. As the side bar on the first page of this chapter indicates, the two disorders are remarkably similar genetically, clinically, and molecularly. Both involve defects in the "Xase" complex in which factors VIIIa and IXa interact cooperatively to activate factor X. Both have an X-linked inheritance pattern. Indeed, the gene encoding factor IX is located quite close to the factor VIII gene on the long arm of the X chromosome. Both disorders have identical clinical presentations, a wide spectrum of diverse mutations spread throughout their respective genes, similar ranges of clinical severity due to variation in factor levels, and shared risks for development of therapy-induced viral infections and neutralizing antibodies.

Recombinant factor IX and ultrapure plasma-derived factor IX are used for treatment of patients with hemophilia B. Both are free of contamination with viruses and activated coagulation factors. The guidelines for treatment with factor IX infusions are very similar to those mentioned earlier for factor VIII. Because factor IX has a half-life of about 24 hours, it requires less frequent infusions to maintain adequate levels in the plasma. However, because of its smaller size, factor IX rapidly equilibrates between the intravascular and extravascular space, so that, on the basis of units administered, twice as much factor IX must be given compared with factor VIII. Patients who develop high-titer inhibitors to factor IX—a very rare occurrence—are treated with recombinant activated factor VII. The prospect of gene therapy for hemophilia B is every bit as promising and as frustrating as that for hemophilia A.

VON WILLEBRAND DISEASE

von Willebrand disease is the most common inherited bleeding disorder, with a prevalence in the United States of about 1 in 90, more than than 50 fold higher than that of hemophilia A. Thus, about 3 million Americans are affected. However, the majority of these individuals escape diagnosis because the defect is so mild it does not come to medical attention. von Willebrand disease can be distinguished from the hemophilias in three major respects: 1) it is inherited in an autosomal dominant manner, 2) bleeding is primarily from mucous membranes, and 3) the bleeding time is prolonged. Additional differences between von Willebrand disease and hemophilia A, as well as important similarities, are listed in Table 15-1.

von Willebrand disease is caused by mutations spread throughout the gene encoding von Willebrand factor (vWF). This protein serves two very different functions: it is the chaperone in the plasma for factor VIII, protecting factor VIII from rapid clearance and degradation. Also, through its binding domains for both collagen and for platelets, vWF acts as a molecular glue that enables platelets to adhere to the wall of injured blood vessels. Further information on the structure and function of this protein is provided in Chapter 13. Because vWF is so large and contains numerous functionally important domains, it has been a challenge to link individual missense mutations to the clinical phenotype in any particular patient. Two other considerations also complicate the pathogenesis of the disease. First, a substantial fraction of individuals with the clinical phenotype of von Willebrand disease lack any detectable abnormality in either vWF allele. Second, the levels of vWF protein and the clinical severity can be significantly affected by genetic factors such as the co-inheritance of modifying genes unlinked to vWF as well as environmental factors including hormones and drugs that affect the synthesis of vWF. Humans with group O blood have lower levels of plasma vWF and are commonly misdiagnosed as having von Willebrand disease.

DIAGNOSIS

A panel of three laboratory tests is used in both the diagnosis and monitoring of von Willebrand disease. Factor VIII activity is measured with the same assay used

---

Von Willebrand Disease

Low or dysfunctioinal vWF

Clinical: Mucosal bleeding, purpura

Genetics: Autosomal

Laboratory:
Ristocetin cofactor <40%
vWF antigen <40%
Factor VIII activity <40%

Function:
Carrier protein for FVIII
Molecular glue
Platelet-vessel wall interaction

TABLE 15-1 Hemophilia A Versus von Willebrand Disease

Factor VIII Deficiency	von Willebrand Factor Deficiency
X-linked	Autosomal
Prolonged partial thromboplastin time	Prolonged partial thromboplastin time
Normal bleeding time	Prolonged bleeding time
Low factor VIII levels	Low factor VIII levels
Normal vWF levels	Low vWF levels
Hemarthrosis and hematomas	Mucosal bleeding

to monitor patients with hemophilia A. vWF antigen is measured with an immunologic assay that detects both normal and mutant vWF proteins. The ristocetin cofactor assay provides a functional assessment of vWF protein. This test measures the agglutination of formalin-fixed normal platelets by the patient's plasma in the presence of ristocetin, which enables vWF multimers to bind to platelet GPIb complex.

von Willebrand disease is divided into three major subtypes, based on a combination of salient clinical features and molecular pathogenesis. Types 1 and 3 are caused by vWF protein deficiency, as measured by vWF antigen levels. Accordingly, the levels of factor VIII activity and ristocetin cofactor activity are decreased in parallel with the vWF antigen level. Type 1 is by far the most common form, accounting for over 70% of affected individuals. The levels of vWF antigen vary widely from 15% to 60% of normal, principally owing to environmental and genetic factors mentioned earlier. As shown in Figure 15-3, the distribution of vWF multimers is normal. In contrast to those of type 1 disease, levels of vWF antigen are less than 5% of normal in type 3 von Willebrand disease (Fig. 15-3). Unlike type 1 and type 2 individuals, patients with type 3 have inherited mutant vWF genes from both parents. Since levels of vWF protein are so low in type 3 patients, they have much more severe bleeding, and indeed, because their factor VIII levels are comparably low, they may develop hemarthroses and other deep tissue bleeding similar to patients with hemophilia A.

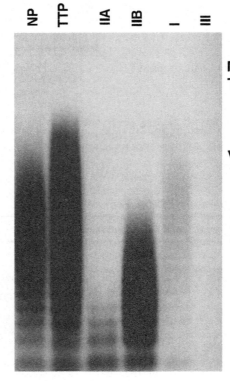

NP: Normal Plasma
TTP: Thrombotic
    thrombocytopenic
    purpura

von Willebrand Disease:
    Type IIA
    Type IIB
    Type I
    Type III

FIGURE 15-3 **Patterns of von Willebrand factor multimers in different types of von Willebrand disease and thrombotic thrombocytopenic purpura (TTP), observed with an electrophoretic technique that separates proteins according to size.**

Type 2 disease, like type 1, is inherited in an autosomal dominant manner and accounts for about 25% of patients with von Willebrand disease. In these patients, the vWF antigen and factor VIII levels are generally normal, but the vWF protein is qualitatively abnormal, leading to a low ristocetin co-factor activity. Type 2 disease includes several subtypes. Most individuals with type 2A disease have defective multimerization of vWF protein, as illustrated in Figure 15-3. Patients with type 2A bleed because of a failure to form large multimers, an abnormality that greatly impairs the ability of vWF to tether platelets to injured endothelium. Two other less common variants of von Willebrand disease merit comment because of their pathophysiologic interest. In type 2B, there is also reduction in the very large multimers (Fig. 15-3), but in this case due to structural mutations that increase the binding of vWF to platelet GPIb/IX. This results in clearance of large multimers from the plasma and sometimes causes a mild thrombocytopenia. Owing to the increased binding of vWF to circulating platelets, platelet agglutination in patients with type 2B disease is unusually sensitive to ristocetin. Also of pathophysiologic interest are rare patients with autosomal recessive type 2N disease, in which patients inherit two defective copies of vWF with mutations within the N-terminal domain that abolish vWF binding to factor VIII. As a result, the vWF antigen and ristocetin cofactor levels are normal, but the factor VIII levels are very low, and the patient has a clinical phenotype very similar to that of hemophilia A.

THERAPY

Patients with severe von Willebrand disease and those requiring optimal hemostasis during and following major surgery should be treated with intravenous infusion of factor VIII concentrates that are enriched in vWF. Patients with less severe disease are often treated quite effectively with desmopressin, a vasopressin analog, which triggers the release into the plasma of vWF protein stored in endothelial cells. However, desmopressin is contraindicated in type 2B von Willebrand disease because it induces severe thrombocytopenia.

OTHER INHERITED BLEEDING DISORDERS

Genetic deficiencies of fibrinogen, prothrombin, and factors V, VII, X, XI, and XIII have been shown to cause abnormal bleeding. All but factor XIII can be diagnosed by a panel of coagulation studies that includes specific factor assays. Factor XIII catalyzes the covalent crosslinking of fibrin, which gives clots greater tensile strength. Deficiency of factor XIII can be demonstrated by testing the stability of the fibrin clot in a chaotropic solution such as 5 M urea. All of these disorders are very rare, except for factor XI deficiency, which is encountered primarily among Ashkenazi Jews. Individuals with factor XI deficiency, even when severe, seldom bleed abnormally unless challenged by trauma or major surgery. Because factor XI has a relatively long half-life, patients can be effectively treated with infusions of fresh frozen plasma.

SELF-ASSESSMENT STUDY QUESTIONS

1. A 14-year-old boy and his 11-year-old sister have each had roughly a dozen episodes of abnormal bleeding, including gastrointestinal hemorrhage and large hematomas following minor trauma or impact. An evaluation revealed that they both have moderately severe von Willebrand disease. Which of the following tests is most likely to be normal in these patients?
   A. Partial thromboplastin time.
   B. Prothrombin time.
   C. Bleeding time.
   D. Ristocetin cofactor.
   E. Factor VIII.

2. A 2-year-old boy was brought to the emergency department by his mother for oozing blood from his mouth following a fall nearly 6 hours earlier. His mother reported that he tended to bleed for prolonged periods from his immunization sites, but there was no history of bruising or hematomas. He was being given antibiotics for a recent ear infection. There was no known family history of a bleeding disorder.

   Physical examination:
   Alert, in no apparent distress, development appropriate for age
   Two small lacerations on the inside of lower lip, oozing blood
   Remainder of examination within normal limits (no petechia, bruises, or joint swelling)

Initial Laboratory Test Values:

Test	Patient Result	Reference Value
Hemoglobin	12.3 g/dL	10.5-13.5 g/dL
Hematocrit	35.4%	33.0%-39.0%
White blood cell count	7900/mm³	6000-17,500/mm³
Platelet count	368,000/mm³	156,000-369,000/mm³
Prothrombin time	11.3 seconds	10.0-12.8 seconds
Partial thromboplastin time (PTT)	49.6 seconds	28.0-38.0 seconds
PTT mixing study	35.7 seconds	28.0-38.0 seconds
Factor VIII	16%	60%-150%
Factor IX	82%	60%-150%
Thrombin time	17.3 seconds	16.0-22.0 seconds
vWF antigen	16%	50%-150%
Ristocetin cofactor	<10%	50%-150%

This clinical presentation and the laboratory test result abnormalities are most consistent with:
   A. Factor VII deficiency.
   B. von Willebrand disease.
   C. Factor X deficiency.
   D. Partial thromboplastin time inhibitor (eg, lupus anticoagulant).
   E. Hemophilia A (factor VIII deficiency).

Acquired Coagulation Disorders

16

H. Franklin Bunn and Bruce Furie

LEARNING OBJECTIVES

After studying this chapter you should:

- Understand the pathogenesis and treatment of vitamin K deficiency.
- Understand the pathogenesis, diagnosis, and treatment of disseminated intravascular coagulation.

One of the most challenging aspects of clinical medicine is the diagnosis and treatment of acquired bleeding disorders. These problems commonly arise in hospitalized patients on medical, surgical, and obstetrical services. The immediate question of whether the bleeding is due to recent trauma or surgery is sometimes difficult to answer with certainty. A careful history may reveal an inherited bleeding disorder or exposure to drugs or toxins that might adversely affect platelet or coagulation functions. A thorough physical examination will usually reveal whether the bleeding is local and restricted to the area of trauma or surgery, rather than widespread. In any case, a patient with unexplained hemorrhage, local or systemic, should be initially evaluated and then closely monitored with baseline screening tests that include a platelet count, prothrombin time, and partial thromboplastin time. Occasionally, additional coagulation tests are needed to delineate the cause of the bleeding and to guide appropriate therapy. Skillful management of these patients, who often have complex illnesses, must be based on a solid understanding of the pathophysiology of hemostasis, as presented in Chapter 13 and amplified in this chapter.

In contrast to inherited conditions such as hemophilia (Chapter 15), acquired bleeding disorders usually involve deficiencies of multiple clotting factors. This chapter will focus primarily on three problems commonly encountered on medical and surgical floors: vitamin K deficiency, severe liver disease, and disseminated intravascular coagulation (DIC).

VITAMIN K DEFICIENCY

Vitamin K is a fat-soluble organic compound found primarily in leafy green vegetables but also in meat and dairy products. It is composed of a bicyclical naphthoquinone backbone and an aliphatic side chain. As shown in Figure 16-1,

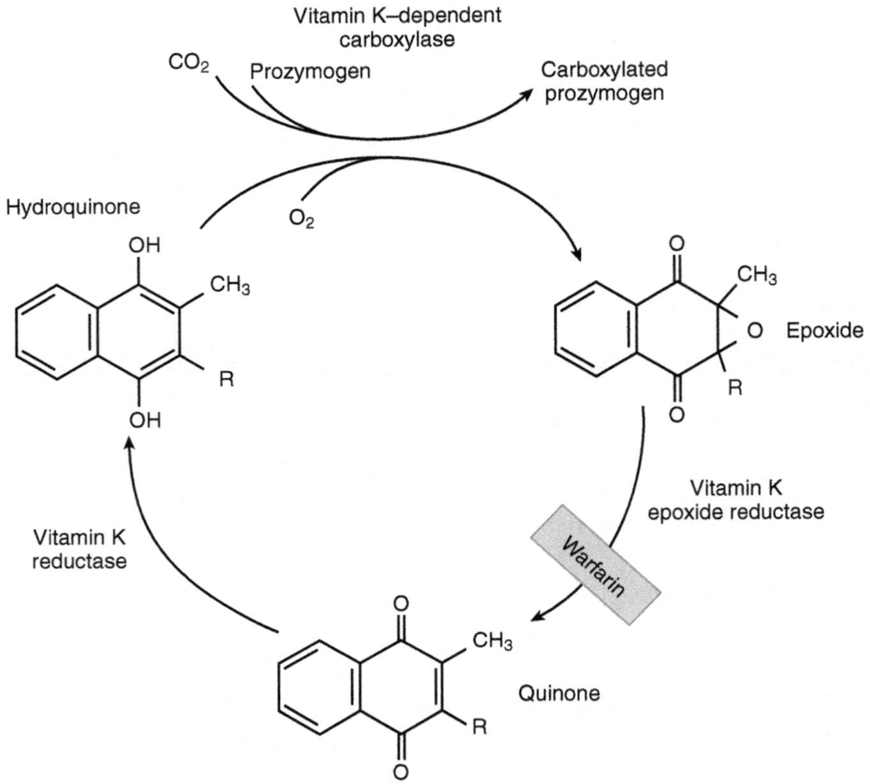

FIGURE 16-1 **The vitamin K cycle.** This figure shows the enzymatic steps that convert vitamin K to the hydroquinone required for participation as a cofactor in γ-carboxylation of glutamic acid residues, and the regeneration of vitamin K by conversion of the epoxide back to the quinone. (Modified with permission from Furie BC and Furie B. Vitamin K metabolism and disorders. In Hoffman R, Benz EJ, Shattil SJ, et al, eds. *Hematology: Basic Principles and Practice*, 3rd Edition. New York, USA, Churchill Livingstone, 2001:1959.)

vitamin K is converted to the hydroquinone by a vitamin K reductase. The hydro-quinone is an essential cofactor utilized by the vitamin K–dependent carboxylase to catalyze the oxidative fixation of carbon dioxide onto specific glutamic acid resi-dues to form γ-carboxyglutamic acid. During this reaction vitamin K is converted to an epoxide, which is then converted back to the quinone by a vitamin K epoxide reductase. This vitamin K–dependent post-translational modification takes place in the Golgi apparatus of many cell types and is restricted to specific domains on a small number of proteins—those known as vitamin K–dependent proteins. In hepatocytes, γ-carboxylation is necessary for the biologic activity of the vitamin K–dependent coagulation factors: the zymogens prothrombin, factors VII, IX, and X (Fig. 16-2), as well as protein C and protein S. In bone, γ-carboxylation is necessary for the synthesis of osteocalcin and matrix Gla protein. In all cases, this structural modification enables binding of divalent calcium. The function of vitamin K–dependent clotting factors requires calcium binding in order to form procoagulant complexes on membrane surfaces.

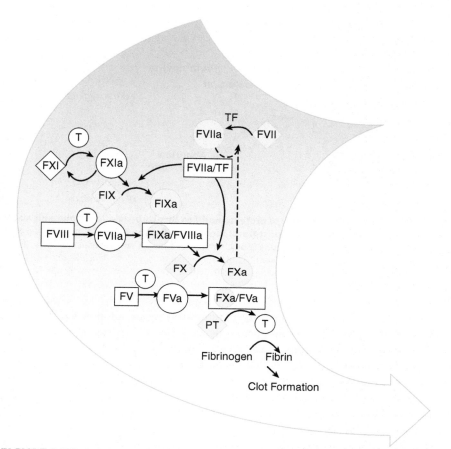

FIGURE 16-2 **The participation of vitamin K–dependent clotting factors highlighted in yellow in the coagulation cascade.** (Modified with permission from Furie B and Furie BC. The molecular basis of blood coagulation. In Hoffman R, Benz EJ, Shattil SJ, et al, eds. *Hematology, Basic Principles and Practice,* 3rd Edition, New York, USA, Churchill Livingstone, 2001:1784.)

Vitamin K is absorbed in the intestine. Sources of vitamin K include food and vitamin K synthesized by flora in the gut. Accordingly, patients who are not eating and who are receiving broad-spectrum antibiotics are at risk for becoming vitamin K deficient. This scenario is commonly encountered, particularly in hospitalized patients, and is often not diagnosed until they develop clinically significant bleeding. Less often, vitamin K deficiency is caused by obstructive liver disease or by disorders of the intestinal mucosa that lead to chronic malabsorption.

Formerly, vitamin K deficiency in newborns sometimes caused ecchymoses, bleeding from venipuncture sites, and, rarely, intracranial hemorrhage. *Hemorrhagic disease of the newborn* arises because plasma levels of vitamin K–dependent clotting factors are relatively low at birth, the gastrointestinal tract of the newborn is relatively sterile, and mother's milk contains very little vitamin K. The risk is enhanced if the mother has been taking antibiotics or anticonvulsant drugs. Fortunately, this complication is now rarely encountered, owing to the routine administration of vitamin K to newborns.

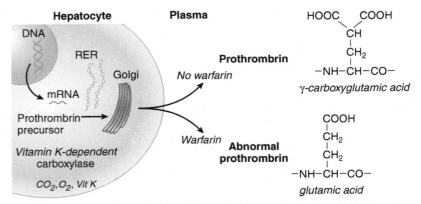

FIGURE 16-3 **The biosynthesis of proteins modified by γ-carboxylation of glutamic acid residues and the inhibition of this post-translational modification by warfarin.** (Modified with permission from Flaumenhaft R and Furie B. Biochemistry of factor IX and molecular biology of hemophilia B. In Hoffman R, Benz EJ, Shattil SJ, et al, eds. *Hematology: Basic Principles and Practice*, 3rd Edition. New York, USA, Churchill Livingstone, 2001:1870.)

An important and common cause of functional "vitamin K deficiency" is overdosage with anticoagulant drugs, primarily warfarin. These drugs are competitive inhibitors of vitamin K epoxide reductase (Fig. 16-1). As shown in Figure 16-3, warfarin administration results in a decrease in γ-carboxylation of prothrombin and other vitamin K–dependent clotting factors. Patients taking warfarin are carefully monitored through regular measurement of the prothrombin time, which allows the dose of warfarin to be adjusted to maintain the patient within a safe and effective anticoagulant range. Patients are at risk of abnormal bleeding when the prothrombin time significantly exceeds this range. Occasionally, mentally disturbed patients develop hemorrhage after self-administration of toxic doses of warfarin or another vitamin K antagonist such as rodent poison.

DIAGNOSIS

In patients with vitamin K deficiency, the prothrombin time is prolonged, often markedly so, owing to functional impairment of prothrombin, factor VII, and factor X. The partial thromboplastin time is also prolonged but to a lesser extent, due to the impairment of prothrombin, factor IX, and factor X. In patients in whom vitamin K deficiency is not apparent from the history or clinical setting, functional assays of specific clotting factors will reveal low levels of prothrombin and factors VII, IX, and X. In contrast, immunologically based assays would demonstrate that the protein levels of these factors are normal or near normal, thereby providing strong evidence for a change in structure that impairs function.

TREATMENT

In many patients, vitamin K deficiency is anticipated and diagnosed prior to any apparent abnormal bleeding. These individuals and those with mild abnormal bleeding can be treated with parenteral administration of vitamin K. The prothrombin time should reach normal levels within about 12 hours of initiating therapy. Patients with severe bleeding should receive not only vitamin K but also infusion of fresh frozen plasma or plasma concentrates that are enriched in prothrombin and factors VII, IX, and X. Concern for the transmission of viral diseases lessens the use of prothrombin concentrates unless they have been prepared free of contaminating viruses.

LIVER DISEASE

The hepatocyte is the only site of synthesis of the vitamin K–dependent coagulation proteins and is the primary, though not the only, site at which factor VIII is produced. Therefore patients with severe liver disease may develop abnormal bleeding due to low levels of these clotting proteins. Moreover, most of these patients develop functionally abnormal fibrinogen due to enhanced glycosylation. The prothrombin time and the partial thromboplastin time are prolonged, and if dysfibrinogenemia is present, the thrombin time is also prolonged.

In patients with liver disease, the risk of abnormal bleeding due to defects in coagulation is often compounded by thrombocytopenia caused either by congestive splenomegaly in patients with cirrhosis or suppression of platelet production in patients with alcoholism. Moreover, patients with impaired liver function fail to clear activated clotting factors from the circulation and therefore are predisposed to developing DIC, discussed in the next section.

In patients with liver disease, abnormal bleeding is primarily from the gastrointestinal tract, due to a combination of low levels of plasma coagulation proteins, thrombocytopenia, and anatomical lesions secondary to the underlying liver disease and its cause. For example, patients with cirrhosis may have esophageal varices, whereas patients with alcoholism often have not only hepatic cirrhosis but also alcohol-induced gastric erosions. Thus, gastrointestinal bleeding is a common problem in patients with liver disease, owing to a complex array of comorbid conditions.

In those patients who are actively bleeding, attention must be directed both to local sites of blood loss as well as correction or amelioration of abnormal hemostasis. Vitamin K should be administered because many of these patients are vitamin K deficient, particularly if they have obstructive liver disease. In most patients, thrombocytopenia can be partially corrected by infusion of platelets. Correction of deficits in plasma coagulation proteins is more challenging, particularly in patients with DIC.

DISSEMINATED INTRAVASCULAR COAGULATION

The most formidable and daunting disorder of hemostasis is DIC. This life-threatening complication is commonly encountered in a variety of medical, surgical, and obstetric settings. The pathophysiology of DIC is complex, but at its core is the release of tissue factor or the exposure of blood to endotoxin in sufficient amounts to activate blood coagulation and overwhelm normal hemostatic regulatory mechanisms. As a result, the coagulation cascade is ignited to such a degree that coagulation factors are consumed along with platelets. This process is accompanied by secondary fibrinolysis due to activation of plasmin, which

TABLE 16-1 Underlying Disorders That Trigger Disseminated Intravascular Coagulation

Vascular Damage Leading to Release of Tissue Factor
Bacterial sepsis
Gram negative organisms
Meningococcus
Pneumococcus
Clostridia
Metabolic stress
Acidosis
Shock
Heat stroke
Release of Tissue Factor from Injured or Pathologic Tissue
Obstetrical complications
Placental abruption
Retained placenta/fetus
Placenta previa
Amniotic fluid embolus
Pre-eclampsia/eclampsia
Malignancies
Solid tumors, mucin-secreting adenocarcinomas
Acute promyelocytic leukemia
Severe burns

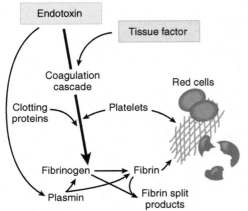

FIGURE 16-4 Scheme summarizing the pathogenesis of disseminated intravascular coagulation.

may digest any fibrin that is formed. Depending on the balance of pro-thrombotic and anti-thrombotic derangements, pathology sections may show widespread deposition of fibrin and platelets throughout the microcirculation accompanied by tissue damage, hemorrhage, or a combination of both.

ETIOLOGY AND PATHOGENESIS

DIC never arises de novo but rather as a consequence of an underlying pathologic process. Further insight into the pathogenesis of DIC can be gained by a consideration of the myriad of disorders that are known triggers, the most important of which are shown in Table 16-1.

In many of these conditions, the release of tissue factor from injured vessels or extravascular cells plays a central role in unleashing the full potential of the blood coagulation pathway (Fig. 16-4). In addition, injury to the endothelium can cause in situ thrombus formation due to both adhesion of platelets and down-regulation of thrombomodulin, which normally converts circulating thrombin into an anticoagulant (Chapter 17). Sepsis is the most common trigger of DIC among medical or surgical in-patients. The production of endotoxin by the offending organism activates monocytes, provoking the release of both endogenous tissue factor and inflammatory cytokines such as tumor necrosis factor and interleukin-1, which in turn induce robust expression of tissue factor. DIC also may be initiated by diffuse vascular injury caused by hypoxia, acidosis, and shock, often coexisting in very sick patients, as well as by antigen-antibody complexes, such as are present in systemic lupus erythematosus.

Intravascular coagulation can also be triggered by release of tissue factor from pathologic tissue. DIC occurs in obstetrical patients as a result of a number of complications listed in Table 16-1. In many of these patients, DIC is induced by the release of fetal cells or fluid into the maternal circulation. Obstetrical DIC usually resolves promptly with surgical correction of the problem. In addition, procoagulant material can be released in certain malignant conditions. In acute promyelocytic leukemia (Chapter 21), the turnover of granule-laden leukemic cells releases procoagulants that often lead to severe DIC. Patients with certain

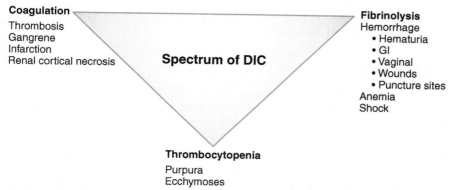

Coagulation
Thrombosis
Gangrene
Infarction
Renal cortical necrosis

Spectrum of DIC

Fibrinolysis
Hemorrhage
 • Hematuria
 • GI
 • Vaginal
 • Wounds
 • Puncture sites
Anemia
Shock

Thrombocytopenia
Purpura
Ecchymoses

FIGURE 16-5 Clinical spectrum of disseminated intravascular coagulation.

solid tumors, particularly mucus-producing adenocarcinomas, sometimes have a more chronic and indolent form of DIC.

Clinical presentation and manifestations are variable, as shown in Figure 16-5. Patients with severe acute DIC commonly have diffuse bleeding, most often ecchymoses in skin and mucous membranes as a result of thrombocytopenia, but occasionally more serious and extensive blood loss. Some patients have profuse gastrointestinal bleeding, usually from multiple sources. Others develop pulmonary or uterine bleeding, hematuria, wound hemorrhage, or spontaneous bleeding from venipuncture sites. The more serious bleeding is due to a combination of thrombocytopenia, deficiency of coagulation factors, and secondary fibrinolysis. A much smaller subset of patients presents with thrombosis, often localized to the fingertips and toes, but sometimes causing necrosis of internal organs such as the renal cortex or bowel. Critically ill patients with the underlying conditions listed in Table 16-1 often have no clinically apparent bleeding or thrombosis but yet have the laboratory abnormalities of DIC. Obviously, these patients require close surveillance.

LABORATORY DIAGNOSIS

Patients with DIC have both thrombocytopenia and global abnormalities in the coagulation profile, as shown in the sidebar. Examination of the peripheral blood smear not only confirms the thrombocytopenia but also reveals relatively large platelets, indicative of enhanced platelet consumption rather than impaired production. In addition, in about one-quarter of patients with DIC, the red cell morphology is abnormal, with fragmented, triangular, and helmet-shaped cells, shown in Figure 16-6B, identical to the morphology encountered in microangiopathic hemolytic disorders such as thrombotic thrombocytopenic purpura (Chapter 14). However, patients with DIC have much less hemolysis than those with thrombotic thrombocytopenic purpura. Abnormal red cell morphology in DIC is due to shear stress as red cells are catapulted through a meshwork of fibrin strands. The markedly abnormal coagulation profile is due in part to low levels of clotting factors, owing to ongoing

DIC: Lab Findings

Prolonged PTT
Prolonged PT
Prolonged TT
Elevated D-dimers
Thrombocytopenia
Fragmented RBCs

consumption. In addition, fibrin degradation products generated by ongoing fibrinolysis are potent inhibitors of thrombin.

TREATMENT

The cardinal mandate in the management of DIC is to first treat the underlying disease. The patient's bleeding, thrombosis, and accompanying laboratory abnormalities may be promptly and fully reversed by effective therapy of the underlying condition—that is, antibiotic treatment of sepsis, surgical debridement of trauma wounds, and removal of fetal and placental tissue from the uterus. Unfortunately, in many (and perhaps most) cases of DIC, it is not possible to effectively treat the underlying disease. In these patients, active bleeding can be controlled by the administration of platelets, fresh frozen plasma, and sometimes coagulation factor concentrates. In patients with thrombosis, careful administration of heparin may be effective. In the absence of either bleeding or thrombosis, close monitoring is crucial because the clinical status of patients with DIC can deteriorate very rapidly.

OTHER ACQUIRED COAGULATION DISORDERS

ACQUIRED INHIBITORS OF COAGULATION FACTORS

Patients may develop profuse and widespread bleeding due to the development of antibodies that specifically inhibit one of the coagulation factors. Factor VIII inhibitors, albeit rare, are encountered more often than those against other coagulation proteins and can cause catastrophic bleeding. This problem may occur de novo but is seen more often postpartum or in patients with lymphoid malignancies or chronic inflammatory disorders. Because the titer of anti-factor VIII antibody is usually very high, the management of these patients is as challenging as that of hemophilia patients who develop a factor VIII inhibitor

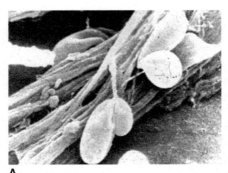
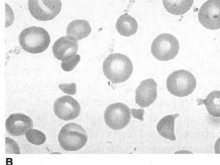

A   **B**

FIGURE 16-6 Disseminated intravascular coagulation. A) Scanning electron micrograph of a microclot showing red cells caught on strands of fibrin. (From Bull BS and Kuhn IN. Production of schistocytes by fibrin strands [an electron microscopic study]. *Blood*, 1968; 35:104-11.) B) Blood film from a patient with disseminated intravascular coagulation showing red cell fragmentation: schistocytes (lower left and center) and a helmet cell (lower right).

(Chapter 15). Even less often encountered are bleeding disorders due to acquisition of antibody inhibitors of other coagulation proteins such as factor V and von Willebrand factor.

Acquired factor X deficiency is sometimes seen in patients with amyloidosis due to binding and rapid clearance of factor X by amyloid.

ANTIPHOSPHOLIPID SYNDROME

Individuals who develop antiphospholipid antibodies often have a slightly prolonged prothrombin time and a significantly prolonged partial thromboplastin time but are at risk of thrombosis rather than bleeding. This entity is discussed in Chapter 17.

SELF-ASSESSMENT STUDY QUESTIONS

1. A 65-year-old dentist presented with fever, weight loss, fatigue, and progressive petechiae and ecchymoses over the last few weeks.

   Laboratory results:
   Hemoglobin 8 g/dL, hematocrit 25%, reticulocyte count 2%
   White blood cell count 40,000/mm³ with 10% neutrophils, 5% band cells, 55% promyelocytes, 10% myeloblasts, 5% monocytes, 15% lymphocytes
   Platelet count 25,000/mm³

   What is the most likely cause of the patient's severe purpura?
   A. Immune thrombocytopenia.
   B. Thrombocytopenia secondary to acute leukemia.
   C. Thrombocytopenia due to gram-negative bacterial sepsis.
   D. Disseminated intravascular coagulation.
   E. Thrombotic thrombocytopenic purpura.

2. A 56-year-old woman was admitted for elective gall bladder surgery. Her preoperative coagulation profile was normal. There was no unexpected bleeding during surgery. During the first week of recovery, she developed a urinary tract infection, treated with broad-spectrum antibiotics. She was anorexic with some nausea and could not eat. On postoperative day 7, the patient sustained a large hematoma in her surgical wound that spread to surrounding subcutaneous tissue. Repeat coagulation test results included a platelet count of 280,000/mm³, prothrombin time of 65 seconds, and partial thromboplastin time of 50 seconds. What is the most likely cause of the patient's bleeding?
   A. Acquired inhibitor to factor VIII.
   B. Acquired inhibitor to factor V.
   C. Vitamin C deficiency.
   D. Vitamin K deficiency.
   E. Disseminated intravascular coagulation.

17 Thrombotic Disorders

H. Franklin Bunn and Kenneth A. Bauer

LEARNING OBJECTIVES

After studying this chapter you should understand:

■ The physiology of the natural anticoagulant mechanisms and how they limit the generation of activated enzymes in the coagulation cascade.

■ How genetic defects in natural anticoagulant mechanisms and abnormalities in procoagulant factors can predispose to venous thrombosis.

■ The interaction of acquired and genetic risk factors in the pathogenesis of venous thrombosis.

As mentioned in the introduction to this section of the book, thrombosis plays a commanding role as a complication of highly prevalent disorders such as obesity, diabetes, and cancer. Myocardial infarction is the leading cause of mortality from arterial thrombosis, whereas pulmonary embolus accounts for most deaths due to venous thrombosis. In this chapter, we will stress the pathophysiologic principles underlying in vivo thrombus formation and the acquired and inherited factors that put patients at increased risk.

Insight into the pathogenesis of thrombotic disorders began with the 19th century pathologist Rudolf Virchow, whose clinical and postmortem observations led him to postulate that the formation of blot clots sufficiently large to occlude major blood vessels was dependent upon three independent processes:

- *Abnormal blood flow*—principally stasis.
- *Irritation of the vessel* wall due to trauma, or a degenerative/inflammatory process such as atherosclerosis.
- *Enhanced blood coagulation*, or what we now call *hypercoagulability*.

Virchow's triad provides a useful framework for evaluating any patient who has developed clinically significant thrombotic disease. The history will often reveal factors that predispose to stasis, such as immobilization of a limb, pregnancy, or prolonged inactivity. Further studies may identify a specific type of vascular pathology as well as abnormalities in blood coagulation. In this chapter, venous thrombosis will be covered in more depth than arterial thrombosis because the former is closely linked to well-defined abnormalities in coagulation, whereas the latter is much more dependent on vascular abnormalities, particularly atherosclerosis, which lie outside the scope of this book.

TABLE 17-1 Risk Factors for Venous Thrombosis

Acquired (Secondary)	Inherited (Primary)
Advancing Age	Factor V Leiden (FVL)
Male Sex	Prothrombin G20210A
Obesity	Antithrombin Deficiency
Prior Thrombosis	Protein C Deficiency
Immobilization	Protein S Deficiency
Pregnancy	
Major Surgery	
Malignancy	
Estrogens (OCP* etc)	
Antiphospholipid Antibody Syndrome	
Heparin-Induced Thrombocytopenia	
Myeloproliferative Disorders	
Inflammatory Bowel Disease	

*Oral contraception pills

As outlined in Table 17-1, both nature and nurture contribute to the development of venous thrombosis. As listed in the left hand column, a wide spectrum of acquired or secondary factors puts individuals at increased risk. Several, such as increasing age, male sex, and obesity, are weak but statistically significant risk factors. In contrast, a history of venous thrombosis is a strong predictor of repeated episodes. Immobilization due to extended bed rest or prolonged air travel leads to blood stasis, particularly in the lower extremities. Immobilization is also an important contributor to the increased risk of venous thrombosis in patients recovering from major surgery. Pregnancy causes stasis in the legs, owing to impairment of venous return by the enlarging uterus. Malignancy and estrogen use will be discussed later in the chapter along with other less common acquired risk factors.

INHERITED DEFECTS THAT ENHANCE THE RISK OF VENOUS THROMBOSIS

During the last 15 years, it has become apparent that inherited abnormalities of blood coagulation play an important role in determining which individuals are at a higher risk for development of venous thrombosis. The right-hand column of Table 17-1 lists monogenic defects linked to the development of venous thrombosis. All consist of mutations in clotting factors or in inhibitors of clotting. Figure 17-1 depicts where these proteins are situated in the coagulation cascade.

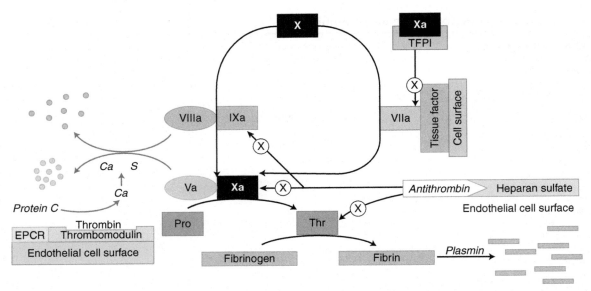

FIGURE 17-1 **Proteins that participate in the control or limitation of clot formation.** Familial thrombophilia can be caused by mutations that affect antithrombin, prothrombin (Pro), factor V, protein C, and protein S. The "a" signifies activation; thus Ca = activated protein C. The circle with the X indicates inhibition or inactivation. EPCR: endothelial protein C receptor.

Two of these genetic variants are mutations in genes encoding clotting proteins—factor V and prothrombin:

- Factor V Leiden is a genetic variant created by a single base change that results in the replacement of arginine by glutamine at position 506. In normal factor Va, Arg506 is the first site cleaved by activated protein C (Fig. 17-2). Subsequent cleavage by this serine protease at Arg306 and Arg679 inactivates factor Va.

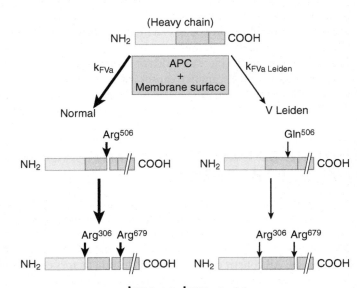

FIGURE 17-2 **Proteolytic degradation of the heavy chain of factor Va by activated protein C. (APC)** Normal factor Va is rapidly cleaved at Arg506 with subsequent cleavage at Arg306 and Arg679. In the factor V Leiden mutation, the absence of the Arg cleavage site at 506 greatly delays subsequent cleavage, K: rate of cleavage.

The absence of the initial cleavage at position 506 in factor V Leiden markedly delays cleavage at the two other sites and thereby results in higher levels of factor Va, which acts as a cofactor for factor Xa.

- Prothrombin G20210A is a single base substitution in the 3' untranslated region of the prothrombin gene that increases the biosynthesis of prothrombin protein. As a result, individuals heterozygous for this mutation have approximately 30% higher plasma levels of structurally normal prothrombin compared with normal individuals. This seemingly modest increase in concentration significantly increases the risk of venous thrombosis.

Both factor V Leiden and prothrombin G20210A mutations are surprisingly common in White populations, with prevalences of about 5% and 2%, respectively. In fact, the high frequency of these two genetic variants suggests that they confer some type of selective advantage. However, their clinical importance lies in the striking finding that one, or sometimes both, of these mutations is encountered in a substantial percentage of individuals who develop deep venous thrombosis either spontaneously or in the presence of acquired risk factors.

Inherited defects that increase risk of deep venous thrombosis also include deficiencies of protein C, protein S, and antithrombin. The mutations in these proteins differ from factor V Leiden and prothrombin G20210A mutations in three major respects:

- They involve inhibitors of coagulation rather than procoagulant factors.
- They are much less common.
- They are located at multiple sites in the respective genes.

The activities of protein C, protein S, and antithrombin also can be decreased in genetically normal individuals by certain conditions or medications.

Because of the low frequency of these mutations, homozygous individuals are very rarely encountered. A functional antithrombin level of less than 10% of normal is incompatible with life. Homozygous individuals with severe protein C or protein S deficiency have a very severe phenotype marked by thrombosis in childhood, adolescence, or even infancy (neonatal purpura fulminans). In contrast, the more frequently encountered heterozygotes are at increased risk of developing thrombosis in adulthood, albeit at low penetrance. The responsible mutations may either suppress expression of the protein (type I) or impair the functional activity of the protein (type II). In the former, both the antigen and activity levels are low, whereas in the latter, the antigen level is normal but the activity level is low.

In contrast to factor V Leiden and prothrombin G20210A mutations, which can be identified unequivocally by DNA analysis, inherited deficiencies of antithrombin, protein S, and protein C are diagnosed by measurements of plasma levels. Interpretation of these levels is often confounded by the fact that they can be lowered by a number of acquired factors (Table 17-2). Of most concern is the impact of acute thrombosis and anticoagulant therapy. Thus, in order to make a convincing diagnosis of an inherited deficiency of antithrombin, protein S, or protein C, measurements should be made after the patient has recovered from the thrombotic episode and is no longer receiving anticoagulants.

An appreciation of the clinical significance of deficiencies in antithrombin, protein C, and protein S requires an understanding of the role of these proteins

TABLE 17-2 Causes of Acquired Deficiencies in Antithrombin, Protein C, or Protein S

Antithrombin	Protein C	Protein S
Pregnancy		Pregnancy
Liver disease	Liver disease	Liver disease
DIC	DIC	DIC
Nephrotic syndrome		
Major surgery		Inflammation
Acute thrombosis	Acute thrombosis	Acute thrombosis
Heparin Rx	Warfarin Rx	Warfarin Rx
Estrogens Rx		Estrogens Rx

in pathways that inhibit clot formation. Figure 17-3 depicts how protein C and protein S limit the extent of clot formation. Thrombomodulin is a transmembrane protein expressed on endothelial cells that has on its extracellular domain a binding site for thrombin. Upon docking onto thrombomodulin, thrombin's substrate specificity becomes restricted to protein C. Protein C, like factors VII, IX, X, and prothrombin, is a vitamin K–dependent zymogen. Protein C binds to a receptor termed *the endothelial protein C receptor* on the endothelial cell surface, where protein C is activated by the thrombin-thrombomodulin complex. The rate of protein C activation is accelerated about 20,000-fold by binding to this complex. Activated protein C cleaves and degrades factors Va and VIIIa, as depicted in

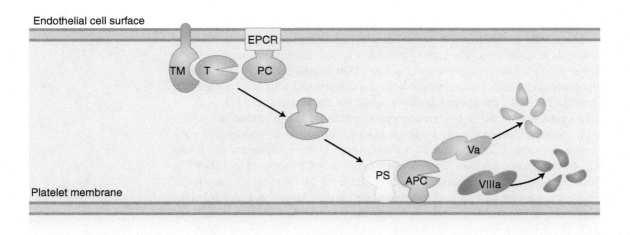

FIGURE 17-3 Activation of protein C on the endothelial cell membrane and assembly of protein Ca and protein S on platelet and other cell membranes, enabling the rapid proteolysis of factors Va and VIIIa.

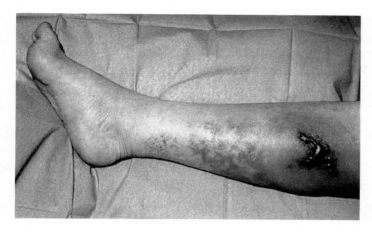

FIGURE 17-4 **Warfarin-induced skin necrosis.**

Figure 17-3. Importantly, the inactivation rate is enhanced by protein S, which is also vitamin K–dependent but not a zymogen.

Individuals with protein C deficiency are at risk for a rare but serious complication termed *warfarin-induced skin necrosis*. When treatment with the anticoagulant warfarin (Chapter 13) is initiated, these patients occasionally develop painful ecchymoses in fat-containing areas of the body such as the breasts or buttocks, which can be quite extensive and debilitating (Fig. 17-4). Microscopically, these lesions contain fibrin thrombi within venules, accompanied by hemorrhagic necrosis. The explanation for warfarin-induced skin necrosis lies in wide differences in the stability of vitamin K–dependent coagulation proteins in the plasma. Factor VII and protein C have the shortest half-lives (6 and 14 hours, respectively), whereas the other vitamin K–dependent proteins have half-lives of 24 to 60 hours. In normal individuals, the fall in protein C activity following the start of warfarin is generally not of clinical significance, but in heterozygotes with levels of protein C that are about half of normal, a further drop in protein C activity during the first day of therapy can trigger thrombosis in the skin.

Antithrombin is a member of a large family of serine protease inhibitors. Although initially described as the primary physiologic inhibitor of thrombin, antithrombin was subsequently shown to also neutralize factors IXa and Xa and, to a lesser extent, factors XIa and XIIa. Antithrombin is also known as heparin cofactor I. In the absence of heparin, antithrombin is a relatively slow inactivator of these activated clotting factors. In contrast, as shown in Figure 17-5, the binding of the heparin polysaccharide to antithrombin changes its conformation in a way that markedly enhances its affinity for thrombin as well as for factors IXa, Xa, XIa, and XIIa. Heparin's binding site to antithrombin has been localized to a sulfated pentasaccharide (Fig. 17-5). This small domain is sufficient to inactivate factor Xa but not thrombin, because thrombin inhibition by heparin requires longer saccharides. This insight has permitted the development of

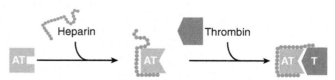

FIGURE 17-5 **Inhibition of thrombin (T) by antithrombin (AT).** The binding of a sulfated pentasaccharide within heparin to antithrombin changes its conformation, enabling it to bind to and inactivate thrombin and other activated clotting factors.

heparin-like drugs that target factor Xa only (such as the synthetic pentasaccharide fondaparinux). Endogenous heparan sulfate polysaccharides on the surface of vascular endothelium also have domains with structures very similar to this pentasaccharide and appear to activate antithrombin, thereby serving as natural anticoagulants.

Individuals with inherited antithrombin deficiency are at an increased risk of developing venous thrombosis, similar to those with protein C and protein S deficiency. Among the inherited thrombotic disorders, the clinical penetrance of venous thromboembolism appears to be highest in families with type I antithrombin deficiency.

IMPACT OF INHERITED AND ACQUIRED FACTORS ON THE DEVELOPMENT OF VENOUS THROMBOSIS

If an individual, particularly a child or young adult, develops venous thrombosis in the absence of any of the acquired factors listed in Table 17-1, he or she may have an inherited defect in one of the proteins discussed earlier. As shown in Figure 17-6, in the presence of one or more of these acquired risk factors, the chance of thrombosis is markedly enhanced by the presence of an inherited defect. The secondary risk factors can be divided into two groups: conditions such as older age, obesity, and cancer and transient precipitating factors such as estrogens, pregnancy, surgery, and immobilization.

The combinatorial impact of inherited and acquired risk factors has been demonstrated by a large, case-control study from Leiden, Holland on the risk and incidence of a first episode of deep venous thrombosis in a previously healthy population (summarized in Table 17-3). It is clear from this table that the risk of venous thrombosis associated with the factor V Leiden mutation and the secondary risk factor, estrogens in the form of oral contraceptives, are synergistic. The combination imposes significantly more risk and a higher incidence than the sum of the two factors alone.

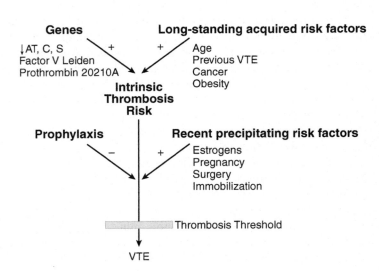

FIGURE 17-6 The impact of genetic defects, along with acquired risk factors, on the development of venous thromboembolism (VTE).

TABLE 17-3 First Episode of Deep Venous Thrombosis

	Risk	Incidence/Year (%)
Normal	1	0.008
Prothrombin 20210A heterozygotes	3 × ⇑	0.02
Oral contraceptives	4 × ⇑	0.03
Factor V Leiden heterozygotes	7 × ⇑	0.06
Oral contraceptives + FVL	35 × ⇑	0.3
Factor V Leiden homozygotes	80 × ⇑	0.5-1

ACQUIRED THROMBOTIC DISORDERS

Antiphospholipid antibody syndrome is characterized by thrombosis in association with an acquired inhibitor directed against proteins bound to membrane phospholipids and/or persistently elevated titers of antibodies against cardiolipin or β_2-glycoprotein I. Patients will often have a prolonged partial thromboplastin time and, less commonly, a prolonged prothrombin time. Mixing studies described at the end of Chapter 13 reveal that the long partial thromboplastin time is not corrected by the addition of normal plasma. Despite this laboratory abnormality, affected individuals almost never have increased bleeding but are at an increased risk for venous as well as arterial thrombosis. In this important respect, antiphospholipid syndrome along with heparin-induced thrombocytopenia and the hypercoagulable state associated with malignancy, described in the following section, differ from the inherited disorders described earlier in this chapter. Other clinical manifestations of antiphospholipid antibody syndrome include immune thrombocytopenia and recurrent fetal loss. Some patients with this syndrome have systemic lupus erythematosus. Indeed, the coagulation abnormality is often called *lupus anticoagulant*. These patients are at a high risk for recurrent thrombosis and should be treated with long-term anticoagulation after an initial, unprovoked thrombotic event.

HEPARIN-INDUCED THROMBOCYTOPENIA

As mentioned in Chapter 13, a small percentage of patients (1%-5%) treated with unfractionated heparin develop a potentially serious complication, heparin-induced thrombocytopenia, owing to development of an autoantibody against a complex of the drug and platelet factor 4 released from platelet alpha granules. As shown in Figure 17-7, the antigen-antibody complex binds to Fc receptors on platelets and triggers their activation. This commonly results in mild or moderate thrombocytopenia, but more importantly, in about 20% to 50% of patients causes both venous and arterial thrombosis. This serious adverse effect is encountered much less often in patients treated with fractionated low-molecular-weight heparin and rarely with the synthetic pentasaccharide fondaparinux.

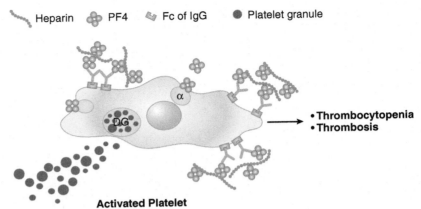

FIGURE 17-7   Platelet activation during heparin-induced thrombocytopenia. The heparin-platelet factor 4 (PF4) antigen binds to antibody. The Fc portion of this complex binds to receptors on the platelet, triggering activation and release of dense granules (DG) and alpha granules (light blue) containing PF4.

MALIGNANCY

There is a high incidence of venous thrombosis in cancer patients. Some evince migratory superficial thrombophlebitis (Trousseau syndrome), often in unusual sites such as the arms. In addition, thrombosis associated with chronic disseminated intravascular coagulation is sometimes encountered in cancer patients (Chapter 15). Those who are terminally ill may develop nonbacterial thrombotic (marantic) endocarditis. The pathogenesis of these thrombotic complications is unclear but probably involves release of thrombogenic agonists from malignant cells, such as microparticles containing tissue factor. Thrombosis also may occur during treatment of cancer with various chemotherapeutic agents, such as L-asparaginase, or estrogen-like drugs such as tamoxifen.

Patients with two types of clonal hematologic disorders, the myeloproliferative disorders and paroxysmal nocturnal hemoglobinuria, are also at a high risk for developing venous and arterial thrombosis. These conditions are discussed in detail in Chapters 20 and 11, respectively.

SELF ASSESSMENT STUDY QUESTIONS

1. Choose the incorrect statement.
   A. Prothrombin 20210 mutation is a polymorphism in the 3' untranslated region that does not affect the structure of prothrombin (factor II) protein but raises its levels in the blood slightly.
   B. Protein S acts as a cofactor with activated protein C.
   C. Factor VIIIa and factor Va are inactivated by antithrombin-heparin complex.
   D. Endogenous heparinoids (glycosaminoglycans) on the luminal surface of endothelial cells are the activators of antithrombin on healthy endothelium downstream from a clot.
   E. Plasma from individuals with the factor V Leiden mutation is resistant to activated protein C.

2. What protein is the physiologic regulator of the level of activated factor V at the site of blood clot formation?
   A. Activated protein C.
   B. Antithrombin.
   C. Thrombin.
   D. Fibrinogen D-dimers.
   E. Fibrin split products.

3. Which of the following conditions primarily involve venous thrombosis (V), arterial thrombosis (A), or both (AV)?
   A. Antithrombin deficiency.
   B. Antiphospholipid antibody syndrome.
   C. Heparin-induced thrombocytopenia.
   D. Factor V Leiden mutation.
   E. Atherosclerosis.
   F. Myeloproliferative disorders.
   G. Prothrombin G20210A mutation.
   H. Protein S deficiency.

PART III White Blood Cell Disorders

Because of their roles as both sentinels and effectors of the innate and adaptive immune system, white blood cells (leukocytes) are frequently measured and monitored in clinical practice. An increased white blood cell count (leukocytosis) is one of the most common signs of infectious and inflammatory diseases.

Neoplasms of immune cells, which include the leukemias, the lymphomas, and the plasma cell tumors, are less common but much more important clinically. Hodgkin lymphoma (the first of these tumors to be described) came to attention in 1832 in a paper entitled "On Some Morbid Appearances of the Absorbent Glands and Spleen" by Thomas Hodgkin. The photograph on the right illustrates the natural history of Hodgkin lymphoma, which includes the inexorable development of massively enlarged lymph nodes and eventual spread of the disease to the liver, spleen, bone marrow, and other tissues. Little could be done for such unfortunate souls.

This sad state has changed dramatically. Beginning in the latter half of the 20th century, white cell neoplasms have been on the leading edge of advances in oncology; indeed, Hodgkin lymphoma was the first human cancer to be cured with radiation and combination chemotherapy. The field now finds itself at the forefront of a genomic revolution that is laying the groundwork for increasingly precise molecular diagnoses and more effective, less toxic targeted cancer therapies.

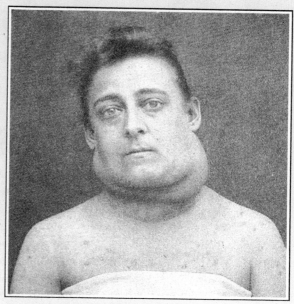

Hodgkin lymphoma, duration 6 months.
From Cabot's "Physical Diagnosis," fifth edition, New York, William Wood and Company, published in 1914.

18 Leukocyte Function and Non-malignant Leukocyte Disorders

Jon C. Aster and Nancy Berliner

LEARNING OBJECTIVES

After studying this chapter you should understand:

- The factors that determine leukocyte counts in the peripheral blood.
- The major causes of granulocytosis (neutrophilia) and other forms of leukocytosis.
- The causes and consequences of leukopenia.
- The mechanisms underlying qualitative disorders of neutrophil function.
- The causes and consequences of hemophagocytic lymphohistiocytosis (macrophage activation syndrome).

Leukocytes constitute the cellular components of the innate and adaptive immune system and are critical for host defense. These cells mediate acute and chronic inflammation, modulate immune responses, and protect the host against numerous pathogens. It is no surprise that defects in leukocyte function predispose to various kinds of infection in proportion to the nature and severity of the defect.

Disorders affecting leukocytes can be divided broadly into malignant disorders (tumors of leukocytes or their progenitors) and non-malignant disorders. The malignant disorders are uncommon but clinically important entities that are covered in subsequent chapters. Here we consider the much more common non-malignant abnormalities that affect leukocytes. These can involve any of the leukocytes (neutrophils, eosinophils, basophils, monocytes, B cells, T cells, and natural killer cells), but the disorders of greatest clinical relevance affect neutrophils; these will be our major focus.

OVERVIEW OF NEUTROPHIL DISORDERS

Like other formed elements of the peripheral blood, neutrophils are the progeny of earlier progenitors that acquire the capacity to function as they mature in the bone marrow (Fig. 18-1). Neutrophils are distributed within the body in several discrete and highly dynamic compartments or pools (Fig. 18-2). In the marrow, mitotically active myeloid progenitors mature over a period of 7 to 10 days to

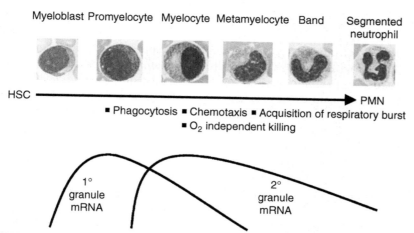

Myeloblast Promyelocyte Myelocyte Metamyelocyte Band   Segmented
                                                                   neutrophil

HSC ⟶ PMN

■ Phagocytosis ■ Chemotaxis ■ Acquisition of respiratory burst
■ O₂ independent killing

1° granule mRNA

2° granule mRNA

FIGURE 18-1 **Myelopoiesis.** As granulocytes develop and mature, they go through a series of recognizable morphologic stages that correlate with the expression of genes that confer the specific functions indicated on the time line. HSC: hematopoietic stem cell (Used with permission from Gaines P and Berliner N. Granulocytopoiesis. In *Clinical Hematology,* Young N, ed, Philadelphia, USA, Mosby/Elsevier, 2006, 62.)

give rise to large numbers of neutrophils. Under steady-state conditions, most of these newly formed neutrophils die without ever being released into the blood, constituting a *storage pool* that can be called upon during times of increased need. Upon release from the marrow, neutrophils enter the *circulating pool,* the only pool that is measured clinically. On average, neutrophils circulate for only 3 to 6 hours before migrating into tissues, where they may survive for up to 3 days. At any given time, roughly half of the neutrophils in the blood are adherent to vessel walls; these cells are referred to as the *marginal pool.* Finally, some circulating neutrophils are sequestered in the spleen. Normally, <5% of the neutrophils in the body are in the circulating pool, which turns over quickly. As a result, stimuli that alter the release of neutrophils from the marrow, neutrophil margination, or the migration of neutrophils into tissues can have rapid and sometimes profound effects on the peripheral blood neutrophil count.

In most clinical laboratories, the normal white blood cell count ranges from 4500 to 11,000/µL, with approximately 60% of the cells being neutrophils. Leukocytosis, an elevation in the white blood cell count, usually stems from a pathologic insult that stimulates a systemic inflammatory reaction. By far the most common form of leukocytosis is granulocytosis, an increase in neutrophils also known as *neutrophilia.*

Acute inflammation of any cause can produce the rapid appearance of granulocytosis by mobilizing neutrophils from the marrow storage pool. In particularly severe bacterial infections, immature granulocytic forms, such as band cells or even earlier progenitors, may be released into the

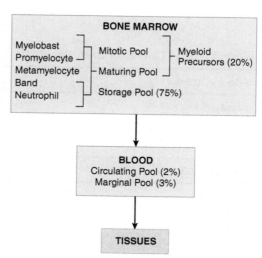

FIGURE 18-2 **Neutrophil pools.** The relative proportions of cells in various pools of neutrophils and neutrophilic progenitors are shown (see text for details).

blood (a finding also called a *left-shift*), and in extreme cases the white blood cell count may rise to >50,000/mm³. In such instances the marked leukocytosis and the presence of immature cells may mimic the appearance of a myeloid leukemia (leukemoid reaction). Occasionally, the inflammatory process may involve the marrow itself and produce marrow fibrosis and distortion, leading not only to the release of immature myeloid elements but also nucleated erythroid progenitors and misshapen tear-drop red cells. This combination of features in a peripheral smear is referred to as *leukoerythroblastosis*. If the marrow involvement is extensive, myelophthisic anemia may result (Chapter 4). It should be emphasized, however, that in the vast majority of cases granulocytosis is a reaction to disorders involving tissues other than the marrow. In contrast, neutropenia, an abnormally low neutrophil count, is often caused by defects in neutrophil production that may require a bone marrow examination for evaluation.

Primary disorders associated with neutrophil dysfunction usually have a genetic basis. Although rare, they are of interest because unraveling of their pathogenesis has led to the identification of genes that regulate normal neutrophil development and function.

GRANULOCYTOSIS

Granulocytosis can be primary or secondary (Table 18-1). Primary disorders associated with granulocytosis include myeloid neoplasms (discussed in subsequent chapters) and a variety of genetic disorders that merit brief mention.

- Hereditary neutrophilia is a rare form of chronic granulocytosis that usually exhibits an autosomal dominant pattern of inheritance. In some families it is caused by gain-of-function mutations in the granulocyte colony-stimulating factor (G-CSF) receptor that lead to marrow hyperstimulation and increased neutrophil production.

- Down syndrome (trisomy 21) is the most common constitutional chromosomal disorder. About 10% of infants with Down syndrome develop a transient myeloproliferative disorder characterized by granulocytosis, circulating immature myeloid precursors, and hepatosplenomegaly. This disorder appears to be caused by acquired mutations in the transcription factor GATA-1 that result in deregulated growth of myeloid progenitors. In approximately 75% of patients, the disorder resolves spontaneously, but the remaining patients develop full-blown acute myeloid leukemia over a period of months to several years.

- Leukocyte adhesion deficiency (LAD) is a rare autosomal recessive disorder that is described later under functional disorders of neutrophils.

Secondary causes of granulocytosis are much more common than primary causes and can be sorted into the following pathogenic categories.

TABLE 18-1   Causes of Granulocytosis

Primary Disorders
Hereditary neutrophilia
Down syndrome (trisomy 21)
Leukocyte adhesion deficiency

Secondary Disorders
Stress
Infection
Inflammation
Drug reactions
Marrow hyperstimulation (elevated growth factor levels)
Splenectomy

- Stress. Acute stress is associated with elevated levels of catecholamines and glucocorticoids, both of which cause rapid demargination of neutrophils. Psychic and physical stress, exercise, seizures, and pain can all cause neutrophilia through this mechanism.

- Infection. Early in infection, factors derived from inflammatory cells such as interleukin-1 and tumor necrosis factor increase the release of neutrophils from the marrow storage pool. When an inflammatory stimulus is sustained, a variety of cells including T cells and macrophages release growth factors such as granulocyte-macrophage colony-stimulating factor (GM-CSF) and G-CSF. These factors enhance the growth and survival of granulocyte progenitors in the marrow and, over a period of 5 to 7 days, increase the rate of neutrophil production. In some instances (eg, disseminated tuberculosis) chronic infections involve the marrow directly and produce a leukoerythroblastic picture in the peripheral blood, owing to marrow inflammation and fibrosis.

- Inflammation of noninfectious etiology can produce neutrophilia through the same mechanisms as those cited under infection.

- Drug reactions can produce neutrophilia through various mechanisms. β-Adrenergic drugs and glucocorticoids cause neutrophils to demarginate, and glucocorticoids also cause a modest increase in the release of neutrophils from the marrow storage pool. Anabolic steroids such as testosterone stimulate hematopoiesis and may cause mild granulocytosis. Lithium used in the treatment of bipolar disorder can cause granulocytosis by stimulating the release of colony-stimulating factors from marrow stromal cells.

- Marrow hyperstimulation. Granulocytosis stemming from elevated levels of hematopoietic growth factors and increased marrow production of neutrophils may be seen in hemolytic anemias and immune thrombocytopenic purpura or following treatment of megaloblastic anemias with folate or vitamin B_{12}. On occasion, cancers produce hematopoietic growth factors such as G-CSF that lead to paraneoplastic neutrophilia.

- Splenectomy. The asplenic state may be associated with mild granulocytosis due to decreased sequestration of neutrophils.

EVALUATION OF THE PATIENT WITH GRANULOCYTOSIS

Neutrophilia is often detected during the evaluation of acutely ill patients suspected of having infections. In patients with acute infections, neutrophils often contain toxic granulation (persistence of primary granules), cytoplasmic vacuoles, and Döhle bodies, pale blue cytoplasmic aggregates of endoplasmic reticulum (Fig. 18-3). In severe sepsis, phagocytosed organisms occasionally may be seen within neutrophils. In acutely ill patients, the primary clinical focus is on the identification of infectious agents and the institution of appropriate antibiotic therapy.

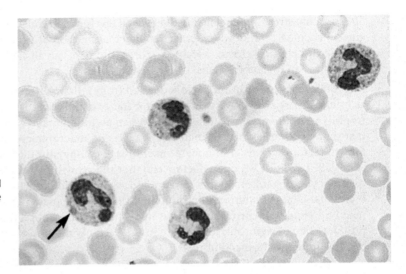

FIGURE 18-3 Döhle bodies and toxic granulation, peripheral smear. An arrow denotes a light blue Döhle body in the cytoplasm of a neutrophil. In addition, several neutrophils contain toxic granulations, coarse purple cytoplasmic granules that are best appreciated in the cell in the upper right part of the field. In many patients with severe infections, neutrophils with both Döhle bodies and toxic granulations may be seen.

The differential diagnosis of neutrophilia in sub-acutely or chronically ill patients is quite broad and includes numerous infectious, inflammatory, and neoplastic disorders. Mild neutrophilia in asymptomatic patients can be related to smoking or subtle inflammatory disease but requires evaluation to rule out important acquired diseases such as chronic myelogenous leukemia.

Neutrophilia is usually reactive and indicative of a normal-functioning bone marrow; consequently, bone marrow evaluation is usually not necessary. The exceptions are neutrophilias associated with either leukoerythroblastosis or the presence of immature myeloid precursors in the peripheral blood. Leukoerythroblastosis is indicative of an infiltrative disorder in the marrow, such as metastatic cancer, primary bone marrow disorders associated with fibrosis, or a disseminated granulomatous disease such as tuberculosis. The presence of immature myeloid precursors (often in concert with eosinophilia and basophilia) is characteristic of myeloid neoplasms such as chronic myelogenous leukemia and polycythemia vera, both of which can be distinguished from reactive processes by molecular tests described in Chapter 20. In unexplained persistent neutrophilia, a bone marrow examination may be informative diagnostically and should always include cultures for tuberculosis and fungal pathogens.

TABLE 18-2 Common Causes of Eosinophilia

Asthma
Allergy (including drug reactions)
Parasite infection
Connective tissue disease (eg, lupus erythematosus)
Neoplasia (may be primary or secondary)

OTHER FORMS OF LEUKOCYTOSIS

The second most common form of leukocytosis is eosinophilia. Like neutrophilia, eosinophilia is much more often secondary than primary (Table 18-2). The most common causes of eosinophilia in the United States are disorders associated with Th2 immune responses, particularly asthma and reactions to allergens such as pollen and drugs. Worldwide, the most common cause of eosinophilia is helminthic worm infections, which are endemic in many parts of the developing world. Other causes of reactive eosinophilia include immune disorders such as systemic lupus erythematosus or vasculitis. Eosinophilia can be seen in some myeloid neoplasms, particularly certain acute myeloid leukemias and myeloproliferative disorders; in such cases, the eosinophils are usually a component of the malignant clone. Marked eosinophilia (absolute eosinophil counts >10,000/mm^3) is particularly likely to be caused by certain types of myeloproliferative disorders, described further in Chapter 20. In other instances, eosinophilia is a reaction to some other kind of tumor. Hodgkin lymphoma (Chapter 23) is one notable example of a tumor that often produces reactive eosinophilia.

Basophilia is uncommon and usually is associated with eosinophilia. Mild basophilia is common in asthma and allergic conditions. More striking basophilia is sometimes seen in association with myeloid neoplasms, particularly chronic myelogenous leukemia and polycythemia vera, in which the basophils are part of the neoplastic clone.

Monocytosis is occasionally seen in association with tuberculosis or myeloid neoplasms, particularly those myeloproliferative disorders in which the monocytes and their precursors are a component of the malignancy.

Lymphocytosis most commonly stems from viral infections, particularly those caused by members of the gamma herpesvirus family, such as Epstein-Barr virus, the causative agent in infectious mononucleosis, and cytomegalovirus. The circulating lymphocytes are predominantly cytotoxic T cells, which are required for an effective immune response against Epstein-Barr virus and other herpesviruses. These T cells characteristically have abundant cytoplasm containing a few azurophilic granules and are sticky, often adhering to surrounding red cells (Fig. 18-4). Among bacterial infections, *Bordetella pertussis* (whooping cough) is unusual in causing lymphocytosis by releasing a toxin that inhibits the migration of lymphocytes out of the blood into lymph nodes. Much less commonly, lymphocytosis is a manifestation of a lymphocytic leukemia.

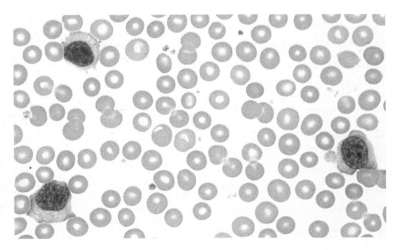

FIGURE 18-4   Mononucleosis, peripheral smear. Large lymphocytes with abundant cytoplasm that sticks to surrounding red cells (kissing cells) are present.

LEUKOPENIA

Leukopenia is defined as a decrease in the white blood cell count below the normal range. The most common and clinically significant form of leukopenia is *neutropenia*, defined as an absolute neutrophil count of <1500 cells/mm³. Patients with marked neutropenia (a state referred to as *agranulocytosis*) are highly susceptible to severe, sometimes fatal infections caused by bacteria and fungi. When neutropenia develops acutely, the risk of infection rises as neutrophil counts fall below 500/mm³; most patients who develop infections in this setting have neutrophil counts of <200/mm³. Chronic neutropenia appears to be compensated through uncertain mechanisms, so that even very low neutrophil counts (50-100/mm³) do not always result in infectious complications.

CAUSES OF NEUTROPENIA

Neutropenia can be divided into congenital forms, which present in infancy or early childhood, and acquired forms, which present at any age (Table 18-3). Neutropenia in infants and very young children often, but not always, stems from genetic defects that cause an insufficiency of neutrophil production, whereas neutropenia in older children and adults may be caused by acquired defects affecting marrow production, neutrophil survival, or both.

The most common forms of congenital neutropenia are the following:

- Constitutional neutropenia. This lifelong neutropenia is usually discovered as an incidental laboratory abnormality and is of no clinical significance. By definition, patients have a modestly decreased neutrophil count (usually 500-1500/mm³) and no evidence of susceptibility to infection. Constitutional

TABLE 18-3 Causes of Clinically Significant Neutropenia

Congenital Disorders
Chronic benign neutropenia (unknown)
Severe congenital neutropenia (elastase mutations, mutations in other genes)
Cyclic neutropenia (elastase mutations)
Other rare inherited types (Chédiak-Higashi syndrome; Shwachman-Diamond-Oski syndrome; reticular dysgenesis)
Acquired Disorders
Drugs (myelosuppressive, idiosyncratic)
Infection (diverse mechanisms)
Autoimmune (increased destruction due to anti-neutrophil antibodies)
Hematologic malignancies (diverse mechanisms)
Nutritional deficiencies (decreased marrow production)

neutropenia is a reflection of genetic variation in the normal absolute neutrophil count, which, in certain ethnic groups, is shifted to a lower mean level. It is most common in people of African descent and in certain Arab populations. These individuals are asymptomatic, usually have other family members with low neutrophil counts, and respond normally to infectious challenges.

- Benign neutropenia of childhood describes a disorder in which neutrophil counts may be quite low (<100 cells/mm^3), but infections nevertheless tend not to be life threatening. Infants typically present at 6 to 12 months of age with an increased number or abnormal persistence of typical childhood infections. The neutrophil count is usually lower than 500 cells/mm^3 and may be near zero, yet patients usually have a surprisingly benign course. They are treated with prophylactic antibiotics and are supported acutely with G-CSF in the setting of severe infection. The disorder likely has an autoimmune basis, as antibodies against neutrophil-specific antigens are often present. This form of neutropenia resolves completely within 2 years in over 95% of these patients.

- Severe congenital neutropenia encompasses a rare group of genetic disorders associated with life-threatening infections. Inheritance may be autosomal dominant, autosomal recessive, or X-linked; a significant fraction of cases are sporadic. Over 60% of the autosomal dominant cases are caused by mutations in neutrophil elastase (also known as ELA2), a serine protease present in azurophilic primary granules that cleaves elastin and many other protein substrates. The pathogenesis of the neutropenia is unknown; it is currently postulated that the mutant elastase folds abnormally and accumulates in the endoplasmic reticulum. This in turn is believed to induce the unfolded protein response, which activates certain intracellular pathways that lead to apoptotic cell death. A bone marrow examination typically reveals a hypercellular marrow with an apparent maturation arrest at the promyelocyte stage of differentiation. A significant percentage of patients with severe congenital neutropenia (20% at 10 years), especially those due to elastase mutations, develop acute myeloid leukemia. These leukemias are usually associated with acquired gain-of-function mutations in the G-CSF receptor, which presumably contribute to the proliferative drive of the neoplasm.

- Cyclic neutropenia is a fascinating disorder in which the neutrophil count in the peripheral blood oscillates from near normal to close to zero over a cycle that averages 21 days. The bone marrow typically shows a decrease in mature granulocytes and a maturation arrest at the myelocyte stage of development during periods of severe neutropenia. Patients are prone to infections, particularly when their neutrophil counts are low, but these tend to be superficial (eg, periodontitis) and less serious than those in severe congenital neutropenia. Cyclic neutropenia is usually inherited in an autosomal dominant fashion and is nearly always caused by mutations in ELA2. It is unknown why elastase mutations produce cyclic neutropenia in some patients and severe congenital neutropenia in others. Patients with cyclic neutropenia do not appear to have any increased susceptibility to myeloid leukemia.

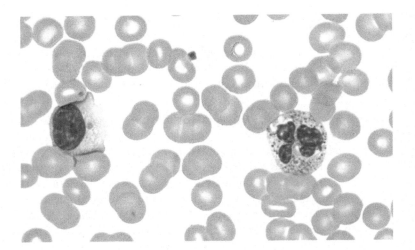

FIGURE 18-5 Chédiak-Higashi syndrome, peripheral smear. This field contains a neutrophil with multiple abnormal blue-gray cytoplasmic granules and a lymphocyte with a single, large, abnormal, red-purple granule.

- Other rare congenital forms of neutropenia are recognized. One that merits brief mention is Chédiak-Higashi syndrome, an autosomal recessive disorder caused by loss-of-function mutations in *LYST*, a gene that is essential for the proper formation of lysosomal granules in cells such as granulocytes, cytotoxic lymphocytes, and melanocytes. A clue to the diagnosis is the presence of abnormal granules in neutrophils and lymphocytes (Fig. 18-5). Patients are prone to bacterial infections due to neutropenia and neutrophil dysfunction. Death often follows an accelerated phase associated with hepatosplenomegaly, pancytopenia, and hemophagocytosis that may be triggered by Epstein-Barr virus infection, which persists because of the dysfunction of cytotoxic T cells.

  Acquired neutropenias are encountered much more frequently than the congenital forms and have diverse causes, including the following:

- Prescription drugs are probably the most common cause of acquired isolated neutropenia. Drugs can produce neutropenia through several mechanisms. Certain chemotherapeutic agents are cytotoxic and cause a predictable transient decrease in neutrophil production that is associated with marrow hypoplasia. In contrast, other drugs suppress the production of neutrophils in an unpredictable, idiosyncratic fashion. In many instances, this second class of drugs appears to induce antibodies that destroy granulocytes and suppress the growth of marrow progenitors. Bone marrow examination often shows a maturation arrest at the promyelocyte or myelocyte stage of granulocyte differentiation.

- Viral and bacterial infections caused by a variety of agents can result in neutropenia. Mild neutropenia may accompany typical childhood viral infections as well as infectious mononucleosis (acute Epstein-Barr virus infection), viral hepatitis, parvovirus B19 infection, and human immunodeficiency virus (HIV) infection. In viral infections, several mechanisms contribute to the neutropenia, including increased margination, increased migration, and decreased production, the latter due to the suppressive effects of cytokines such as interferon-gamma on the marrow. On occasion, Epstein-Barr virus, hepatitis, or HIV infections cause prolonged severe neutropenia, sometimes by inducing autoantibodies. Bacterial infections generally cause neutrophilia, but exceptions to this rule include typhoid fever (*Salmonella typhi*), brucellosis, rickettsial infections, and disseminated tuberculosis. These infections are commonly associated with neutropenia through a variety of mechanisms. Sepsis may be associated with neutropenia, particularly in infants, the elderly, and patients with severe alcoholism. Neutropenia in the setting of sepsis may stem from increased peripheral destruction or decreased marrow production (marrow exhaustion) and is understandably associated with a poor prognosis.

- Autoimmune neutropenia may be isolated or occur as part of a generalized autoimmune disorder, particularly systemic lupus erythematosus. The basis of the neutropenia is not clear, because many patients with anti-neutrophil antibodies have normal neutrophil counts, suggesting that cell-mediated neutrophil destruction also plays a role. The neutropenia is often mild and benign and serves mainly as a marker of the activity of the underlying disease.

- Hematologic malignancies can produce neutropenia in several ways. Acute leukemias, myelodysplastic syndromes, and other marrow-based neoplasms often displace normal marrow progenitors, leading to insufficient marrow production. Certain lymphoid neoplasms (eg, chronic lymphocytic leukemia) may be associated with the production of autoantibodies directed against neutrophils and marrow progenitors. One uncommon neoplasm associated with isolated neutropenia is large granular lymphocyte leukemia, a neoplasm of cytotoxic T cells that suppresses granulocytic progenitors in the bone marrow through uncertain mechanisms.

- Nutritional deficiencies of folate and vitamin B_{12} are often associated with neutropenia that is generally not as severe as the megaloblastic anemia seen with these deficiencies.

- Hypersplenism may cause mild neutropenia due to sequestration of neutrophils.

- Adult patients sometimes present with neutropenia of uncertain etiology (idiopathic neutropenia). Some with very mild neutropenia (1000-1500 neutrophils/mm³) may have an underlying inflammatory disorder associated with cytokine production that suppresses neutrophil production. In others, the neutropenia is severe (50-100 neutrophils/mm³). These patients should have a bone marrow examination and cytogenetic studies to rule out a myelodysplastic syndrome (Chapter 20). If the marrow is normal, the disorder tends to follow a benign course.

EVALUATION OF NEUTROPENIA

It is often helpful to obtain serial neutrophil counts, both to confirm the presence of neutropenia and to follow trends in the neutrophil count over time. A careful history can determine whether the neutropenia is likely to be acute or chronic.

In the pediatric age group, it is important to ask parents about a family history of neutropenia or increased susceptibility to infection. The patient should be examined for evidence of infection, with particular attention paid to the oropharynx, lymph nodes, spleen, and perianal region.

In those with severe bacterial infections and sepsis, the clinical focus is on identifying the organism and its likely source and treatment with broad-spectrum antibiotics. In other settings, certain laboratory tests may be helpful. The peripheral smear sometimes contains clues; for example, the presence of increased numbers of large lymphocytes with cytoplasmic granules should raise suspicion of acute viral infection or large granular lymphocytic (LGL) leukemia, a neoplasm usually of cytotoxic T cell origin, both of which can be evaluated with additional tests. Bone marrow examination often reveals findings that point to particular etiologies. Drug-related and autoimmune neutropenias are frequently associated with a maturation arrest in the marrow. Dysplasia (abnormal and disordered maturation of bone marrow progenitors) might be evidence of a myelodysplastic syndrome (see Chapter 20), which can be evaluated further by cytogenetic analysis of marrow cells. In newborns, infants, and young children, special genetic tests may reveal elastase mutations or other inherited defects associated with congenital neutropenias.

TREATMENT OF NEUTROPENIA

Initial treatment is directed toward mitigating the complications of neutropenia. In patients with severe neutropenia, fever is an indication for prompt treatment with broad-spectrum antibiotics that cover bacterial and fungal infections, following appropriate diagnostic cultures. It is important to remember that neutrophils are responsible for many of the clinical manifestations of infection and that infected neutropenic patients cannot produce pus or characteristic localizing signs. Therefore, fever may be the only manifestation of infection. Even if cultures are negative, patients should continue receiving antibiotics until the neutrophil count recovers (in drug-induced or other acute neutropenias) or for a full 7 to 10 day course (in the setting of refractory neutropenia).

Other treatment options aim to restore the neutrophil count and vary depending on the underlying cause. Drugs are always chief suspects and should be stopped unless essential. Drug-induced neutropenia usually resolves about 7 to 10 days after the drug is stopped, although some drugs can cause prolonged neutropenia that persists for several weeks. In those with severe drug-related neutropenia, recovery can be speeded by administration of G-CSF. With symptomatic congenital neutropenias, the two main therapeutic options are G-CSF and bone marrow transplantation. Before the advent of G-CSF, nearly all patients with severe congenital neutropenia died in infancy. High-dose therapy with G-CSF now allows these patients to survive to adulthood but has revealed a propensity for the development of myeloid leukemia. The majority of patients with chronic benign neutropenia are managed without G-CSF, except in the setting of severe infections. Autoimmune neutropenia can be treated with a variety of immunosuppressive agents such as glucocorticoids. Large granular lymphocyte leukemia often responds very well to treatment with glucocorticoids or low-dose methotrexate.

LYMPHOPENIA

Lymphopenia is the second most common form of leukopenia. Most of the normal lymphocytes found in peripheral blood are T cells, mainly CD4-positive helper cells and smaller numbers of CD8-positive cytotoxic cells. Lymphopenia may be generalized (affecting B and T cells) or involve only T cells or T-cell subsets.

The most common forms of lymphopenia are acquired. One of the most important causes is infection with human immunodeficiency virus (HIV), which has a specific tropism for T-helper cells expressing CD4. In advanced HIV (acquired immunodeficiency syndrome, or AIDS), this leads to a profound deficiency of CD4-positive T-helper cells, lymphopenia, and frequent secondary infections by opportunistic pathogens. Another common acquired cause is treatment with glucocorticoid-type steroids, which are often used to treat autoimmune diseases, inflammatory conditions, and lymphoid neoplasms. At high doses, glucocorticoids induce the apoptosis of lymphocytes and their progenitors through mechanisms that remain poorly understood.

Primary causes of lymphopenia include rare congenital immunodeficiency states such as severe combined immunodeficiency, in which the production of both T and B cells is markedly compromised. Severe combined immunodeficiency may be inherited in an autosomal dominant or X-linked fashion. It is caused by loss-of-function mutations in several different genes, including those needed for antigen receptor gene rearrangement (such as the recombination activating genes *RAG-1* and *RAG-2*). Primary causes of isolated T-cell lymphopenia include thymic aplasia (DiGeorge syndrome), which is usually associated with germline deletions involving chromosome 22q11.

QUALITATIVE DISORDERS OF NEUTROPHIL FUNCTION

The susceptibility of neutropenic patients to bacterial and fungal infections highlights the importance of neutrophils in killing these pathogens. To do their job properly, circulating neutrophils must be able to execute a sequential series of tightly regulated cellular functions.

- Adhesion to endothelium and migration into tissues. A variety of substances released from affected tissues, including histamine (from mast cells), components of microorganisms, and inflammatory mediators released from tissue macrophages initiate this process by activating the endothelial cells that line blood vessels. Inflamed endothelium expresses surface molecules that promote the adhesion of neutrophils, such as E-selectin and other ligands for β_2-integrins (Fig. 18-6). Once firmly adherent, neutrophils migrate into tissues through gaps that appear between endothelial cells.

- Chemotaxis. To find their prey, neutrophils actively move in response to chemoattractants such as bacterial products, proteolytic fragments of complement (C5a), and mediators such as the cytokine interleukin-8 that are released from inflammatory cells already on the scene, all of which bind to G-coupled receptors expressed on neutrophils. These receptors produce

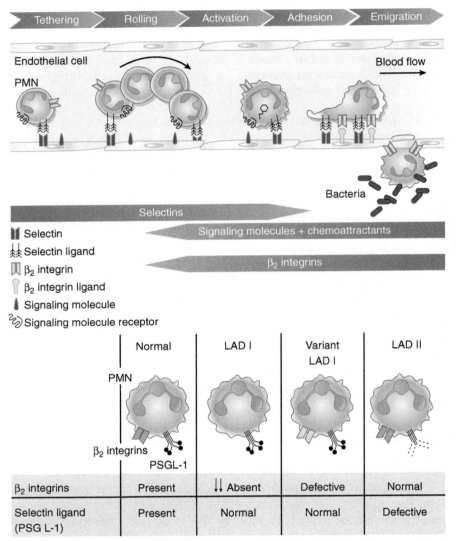

FIGURE 18-6 Leukocyte adhesion and leukocyte adhesion deficiency. Normal adhesion of leukocytes such as neutrophils (PMNs) to vessel walls (upper panel) is initiated by weak interactions between selectins on endothelial cells and selectin ligands on neutrophils. When stimulated by inflammatory mediators, leukocytes up-regulate the expression of β_2 integrins on their surfaces. These integrins bind strongly to ligands on endothelial cells, allowing leukocytes to firmly adhere and extravasate into tissues. In leukocyte adhesion deficiency (LAD), genetic defects in either β_2-integrins (LAD I) or selectin ligands (LAD II) disrupt this process. As a result, leukocytes are incapable of extravasation from the blood into tissues. (Modified with permission from Bunting M, Harris ES, McIntyre TM, et al. Leukocyte adhesion deficiency syndromes: adhesion and tethering defects involving [beta] 2 integrins and selectin ligands. Curr Opin Hematol 2002; 9: 30-35.)

signals that orient the cytoskeletal machinery of the neutrophil, allowing the cell to move toward the site where the pathogens are located.

- Recognition and phagocytosis of pathogens. Neutrophils express receptors for bacterial products (eg, endotoxin) and opsonins, host proteins such as antibodies, and proteolytic fragments of complement (eg, C3b) that are deposited on bacteria. Of these, opsonins are particular effective at inducing phagocytosis, the process by which the pathogen is engulfed in a plasma membrane vesicle known as a phagosome and taken up into the neutrophil.

- Degranulation. Newly formed phagosomes rapidly fuse with the neutrophil's cytoplasmic granules, a type of specialized lysosome, to create phagolysosomes.

- Pathogen killing. Pathogens consumed and transferred into phagolysosomes are killed through several mechanisms. One involves the direct action of preformed factors found in granules, such as proteases (eg, elastase) and lysozyme, an enzyme that digests bacterial cell walls. However, the most important mechanism of pathogen killing is the generation of reactive oxygen and nitrogen species within the phagolysosome. This so-called respiratory burst depends on the assembly of a multiprotein enzyme, NADPH oxidase, which reduces O_2 to superoxide (O_2^-). Additional reactions involving O_2^- in turn produce hypochlorite (OCl^-, the active ingredient in bleach) and other highly reactive free radicals that damage the membranes and cell walls of phagocytosed pathogens, inducing sufficient injury to kill them.

The importance (and many of the molecular details) of these processes were made clear by rare patients who suffer recurrent bacterial and fungal infections despite apparently normal or even increased numbers of circulating neutrophils. Studies of such patients led to the identification of specific defects in neutrophils stemming from loss-of-function mutations in genes required for one or more of the steps outlined earlier. Several of these disorders are of pathophysiologic interest.

- Disorders of leukocyte adhesion. Leukocyte adhesion deficiency (LAD) (Fig. 18-6) is an autosomal recessive disorder caused by mutations that have deleterious effects on the function of β_2 integrin (LAD I) or the selectin ligand PSGL-1 (LAD II). Patients often have elevated neutrophil counts, particularly in the face of infection, due to an inability of neutrophils to adhere to endothelium and migrate into infected tissues.

- Disorders of phagolysosome function. One of the best known of these disorders is chronic granulomatous disease, which is caused by mutations that impair the activity of NADPH oxidase, the enzyme required for the respiratory burst. The failure to kill phagocytosed bacteria or fungi effectively allows infections to persist. As infections become chronic, activated macrophages accumulate and cluster into poorly formed granulomas, a feature that gives this disorder its name.

- Disorders affecting neutrophil granules. The prototype of these rare diseases is Chédiak-Higashi syndrome, which has already been discussed under *neutropenia*. The abnormal granules in this disorder result in impaired bacterial killing.

HISTIOCYTIC DISORDERS—HEMOPHAGOCYTIC LYMPHOHISTIOCYTOSIS

Histiocyte (literally *tissue cell*) is an archaic term still applied to tissue macrophages. Disorders associated with macrophage dysfunction are uncommon. One that deserves mention due to its severity bears the unfortunate name *hemophagocytic lymphohistiocytosis* (HLH). HLH occurs in a variety of settings and has a number of triggers. The common feature in all is the activation of macrophages throughout the body due to overstimulation by factors released by T effector cells. The activated macrophages phagocytose hematopoietic cells and release additional cytokines and chemokines, producing a systemic inflammatory state associated with cytopenias.

HLH occurs in both familial and acquired forms. The familial forms usually present in infants and are caused by autosomal recessive mutations in at least four different genes. One of the most commonly mutated genes encodes perforin, a component of the granules of cytotoxic T cells. The acquired forms can occur in children or adults and may be a complication of autoimmune disorders (where it has been termed *macrophage activation syndrome*), T-cell lymphoma, or infection, especially with Epstein-Barr virus. Regardless of the cause, patients with HLH typically present with fever, splenomegaly, and pancytopenia. An examination of the bone marrow reveals macrophages phagocytosing both mature and immature marrow elements (Fig. 18-7). Laboratory abnormalities typically include a very high ferritin level (>10,000 μg/L), a finding that is quite sensitive and specific for HLH.

Primary forms of HLH often respond to chemotherapy and immunosuppressive agents but inevitably recur and are ultimately fatal unless bone marrow transplantation is performed. Secondary forms of HLH may be treated with therapy for the underlying illness (eg, chemotherapy for a patient with T-cell lymphoma) but often also require regimens directed at the HLH, which are similar to those used in

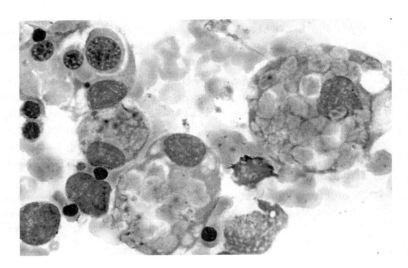

FIGURE 18-7 **Hemophagocytic lymphohistiocytosis, bone marrow aspirate.** Three macrophages in this field contain multiple phagocytosed red cells.

primary disease. Recognition and treatment of cases of secondary HLH (eg, those associated with Epstein-Barr virus) with chemotherapy regimens that include the topoisomerase II inhibitor etoposide appear to increase survival, particularly in pediatric patients.

SELF-ASSESSMENT STUDY QUESTIONS

1. Findings consistent with infection include:
   A. Persistence of primary granules in circulating neutrophils.
   B. Large circulating lymphocytes containing azurophilic granules.
   C. The appearance of band cell forms in the peripheral blood.
   D. Neutrophilia.
   E. Neutropenia.
   F. All of the above.

2. The most frequent cause of clinically significant neutropenia is:
   A. Large granular lymphocytic leukemia.
   B. Congenital abnormalities.
   C. Severe viral infections.
   D. Iatrogenic.
   E. Idiopathic.

3. A 21-year-old African-American college student applies for a Rhodes scholarship, which he is granted. Before leaving for England, he is required to have a health form completed. During his evaluation at the University Health Services a CBC is obtained. Results show that he has a WBC of 3200, with 35% neutrophils. His primary physician tells him to consider holding off on accepting the Rhodes, and refers him to you for further evaluation. He has no history of excessive infections, and has been healthy all his life. His physical exam is normal. His CBC today shows a WBC of 3400 with 30% neutrophils, a Hct of 41, and platelets of 200K.

   What should you advise him regarding his scholarship?
   A. He should have a bone marrow examination to rule out a bone marrow process causing neutropenia.
   B. He should go to England without any further evaluation.
   C. He should have serial blood counts to rule out cyclic neutropenia.
   D. He should have chromosome analysis of his peripheral blood.

4. A patient is diagnosed with hyperthyroidism and has been started on propylthiouracil (PTU). Six weeks later he comes to the emergency room complaining of fever and a sore throat. He has a temperature of 102° and a tonsillar exudate. A CBC is performed and shows a WBC of 1500 with 5% neutrophils, a hematocrit of 38, and a platelet count of 200K. The PTU is stopped.

   Appropriate therapy is:
   A. Start the patient on amoxicillin and schedule him to return to clinic the following day for follow-up of his throat culture.
   B. Admit the patient to the hospital and begin on broad-spectrum antibiotics.
   C. Start the patient on amoxicillin and admit for observation.
   D. Admit the patient to the hospital and begin broad-spectrum antibiotics and G-CSF.

19 Introduction to Hematologic Malignancies

Jon C. Aster and Mark Fleming

LEARNING OBJECTIVES

After studying this chapter you should know:
- The major categories of hematologic malignancies.
- The types of tests that are used to diagnose hematologic malignancies.
- The importance of clonality as a defining feature of these diseases.

Just as studies of hematopoiesis have been at the forefront of stem cell biology, rapid advances in our understanding of the pathogenesis of hematopoietic and lymphoid tumors have brought us to the dawn of a new molecular era of cancer diagnosis and therapy. Remarkably, in the not-too-far distant future it will become possible to routinely sequence the entire genome of blood cancers, providing us with a detailed view of the genetic changes that underlie these tumors. These advances will undoubtedly revolutionize how we diagnose and treat patients with these diseases and other cancers as well.

This accelerating rate of progress is exhilarating for workers in the field, but it creates challenges for students who are trying to grasp the basics (and authors who are trying to help them do so!). With this in mind, this chapter and the following one are meant to serve as a primer for students new to these fascinating and clinically important diseases. Here, we provide an overview of the classification and diagnosis of hematologic malignancies. In Chapters 20-24, we delve into the pathogenesis of these malignancies, emphasizing molecular insights that have already impacted the diagnosis and treatment. In these chapters we provide a more detailed look at the pathophysiology, clinical features, and treatment of the major types of hematologic malignancy, which include some of the most common cancers of children and adults.

NOMENCLATURE OF HEMATOLOGIC MALIGNANCIES

The names and descriptive terms used for the various hematologic malignancies reflect their origin and usual clinical behavior. Tumors composed of cells of the myeloid series (granulocytes, red cells, platelets, and their progenitors) are referred to as *myeloid*, *myelogenous*, or *myeloproliferative*, whereas tumors composed of lymphocytes or their progenitors are variously termed *lymphoid*, *lymphocytic*, *lymphoblastic,* or *lymphoproliferative. Leukemia* (literally, *white blood*) is applied to neoplasms that typically involve the bone marrow and the peripheral blood, whereas *lymphoma* is used to describe lymphoid tumors that commonly present as masses within lymph nodes or other soft tissues. Some lymphomas are named based on the resemblance of the tumor cells to a normal counterpart; for example, the malignant B cells of follicular lymphoma closely resemble the normal cells found within the B-cell follicles (also commonly referred to as germinal centers) of lymph nodes. Other descriptors relate to the natural history of the disease in question. Acute leukemias, if untreated, are lethal within weeks to several months, whereas chronic leukemias may be compatible with survival for many years without treatment.

CLASSIFICATION OF HEMATOLOGIC MALIGNANCIES

Classification systems are meant to provide a common language for the diagnosis and treatment of specific disease entities. As recently as 20 years ago, few areas of medicine were as contentious and confused as the classification of hematologic malignancies. Diagnoses were then based largely on clinical features and the morphologic appearance of tumor cells, criteria that are inadequate for classifying the diversity of hematologic malignancies that we now recognize molecularly.

In 1994, this picture began to change with the advent of classification that subdivided lymphoid tumors into distinct entities based on clinical features, microscopic appearance, and objective markers, including lineage-specific proteins and tumor-specific genetic aberrations. This proved so successful that the same approach was subsequently extended to myeloid neoplasms. There is now wide acceptance of a classification system, shown in Table 19-1, that sorts hematologic neoplasms based on their lineage and presumed cell of origin. The "cell of origin" concept is particularly important in the classification of lymphoid neoplasms, many of which are composed of cells that appear to be the malignant counterparts of some normal stage of B or T lymphocyte differentiation.

The neoplasms recognized in the World Health Organization classification of hematologic malignancies fall into five broad clinicopathologic categories, each containing a number of entities:

- Acute leukemias are tumors in which early myeloid or lymphoid progenitors (blasts) accumulate in the bone marrow and to varying degrees spill into the peripheral blood and infiltrate other tissues. They are believed to arise from early myeloid or lymphoid progenitors. Leukemic blasts are so primitive as to be nonfunctional and tend to displace or suppress the production of normal hematopoietic elements in the marrow. As a result, most patients present with symptoms related to pancytopenia.

- Chronic myeloproliferative disorders are tumors that arise in the bone marrow and most commonly lead to the increased production of one or more types of mature myeloid cells. They may arise from early myeloid progenitors or hematopoietic stem cells. Most symptoms initially stem from the hyperproliferation of bone marrow progenitors and increased numbers of red cells, granulocytes, and/or platelets in the peripheral blood and the spleen.

TABLE 19-1 World Health Organization Classification of Hematologic Malignancies (Abridged Version)

Myeloid neoplasms	
Subtype	Putative cell of origin
Acute myeloid leukemia (AML)	Early myeloid progenitor
AML with recurrent genetic aberrations	
AML without recurrent genetic aberrations	
AML following cytotoxic therapy	
Chronic myeloproliferative disorders	Hematopoietic stem cell or early myeloid progenitor
Chronic myelogenous leukemia	
Polycythemia vera	
Essential thrombocythemia	
Chronic eosinophilic leukemia	
Primary myelofibrosis	
Myelodysplastic syndromes	Early myeloid progenitor
Lymphoid neoplasms	
Immature B-cell and T-cell tumors	
B-cell acute lymphoblastic leukemia/lymphoma	Early B-cell progenitor
T-cell acute lymphoblastic leukemia/lymphoma	Early T-cell progenitor
Mature B-cell tumors	
Chronic lymphocytic leukemia/small lymphocytic lymphoma	Post-germinal center B cell
Mantle cell lymphoma	Naïve B cell
Follicular lymphoma	Germinal center B cell
Burkitt lymphoma	Germinal center B cell
Diffuse large B-cell lymphoma	Germinal center or post-germinal center B cell
Plasma cell tumors and related entities	
Multiple myeloma	Post-germinal center B cell
Lymphoplasmacytic lymphoma	Mature B-cell
Mature T-cell and natural killer cell tumors	Mature T-cell or natural killer cell
Hodgkin lymphoma	Germinal center or post-germinal center B cell

- Myelodysplastic syndromes are a poorly understood, heterogeneous group of myeloid tumors in which the maturation of bone marrow progenitors is abnormal (dysplastic) and ineffective. The cell of origin is believed to be an early myeloid progenitor. Patients present with symptoms related to one or more cytopenias and follow a highly variable course.

- Lymphomas and related lymphoid neoplasms are a large, diverse group of tumors derived from mature lymphocytes or their progenitors. These disorders are the most common types of hematologic malignancy. In the United States, roughly 100,000 people per year are newly diagnosed with one of these disorders. The lymphomas are divided into two broad classes: 1) Hodgkin lymphoma, a group of B-cell neoplasms linked by the presence of highly unusual tumor giant cells referred to as Reed-Sternberg cells, and 2) all of the other lymphomas, which are called the non-Hodgkin lymphomas. Non-Hodgkin lymphomas may be derived from cells at any stage of lymphocyte development, which explains in part their remarkable diversity. Overall, tumors of B-cell origin make up 85% to 90% of non-Hodgkin lymphomas in the United States, with most of the remaining tumors being of T-cell origin; natural killer cell lymphomas also occur, but are very rare. The variation in clinical behavior among these tumors is enormous, ranging from some of the most rapidly growing, aggressive tumors of man to neoplasms that are so indolent that for years they were referred to as pseudolymphomas. As will be discussed in the chapters covering specific lymphoid neoplasms, the clinical approach to these diseases is dictated in part by their behavior; aggressive lymphoid neoplasms must be treated as quickly as possible, whereas indolent tumors may wax and wane for years even in the absence of therapy.

- Plasma cell neoplasms and related entities are tumors composed at least in part of terminally differentiated B cells (plasma cells). These relatively common tumors occur mainly in older adults and often present with symptoms related to the production of complete or partial immunoglobulins by the tumor cells. The most important of these tumors are 1) multiple myeloma, which characteristically causes destructive bone lesions and 2) lymphoplasmacytic lymphoma, in which the tumor cells often produce immunoglobulin M (IgM), sometimes in quantities sufficient to produce a hyperviscosity state called Waldenström macroglobulinemia.

These categories provide a very helpful means for organizing the hematologic malignancies, but it must be recognized that the boundaries between specific entities sometimes blur. All of the tumors that are called lymphomas and even plasma cell tumors occasionally present as leukemias with peripheral blood involvement; conversely, virtually all of the tumors called *leukemias* may on occasion present as a tissue mass without involvement of the bone marrow or blood. This variation in clinical presentation is reflected in the names of some of the entities of the classification (Table 19-1). For example, tumors of immature lymphoid cells (lymphoblasts) may be referred to as *acute lymphoblastic leukemia* or *lymphoblastic lymphoma* depending on their clinical presentation; the same is true of a tumor of mature B cells that is variously referred to as *chronic lymphocytic leukemia* or *small lymphocytic lymphoma*. For the student, the important thing to remember is that these pairs of names refer to different clinical manifestations of the same tumor.

A second complication that must be appreciated is that some indolent forms of leukemia and lymphoma commonly transform into more aggressive forms of disease that fall into a different diagnostic category. In hematologic malignancies where the cell of origin is a hematopoietic stem cell (eg, chronic myelogenous leukemia), the transformed tumor may not only have a different morphology but also have an immunophenotype that is very different from the tumor that preceded it. Specific examples of transformation events will be discussed in subsequent chapters.

DIAGNOSIS OF HEMATOLOGIC MALIGNANCIES

Diagnosis of each of the hematologic malignancies requires a tissue biopsy or examination of a peripheral blood smear. In leukemias, the diagnosis typically can be made by examination of a peripheral blood smear and/or bone marrow biopsy and aspirate. For plasma cell neoplasms, the diagnosis is usually based on a bone marrow biopsy, whereas lymphomas are most commonly diagnosed by biopsy of a lymph node or another soft tissue site.

At the time of the initial biopsy, it is usually unknown whether a patient has a malignancy or a benign disorder leading to hyperplasia of myeloid or lymphoid cells, such as an infection or an inflammatory condition. The key to distinguishing between benign and malignant processes is *clonality*. Neoplasms originate from a single transformed cell and are therefore monoclonal. In contrast, reactive processes stem from the response of many different cells and are polyclonal.

Sometimes all that is required to make the distinction between benign and neoplastic processes is a glance at the tissue under the microscope; for example, replacement of normal tissue by a monomorphous population of abnormal cells is a hallmark of certain neoplasms (Fig. 19-1A). However, the make-up of other

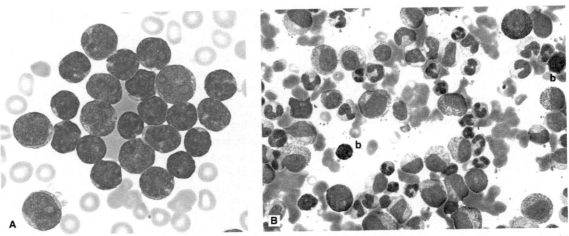

FIGURE 19-1 Varied morphology of hematologic malignancies. A) Acute lymphoblastic leukemia (bone marrow aspirate) is an example of a relatively monomorphic tumor composed of a population of lymphoblasts that are arrested at early stages of B-cell differentiation. B) Chronic myelogenous leukemia (CML, bone marrow biopsy), in contrast, is a tumor derived from hematopoietic stem cells in which maturation is preserved. As a result, marrow involved by CML is replaced by a heterogeneous tumor cell population that mimics the appearance of hyperplastic non-malignant bone marrow. As is typical of CML, most of the cells in this field consist of granulocytes at various phases of differentiation, including neutrophils, eosinophils, and several dark-staining basophils (b).

hematologic tumors is quite heterogeneous, mimicking the appearance of an exuberant reactive process (Fig. 19-1B). In such instances, molecular tests of clonality (described in a following section) play a critical role in establishing the diagnosis of a hematologic malignancy.

The mainstay of diagnosis remains the microscopic examination of tumor cells in smears or tissue sections, but morphology alone is insufficient to accurately diagnose and classify most hematologic malignancies. Thus, tumor samples are routinely examined by using several of the following complementary approaches:

- Morphology. The appearance of tumor cells usually allows a diagnostician (typically a pathologist with training in hematopathology) to generate a short list of diagnostic possibilities. For example, the presence of blasts containing Auer rods, abnormal needle-like azurophilic granules (Fig. 19-2A), is diagnostic

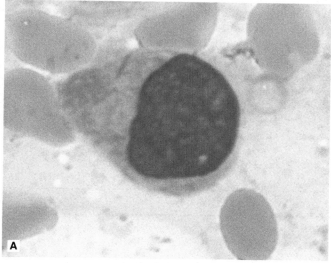

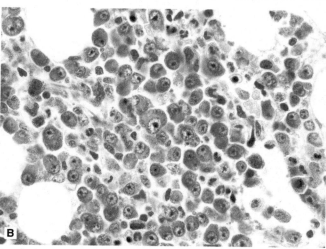

FIGURE 19-2 Examples of characteristic morphologies in hematologic malignancies. A) Auer rods (bone marrow aspirate). A myeloblast is shown that contains a single Auer rod, a needle-like, cytoplasmic, azurophilic granule that is pathognomonic of myeloid malignancies, most notably acute myeloid leukemia. B) Multiple myeloma (bone marrow biopsy). The marrow is largely replaced by a sheet of plasma cells with abnormally prominent, centrally placed nucleoli.

of an acute myeloid leukemia and would trigger the performance of other tests needed to further classify this type of tumor. Similarly, replacement of the marrow by an abnormal population of plasma cells would strongly support the diagnosis of multiple myeloma (Fig. 19-2B). However, it is often impossible to determine the lineage of a hematologic malignancy with certainty by morphology. For example, many B-cell and T-cell lymphomas cannot be reliably distinguished by appearance alone, and (as mentioned earlier) it may not even be possible to tell a reactive hyperplasia from a malignancy without additional tests.

- Immunophenotyping refers to the staining of tumor cells with antibodies specific for antigens (mostly proteins) that are useful in the classification of hematologic malignancies. Some of the antigens that are particularly useful are summarized in Table 19-2. When fresh, unfixed tumor cells are available, antigens are often detected by flow cytometry (described in Chapter 1). In flow cytometry, cells are identified and enumerated based on their light scattering properties and their expression of various antigens, which are detected with antibodies tagged with fluorescent dyes. Flow cytometry is widely used in the diagnosis of acute leukemias and non-Hodgkin lymphomas. It is often also used to establish the clonality of mature B-cell tumors (Fig. 19-3). Mature B cells express only one type of immunoglobulin (Ig), which is composed of two heavy chains paired with either kappa or lambda light chains.

TABLE 19-2 Commonly Used Markers in the Diagnosis of Hematologic Malignancies

Markers	Cells
CD34	Hematopoietic stem cells, early myeloid and lymphoid progenitors
CD117 (c-*KIT*)	Early myeloid progenitors
CD13, CD33	Early and late myeloid forms
Terminal deoxyribonucleotidyl transferase	Lymphoid progenitors
CD10, CD19	Early B-cell progenitors
CD20, surface immunoglobulin	Mature B cells
CD10, BCL6	Follicular B cells
Cytoplasmic immunoglobulin	Plasma cells
CD3, CD4, CD8	T-cell progenitors and mature T cells
CD5	T cells, certain B-cell tumors
CD15, CD30	Reed-Sternberg cells

CD, cluster designation.

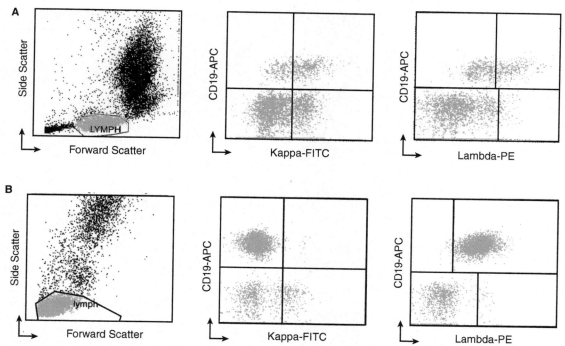

FIGURE 19-3   Use of flow cytometry to evaluate B-cell clonality. Cell suspensions prepared from two lymph node biopsy specimens obtained from patients suspected of having lymphoma were "gated" based on forward and side scatter (left hand panel), and the cells in the lymphocyte gate were then further characterized based on staining with antibodies specific for CD19 (tagged with the fluorescent dye APC), kappa immunoglobulin light chain (tagged with fluorescent dye FITC), and lambda immunoglobulin light chain (tagged with the dye PE). In A) roughly equal numbers of CD19-positive B cells expressing kappa and lambda light chain are present, a result consistent with the presence of a reactive polyclonal B-cell population. In B) there is a predominant population of cells expressing lambda light chain, indicating the presence of a monoclonal B-cell proliferation. Additional features of this population, including the expression of other markers and the morphology of the cells, would then be used to arrive at a specific diagnosis.

In polyclonal B-cell proliferations, the ratio of kappa- to lambda-expressing cells is usually close to 1:1. However, because malignancies are derived from single transformed cells, in mature B-cell tumors, all of the cells express only kappa or lambda light chain. Due to its ability to quantify multiple markers on single cells, flow cytometry also can be used to detect cells expressing unusual combinations of antigens (another hallmark of certain hematologic malignancies), even within large populations of normal cells. Its chief limitation is that it must be done on fresh, unfixed cells, which are available only if a hematologic malignancy is suspected at the time the biopsy is obtained. A second method that avoids this limitation is immunohistochemistry (Fig. 19-4). Here, sections of tissues fixed in formalin and embedded in paraffin (the standard method of handling tissues in pathology departments) are placed on slides and incubated with specific antibodies. Staining is then developed by incubation with secondary antibodies linked to an enzyme such as horseradish peroxidase and a substrate that is converted by the enzyme to an insoluble colored precipitate. This method is widely used in

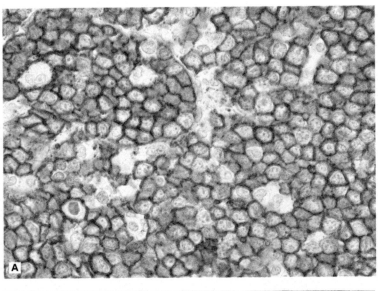

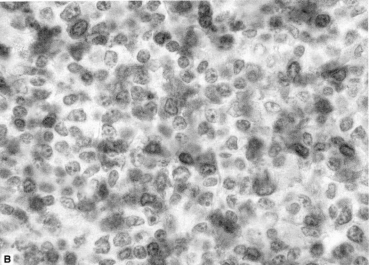

FIGURE 19-4 **Use of immunohistochemistry to detect lineage-specific antigens.** A diffuse large B-cell lymphoma is shown that has been stained with antibodies specific for CD20 (A), a surface protein that is expressed only by B lymphocytes, or CD3 (B), a marker that is restricted to T lymphocytes. The staining reaction is developed with a chromogenic substrate that produces a brown color; the nuclei of the cells have been counterstained with the blue dye hematoxylin. The tumor cells are positive for CD20, whereas a few reactive intermixed T cells are positive for CD3.

the diagnosis of hematologic malignancies, particularly non-Hodgkin and Hodgkin lymphomas.

- Histochemistry is used mainly in the diagnosis of acute leukemias. It is performed by incubating smears of marrow or blood with chemicals that differentially stain bone marrow cells of various lineages. Some stains involve the use of dyes that change color in the presence of specific leukocyte enzymes. Examples include stains for myeloperoxidase and specific esterase (both expressed by myeloblasts and more mature granulocytes) and nonspecific esterase (expressed by monoblasts and monocytes). Other stains react with non-enzymatic cellular constituents. The periodic acid–Schiff stain is used to detect glycogen, which is frequently present in the lymphoblasts of acute lymphoblastic leukemias and occasionally found in erythroblasts in myeloid neoplasms. The Prussian blue stain is used to detect non-heme iron, which accumulates in the mitochondria of red cell progenitors in certain myelodysplastic syndromes.

• Cytogenetics. Tumor-specific cytogenetic aberrations can serve to establish the clonality of myeloid or lymphoid proliferations and in some instances are so characteristic of particular hematologic malignancies that they are required for the diagnosis. For example, all cases of chronic myelogenous leukemia are associated with chromosomal rearrangements that juxtapose the 3' portion of the *ABL* gene (normally on chromosome 9) with the 5' portion of the *BCR* gene on chromosome 22, thereby creating a chimeric *BCR-ABL* fusion gene with oncogenic activity. In most instances, this event occurs by way of a reciprocal translocation between chromosomes 9 and 22 that causes the formation of two abnormal chromosomes, one derived from chromosome 9 and the other from chromosome 22. The derivative chromosome 22 that bears the *BCR-ABL* fusion gene is often referred to as the Philadelphia chromosome (named for the city of its discovery). When fresh samples of marrow or blood are available, the Philadelphia chromosome usually can be directly visualized by determining the karyotype of tumor cells harvested in metaphase, the time in mitosis when chromosomes condense and can be recognized by their appearance (Fig. 19-5A). However, sometimes metaphases are not obtained, or complex rearrangements involving chromosomes 9 and 22 are present. In such instances, the *BCR-ABL* fusion gene and its reciprocal partner, an *ABL-BCR* fusion gene, can be detected directly by fluorescence in situ hybridization (FISH), in which DNA probes spanning the *BCR* and *ABL* loci are hybridized to interphase nuclei from tumor cells. In the example shown (Fig. 19-5B), the reciprocal rearrangement of *BCR* and *ABL* causes two abnormal fusion signals to appear, one due to the presence of the *BCR-ABL* gene on chromosome 22 and the second due to the nonfunctional *ABL-BCR* fusion gene on chromosome 9.

• Molecular genetics. Sequence analysis of DNA or RNA isolated from tumor cells is playing an increasing part in the diagnosis of hematologic malignancies. For example, the diagnosis of polycythemia vera, a type of myeloproliferative disorder, requires the detection of activating mutations in the gene encoding the tyrosine kinase JAK2. Another common use of molecular genetics is the assessment of clonality in lymphoid proliferations. Rearrangement and assembly of the immunoglobulin genes in B cells and the T-cell receptor genes in T cells create unique DNA sequences that are specific for that cell and all its progeny. Polyclonal, reactive lymphoid proliferations are composed of cells with many different sets of rearranged antigen receptor genes, whereas in lymphoid neoplasms all tumor cells share the same clonal rearrangements. Polymerase chain reaction (PCR)-based tests that involve the amplification of rearranged antigen receptor genes can

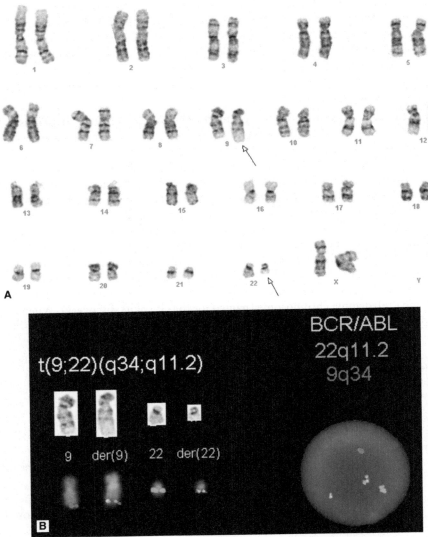

FIGURE 19-5 Cytogenetic analysis of hematologic malignancies. A) Karyotype, chronic myelogenous leukemia. Metaphase chromosomes stained with Giemsa dye are shown. The arrows denote two derivative chromosomes, a derivative 9 (der 9) and a derivative 22 (der 22), produced by a balanced translocation involving the *BCR* gene on chromosome 22 and the *ABL* gene on chromosome 9. The small der 22 chromosome, also known as the Philadelphia chromosome, contains the *BCR-ABL* fusion oncogene. B) Detection of a *BCR-ABL* fusion gene by fluorescence in situ hybridization (FISH). Interphase nuclei have been hybridized to fluorescently labeled probes specific for *ABL* and *BCR*. Cells containing a balanced (9;22) translocation have chimeric *BCR-ABL* and *ABL-BCR* genes that produce two fusion signals as well as one normal copy of *ABL* and one normal copy of *BCR*, each of which produce a normal signal.

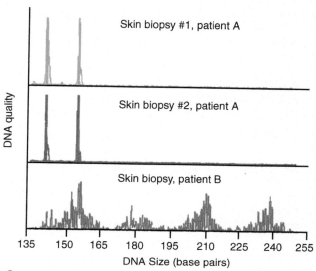

FIGURE 19-6 **Molecular detection of clonality by using antigen receptor gene rearrangements.** Consensus oligonucleotide DNA primers that are complementary to TCRgamma V and J regions were used to perform the polymerase chain reaction (PCR) on DNA prepared from three different skin biopsy specimens suspected of being involved by cutaneous T-cell lymphoma, two of which were obtained from the same patient. The PCR products were then subjected to capillary electrophoresis, which can separate DNA fragments differing in size by as little as a single base pair. The sample from patient B produced multiple amplification products of differing sizes, a pattern that is consistent with a polyclonal reactive process. Differences in the sizes of the various V and J region segments in the TCRgamma gene produce a series of peaks and valleys in the normal sample. The individual products within each peak result from the random removal of bases by exonuclease and addition of bases by the enzyme terminal deoxyribonuclease at the time of joining of Vgamma and Jgamma segments in early T cells. In contrast, the two skin biopsy specimens from patient A produced two identical major PCR products, a result consistent with involvement of both sites by a single T-cell tumor that has rearranged both of its TCRgamma genes. (With permission from Dr. Janina Longtine.)

distinguish between polyclonal and monoclonal lymphoid proliferations with a high degree of sensitivity and specificity and are now in wide clinical use (Fig. 19-6). PCR analysis of reverse-transcribed messenger RNA (mRNA) from chronic myelogenous leukemia cells offers a reliable and sensitive means of detecting the BCR-ABL transcript.

In addition to these tissue-based tests, other clinical and laboratory test findings weigh in on the diagnosis of certain hematologic malignancies. For example, tests that detect and quantify monoclonal antibodies or fragments of antibodies within the serum and the urine are important adjuncts in the diagnosis of plasma cell neoplasms, and radiologic studies to identify destructive bone lesions are part of the work-up of patients suspected of having multiple myeloma. The diagnosis of T-cell lymphoma is based in part on the pattern of tissue involvement, because specific subtypes of these diseases preferentially involve the skin, adipose tissue, gut, or spleen. It is believed that this behavior recapitulates the ability of normal T lymphocytes to home to specific tissues.

SELF-ASSESSMENT STUDY QUESTIONS

1. Which of the following is currently used to diagnose and classify hematopoietic neoplasms?
   A. Morphology.
   B. Histochemistry.
   C. Immunophenotyping (flow cytometry and/or immunohistochemistry).
   D. Cytogenetics (karyotyping and/or fluorescence in situ hybridization).
   E. DNA sequence analysis.
   F. All of the above.

2. Which of the following is most important in distinguishing between a benign and malignant lymphoid proliferation?
   A. Morphology.
   B. Physical examination.
   C. Immunophenotype.
   D. Clonality.
   E. Histochemistry.

3. Match the tumor to the laboratory test finding.

   A. Acute myeloid leukemia   a. Periodic acid–Schiff stain positivity
   B. Lymphoblastic leukemia/lymphoma   b. Abnormal plasma cells
   C. Multiple myeloma   c. Auer rods
   D. B-cell lymphoma   d. JAK2 mutation
   E. Chronic myelogenous leukemia   e. *BCR-ABL* fusion gene
   F. Polycythemia vera   f. Surface Ig light chain restriction

Myeloproliferative Disorders and Myelodysplastic Syndromes

Jon C. Aster and Daniel J. DeAngelo

L E A R N I N G   O B J E C T I V E S

After studying this chapter you should understand:

- The pathogenic role of specific tyrosine kinase mutations in various myeloproliferative disorders.
- The role of BCR-ABL in the diagnosis and targeted therapy of chronic myelogenous leukemia.
- The diagnostic and pathogenic role of JAK2 mutations in polycythemia vera.
- The pathophysiology and clinical features of the myelodysplastic syndromes.

CANCER AS A GENETIC DISEASE

Like other cancers, hematologic malignancies are caused by acquired somatic mutations that activate proto-oncogenes or inactivate tumor suppressors. Remarkably, we now know that at least some of these potentially oncogenic events occur from time to time in the hematologic cells of most if not all healthy people, the vast majority of whom will not suffer from a hematologic malignancy during their lifetimes. It follows that no single mutation is sufficient to create these cancers. Instead, they appear to result from the interplay of multiple mutations that collaborate to create a transformed phenotype. Molecular analyses have proven that although tumor cells within an individual cancer demonstrate some degree of genetic heterogeneity, all share a core set of identical mutations, indicating that they originate from a single, transformed cell.

The appearance and behavior of specific hematologic malignancies stem from two major factors: 1) the identity of the oncogenic mutations found in the tumor cells and 2) the cellular context, which is to say the identity of the founding cell from which the tumor originates. The latter dictates the effects of the former on cellular proliferation, survival, and differentiation. These two themes—acquired mutations and cellular context—will be woven through our discussion of all of the hematologic malignancies. In this chapter, we discuss the myeloproliferative disorders and myelodysplastic syndromes, tumors that originate in early hematopoietic progenitors that primarily affect marrow function and give rise to differentiated progeny. Subsequent chapters will cover the acute leukemias, aggressive tumors of early myeloid or lymphoid progenitors, and the diverse collection of tumors that are derived from mature lymphocytes and plasma cells.

MYELOPROLIFERATIVE DISORDERS

The molecular hallmark of the myeloproliferative disorders is the presence of gain-of-function mutations that activate tyrosine kinases, enzymes that phosphorylate proteins on tyrosine residues. In general, these aberrant tyrosine kinases turn on the same pathways that are normally activated by hematopoietic growth factors, but they do so in a growth factor–independent fashion. In Chapter 2, we noted that the pathways activated by hematopoietic growth factors enhance the growth and survival of myeloid progenitors in the bone marrow. As a result of constitutive activation of pro-growth and pro-survival signaling pathways, the bone marrow in the myeloproliferative disorders is hypercellular, and early in the course of the disease there is an increase in one or more of the formed myeloid elements (granulocytes, platelets, and/or red cells) in the peripheral blood. Differentiation is initially unaffected or altered in relatively subtle ways, such that patients tend to suffer from symptoms related to an increase in myeloid progenitors and formed elements. Some myeloproliferative disorders are associated with striking increases in basophil counts (basophilia) or eosinophil counts (eosinophilia), features that can serve as important diagnostic clues.

Unfortunately, as with virtually all cancers, the myeloproliferative disorders are prone to acquire additional mutations during their course that lead to more aggressive behavior and a worsening of the clinical picture. Disease progression can take one of two forms: 1) transformation to acute leukemia, in which the marrow is replaced by undifferentiated cells called *blasts*, and 2) progression to myelofibrosis, in which the marrow is replaced by collagen deposited by reactive fibroblasts. Both of these events are understandably associated with the development of low blood counts (cytopenias) due to marrow dysfunction.

Diagnosis of the major subtypes of myeloproliferative disorders is based on the detection of mutations in specific tyrosine kinases combined with clinical features and laboratory findings (summarized in Table 20-1). The myeloproliferative disorders are not common, but they are of more than passing interest because an understanding of their pathogenesis has led to the development of effective, relatively nontoxic therapies that specifically target the underlying causative molecular lesions. In the section that follows, we describe the important myeloproliferative disorders.

CHRONIC MYELOGENOUS LEUKEMIA

Chronic myelogenous leukemia (CML) is always associated with a somatic mutation that produces a *BCR-ABL* fusion gene, usually a balanced translocation between chromosomes 9 and 22 (the so-called Philadelphia chromosome; see Chapter 19). The fusion gene encodes a chimeric BCR-ABL tyrosine kinase that self-associates through its BCR moiety, leading to constitutive activation of the ABL kinase. In most instances, the positions of the chromosomal breakpoints are

TABLE 20-1 **The Myeloproliferative Disorders**

Entity	Cell of Origin	Tyrosine Kinase Mutation	Typical Peripheral Blood Findings	Clinical Features
Chronic myelogenous leukemia	Hematopoietic stem cell	*BCR-ABL* fusion gene	Neutrophilia, eosinophilia, basophilia, left-shift, thrombocytosis, mild anemia	Symptoms related to extensive extramedullary hematopoiesis; transformation to acute leukemia in 100% of cases; infrequent progression to myelofibrosis
Polycythemia vera	Early myeloid progenitor	*JAK2* point mutations	Pancytosis (erythrocytosis, neutrophilia, basophilia, and thrombocytosis)	Symptoms related to high red cell counts; rarely transforms to acute leukemia; progresses to myelofibrosis in 10%-20% of cases
Essential thrombocytosis	Early myeloid progenitor	*JAK2* or *MPL* point mutations	Thrombocytosis	Symptoms related to high platelet counts; rarely transforms to acute leukemia; progresses to myelofibrosis in 10%-20% of cases
Primary myelofibrosis	Early myeloid progenitor	*JAK2* or *MPL* point mutations	Anemia, leukoerythroblastosis	Symptoms related to early-onset myelofibrosis, which leads to anemia and extensive extramedullary hematopoiesis; rarely transforms to acute leukemia
Chronic eosinophilic leukemia	Early myeloid progenitor or hematopoietic stem cell	PDGFR-α or PDGFR-β fusion genes	Leukocytosis, eosinophilia, monocytosis (particularly with PDGFR-β rearrangements)	Symptoms related to fibrosis of tissues infiltrated by eosinophils, including the heart and skin
Systemic mastocytosis	Early myeloid progenitor	*c-KIT* point mutations	None	Symptoms related to mediators released from mast cells, including pruritus, diarrhea, flushing, diaphoresis, syncope, and osteopenia
Myeloproliferative disorder associated with *FGFR1* rearrangement	Hematopoietic stem cell	Rearrangements of *FGFR1* (usually translocations)	Leukocytosis, eosinophilia	Initial symptoms related to myeloproliferative disease; however, usually progresses to acute lymphoblastic leukemia/ lymphoblastic lymphoma; may recur after therapy as acute myeloid leukemia.

FGFR1, fibroblast growth factor receptor 1 gene.

such that the BCR-ABL protein is 210 kDa in size. The cause of the translocation is not known. The incidence of CML was increased in survivors of the atomic bombs in Nagasaki and Hiroshima, possibly indicating that radiation-induced DNA damage can promote the formation of the 9-22 translocation, or t(9;22). However, very sensitive polymerase chain reaction (PCR) assays have enabled detection of low levels of *BCR-ABL* fusion transcripts in a high percentage of normal blood donors, the vast majority of whom will never develop CML. It therefore appears that the *BCR-ABL* fusion gene is necessary but not sufficient for CML development.

The BCR-ABL kinase activates the RAS, JAK-STAT, and PI-3 kinase/AKT pathways, the same pathways that are stimulated by hematopoietic growth factors in normal progenitors. As a result, there is an overgrowth of granulocytic and megakaryocytic precursors in the bone marrow (Fig. 20-1). For unclear reasons, erythroid elements are not as responsive to the effects of the BCR-ABL kinase, and, as a result, the ratio of granulocytic to erythroid progenitors in the marrow is markedly elevated. Seeding of neoplastic hematopoietic stem cells and marrow progenitors to the spleen and liver results in extramedullary hematopoiesis, which often produces organomegaly (Fig. 20-2). The peripheral blood smear typically

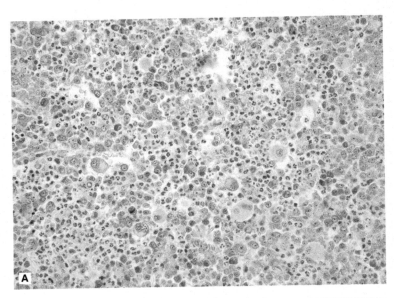

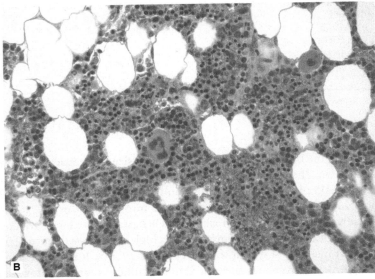

FIGURE 20-1 Chronic myelogenous leukemia (bone marrow biopsy).
A) The biopsy is hypercellular (no fat) due to the presence of excess granulocytes and granulocytic precursors, including eosinophilic forms, and increased numbers of megakaryocytes. Compare its appearance to a normal bone marrow biopsy B), which is roughly 50% cellular and contains normal proportions of cells from the erythroid, myeloid, and megakaryocytic lineages.

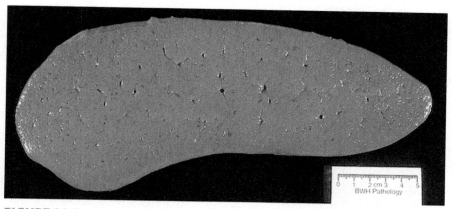

FIGURE 20-2 **Splenomegaly, chronic myelogenous leukemia.** The expansion of the red pulp by extramedullary hematopoiesis effaces the white pulp, producing a homogeneous beefy red appearance.

shows neutrophilia with a left-shift (the presence of immature granulocytic forms) and varying degrees of eosinophilia, basophilia, monocytosis, and thrombocytosis plus mild anemia (Fig. 20-3).

CML differs from most of the other myeloproliferative disorders in two important ways: 1) virtually all untreated patients progress to a phase identical to acute leukemia (blast crisis), usually over a period of 3 to 5 years, and 2) the acute leukemia may resemble an acute myeloid leukemia or an acute lymphoblastic leukemia. The ability of CML to progress to either acute myeloid or lymphoid leukemia is good evidence that the tumor originates in a multipotent hematopoietic stem cell. Prior to blast crisis, some patients experience an accelerated phase heralded by increased resistance to therapy, falling platelet counts, and increasing

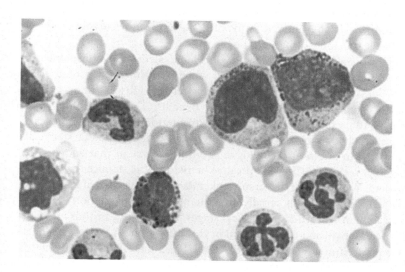

FIGURE 20-3 **Chronic myelogenous leukemia, peripheral blood.** Note the leukocytosis, the presence of immature granulocytic precursors (promyelocytes), the abnormal nuclear segmentation of the neutrophils, and the presence of a basophil, all of which are characteristic. (Courtesy of Lichtman MA, Shafer MS, Felgar RE, Wang N, Lichtman's Atlas of Hematology ([Online via Access Medicine], McGraw-Hill.)

numbers of basophils and blasts. Uncommonly, CML progresses to a stage that is identical to primary myelofibrosis (described in a later section).

The diagnosis is established by detection of a *BCR-ABL* fusion gene (usually by PCR-based analysis of mRNA or by fluorescence in situ hybridization; see Fig. 19-5) in the context of the typical clinical and laboratory findings. These methods are more sensitive, more reliable, and less labor intensive than karyotypic analysis of chromosome morphology. Roughly 5000 new CML cases are seen in the United States yearly. It can occur in children but is much more common in older adults and the elderly. The median age is 67 years at the time of diagnosis, and both sexes are equally likely to be affected. Patients often present with symptoms related to splenomegaly (early satiety due to compression of the stomach or pain related to splenic infarction) and hypermetabolism (fatigue, weight loss, sweats), but about half of newly diagnosed patients are asymptomatic, being identified by routine screening blood work.

The treatment of CML has been revolutionized by the development of imatinib mesylate, an adenosine triphosphate (ATP) analog that inhibits BCR-ABL. More than 99% of patients who present with stable-phase CML experience a complete hematologic remission when treated with imatinib, an agent designed to selectively target the active site of the kinase. Most (but not all) patients, however, show low-level persistence of the *BCR-ABL* fusion transcript, as detected by very sensitive PCR-based tests. Some of these patients will relapse on imatinib therapy, and when this occurs it is often associated with outgrowth of a clone in which there is a mutation in BCR-ABL that prevents imatinib from binding. Retrospective analyses have shown that these resistant clones are already present at the time therapy commences. Some experimental data suggest that BCR-ABL signaling causes an increased rate of mutation (a mutator phenotype) and that suppression of BCR-ABL with imatinib not only lowers the proliferative drive of the *BCR-ABL*–positive clone but also prevents the acquisition of mutations that lead to drug resistance and blast crisis. According to this view, patients diagnosed early in the course of the disease may remain in remission on imatinib indefinitely. The picture is different for those whose CML recurs while they are receiving imatinib. These patients can be treated for a time with other drugs that are capable of targeting imatinib-resistant mutated forms of *BCR-ABL*, but eventual outgrowth of new drug-resistant clones appears to be the rule.

The only proven cure for CML is allogeneic stem cell transplantation (described in Chapter 26), which works well when performed on patients with stable disease but is less successful in those with accelerated disease or blast crisis. Stem cell transplantation has two therapeutic benefits. The conditioning regimen that is used to prepare the patient for transplantation involves high doses of chemotherapy, which kill most of the *BCR-ABL*–positive hematopoietic stem cells and their progeny. In addition, the allogeneic immune system that engrafts the patient recognizes residual *BCR-ABL*–positive hematopoietic stem cells as foreign and attacks them, a so-called graft-versus-leukemia effect. The level of *BCR-ABL*–positive cells can be monitored serially after stem cell transplantation to detect evidence of relapse at its earliest preclinical stages. Remarkably, in those in early stages of relapse, transfusion of donor leukocytes can augment the graft-versus-leukemia effect and eliminate the *BCR-ABL* clone (Fig. 20-4). The downside of this maneuver is an increased incidence of graft-versus-host disease, which can have

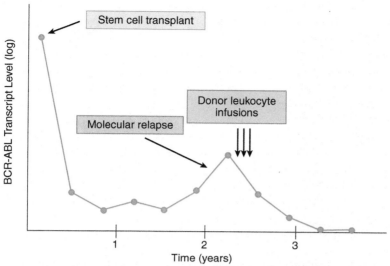

FIGURE 20-4 Response of relapsed chronic myelogenous leukemia (CML), post-stem cell transplant, to donor leukocyte infusion. The CML tumor burden can be monitored by using a quantitative reverse-transcriptase polymerase chain reaction (qRT-PCR) assay in which the signal is proportional to the level of *BCR-ABL* fusion mRNA. In this case, the samples were peripheral blood, but bone marrow cells also can be used. After initially decreasing following stem cell transplantation, the level of *BCR-ABL* fusion transcripts in this patient began to increase, a molecular finding that is a reliable early harbinger of CML relapse. Infusion of donor leukocytes from the allogeneic transplant donor was used to produce a graft-versus-leukemia response, which reduced the burden of the leukemic clone to an undetectable level.

serious or even fatal consequences. It is hoped that more sophisticated approaches to transplantation can be developed that will maintain the beneficial graft-versus-leukemia effect while minimizing graft-versus-host disease.

POLYCYTHEMIA VERA

Polycythemia vera (PCV) is associated with acquired activating point mutations in *JAK2*, a gene that encodes a tyrosine kinase, and a clinical picture that is dominated by signs and symptoms related to the overproduction of red cells. The primary effect of the mutated *JAK2* is to activate JAK/STAT signaling; the RAS and PI-3 kinase/AKT pathways are also stimulated but to a lower degree than by BCR-ABL. Nevertheless, the net effect is to greatly diminish the requirements of marrow myeloid progenitors for growth factors such as erythropoietin, as shown in Figure 20-5.

The diagnosis of PCV requires the molecular identification of a *JAK2* mutation and an increased hemoglobin level. The hemoglobin is usually >18.5 g/dL in affected men and >16.5 g/dL in affected women. The bone marrow is moderately hypercellular, and the peripheral blood characteristically shows not only erythrocytosis but also granulocytosis (often with basophilia) and thrombocytosis. Erythropoietin levels are low, a finding that distinguishes PCV from secondary forms of erythrocytosis (Chapter 12). Diagnosis can be difficult in those with concomitant blood loss, which

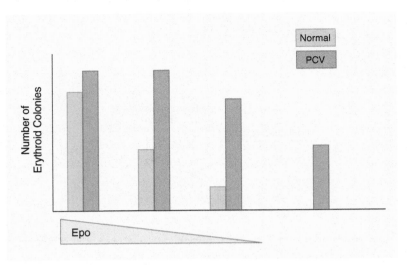

FIGURE 20-5 **Erythropoietin-independent growth of erythroid progenitors in polycythemia vera (PCV).** Bone marrow cells from a normal donor and a patient with PCV were plated in semi-solid media in the presence of decreasing amounts of erythropoietin. PCV progenitors produce colonies of erythroid cells in the absence of erythropoietin, whereas normal progenitors do not.

may reduce the hematocrit to the normal range. Marrow iron stores are typically decreased, due to uptake of iron by the proliferating erythroid progenitors.

PCV is an uncommon disease of older adults with a slight male predominance. Most symptoms are related to the increased red cell mass, which makes the blood abnormally viscous. Distention of the venous side of the circulation results in a plethoric complexion. The abnormal blood flow and acquired defects in platelet function often lead to bleeding or thrombotic complications. The latter include myocardial infarction, deep vein thrombosis, stroke, and thrombosis of the mesenteric, portal, or hepatic veins, all of which can be fatal. Pruritus, often exacerbated by hot showers (aquagenic pruritus), is a common complaint. A more serious problem is erythromelalgia, a burning sensation in the hands or feet that is caused by microvascular occlusion. Splenomegaly is usually present but typically modest. Transformation to acute leukemia may occur late in the course of the disease but is uncommon (5-10% of cases) and always takes the form of acute myeloid leukemia, suggesting that the cell of origin is an early myeloid progenitor. Roughly 20% to 40% of cases progress to a phase of bone marrow fibrosis that is indistinguishable from primary myelofibrosis.

The median survival time of untreated symptomatic PCV patients is less than 1 year, but this dismal prognosis is improved dramatically by simply lowering the hematocrit to the low normal range. This is usually achieved by periodic blood removal (phlebotomy) or gentle chemotherapy (hydroxyurea). Low-dose aspirin is given in an effort to lessen the risk of thrombotic complications. Progression to myelofibrosis is associated with severe anemia and increasing splenomegaly; once this occurs, the disease becomes very difficult to treat. Cure of PCV can be achieved only with stem cell transplantation, a treatment generally reserved for patients with leukemic or myelofibrotic complications.

ESSENTIAL THROMBOCYTOSIS

Essential thrombocytosis may be associated with acquired activating point mutations in *JAK2* (about 50% of cases) or *MPL* (5%-10% of cases). MPL encodes the receptor for thrombopoietin, the major growth factor for megakaryocyte progenitors. *MPL* is a member of a family of cytokine receptors that activate several downstream pathways, particularly the JAK/STAT pathway. Thus, both types of mutations found in essential thrombocytosis cause growth-factor-independent hyperactivation of *JAK2*. It is likely that most of the remaining 40% to 45% of essential thrombocytosis cases harbor mutations that also lead to hyperactivation of pathways involving tyrosine kinases.

The pathogenesis of essential thrombocytosis involves the excessive proliferation of megakaryocytic progenitors, which results in a striking increase in the number of marrow megakaryocytes and thrombocytosis, sometimes associated with the presence of exceptionally large platelets in the peripheral blood (Fig. 20-6). It is not understood why some patients with *JAK2* mutations present with PCV and others with essential thrombocytosis; it may be that these two disorders originate in different early myeloid progenitors with distinct differentiation potentials or that germline variation or somatic mutations in other genes modify the phenotype produced by *JAK2* mutations.

Like other myeloproliferative disorders, the diagnosis of essential thrombocytosis depends on a combination of clinical and laboratory test findings. By definition, patients with essential thrombocytosis have sustained platelet counts of >450,000/mm³ and lack features of other myeloproliferative disorders such as CML and PCV. The diagnosis can be established by detection of *JAK2* or *MPL* mutations; in the absence of these genetic findings, the diagnosis is made only after excluding causes of reactive thrombocytosis, such as chronic inflammation and iron deficiency.

Most symptomatic patients are over age 50. Younger patients with essential thrombocytosis often remain free of any clinical manifestations for years, except

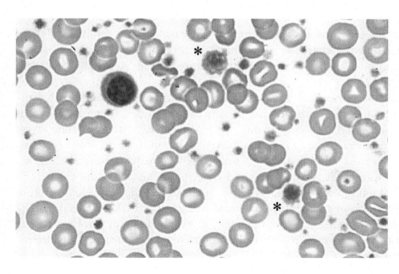

FIGURE 20-6 **Essential thrombocytosis (peripheral smear).** Several giant platelets (denoted by asterisks) are present, along with thrombocytosis.

for a persistently elevated platelet count. Symptoms are often related to abnormal platelet function and take the form of thrombosis or bleeding complications similar to those seen in PCV. Patients occasionally report pruritus or erythromelalgia but less often than those with PCV. A minority of patients progress to myelofibrosis. Transformation to acute myeloid leukemia is rare.

Treatment is centered on lowering the risk of thrombotic complications. All patients should receive low-dose aspirin. Those with very high platelet counts (>1,500,000/mm^3), a history of thrombosis, or advanced age (>60) appear to benefit from gentle chemotherapy with hydroxyurea, which lowers platelet counts.

PRIMARY MYELOFIBROSIS

Like essential thrombocytosis, primary myelofibrosis is associated with acquired activating point mutations in *JAK2* (about 50% of cases) or *MPL* (5%-10% of cases). Very early in its course, before marrow fibrosis becomes established, primary myelofibrosis may be associated with leukocytosis and thrombocytosis in the peripheral blood and marrow hypercellularity due to increased numbers of granulocytic precursors and megakaryocytes. However, as the disease progresses, the marrow is replaced by a fibrous matrix deposited by reactive fibroblasts, which are stimulated by factors such as platelet-derived growth factor (PDGF) and tumor-derived growth factor-β secreted from the abnormal megakaryocytes. The fibrosis distorts and effaces the marrow space, causing hematopoiesis to shift from the marrow to extramedullary sites such as the spleen and liver. Full-blown primary myelofibrosis is marked by anemia that is often severe enough to require transfusions and leukoerythroblastosis (tear-drop red cells, nucleated erythroid progenitors, and early granulocytic elements) that stems from the abnormal release of formed elements from the fibrotic marrow and sites of extramedullary hematopoiesis. Platelet and leukocyte counts vary widely. About one-third of patients are thrombocytopenic, but a roughly equal number have thrombocytosis. Mild to moderate leukocytosis is seen in about 50% of those affected, whereas leukopenia is uncommon.

Primary myelofibrosis is an uncommon disease of older adults. The diagnosis is based on the characteristic clinical picture and bone marrow biopsy, which is required to demonstrate the marrow fibrosis (Fig. 20-7). The distortion of the marrow causes progenitors to "herniate" into dilated sinusoids and be released into the peripheral blood, often contributing to leukoerythroblastosis (Chapter 18). Megakaryocytes are usually increased in number and present in abnormal clusters. Late-stage primary myelofibrosis is often associated with massive splenomegaly due to extramedullary hematopoiesis. In some patients, the fibrotic marrow is converted to bone (osteosclerosis), whereas a minority of others transform to acute myeloid leukemia, which may appear first in extramedullary sites such as lymph nodes. The overall clinicopathologic picture is identical to that seen when myelofibrosis arises out of PCV, essential thrombocytosis, or CML, suggesting that primary myelofibrosis may not be a unique entity but rather a common pathway of progression among different myeloproliferative disorders.

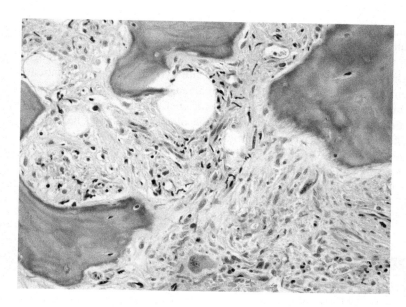

FIGURE 20-7   **Primary myelofibrosis, bone marrow biopsy.** The marrow space is replaced by fibrosis, producing a hypocellular appearance.

The prognosis varies depending on the presentation. Patients with leukopenia (white cell count <4000/mm³) or marked leukocytosis (white cell count >30,000/mm³) together with anemia (hemoglobin <10 g/dL) have a median survival time of around 2 years; the average overall survival is 5 to 8 years. Treatment options are limited. Splenectomy is sometimes performed to relieve symptoms related to massive splenomegaly (pain, early satiety, weight loss) but at the risk of eliminating an important source of blood cells and increasing the platelet count with the threat of thromboembolism. Bone marrow transplantation is an option for younger patients. JAK2 inhibitors are being evaluated as a potential targeted therapy in those with disease associated with *JAK2* mutations.

CHRONIC EOSINOPHILIC LEUKEMIA

Chronic eosinophilic leukemia is a rare disorder that merits mention due to its unusual pathogenesis and its response to targeted therapy. Chronic eosinophilic leukemia is usually associated with activating mutations in the PDGF receptor (PDGFR)-α or -β genes, which are also receptor tyrosine kinases. For reasons that are unclear, these mutations have their greatest effect on eosinophilic progenitors. Chronic eosinophilic leukemia is characterized by an increase in eosinophilic precursors in the marrow, eosinophilia in the peripheral blood, splenomegaly, and tissue dysfunction due to fibrosis. There is sometimes an accompanying increase in the number of mast cells, which can be striking; in such cases, the mast cells are also part of the neoplastic clone. The tissue fibrosis is a direct response to fibrogenic substances released from the neoplastic eosinophils, which infiltrate many tissues. One frequently affected organ is the heart. Cardiac involvement takes the form of endomyocardial fibrosis, which may be of sufficient severity to cause a restrictive cardiomyopathy called *Loeffler endocarditis*. Scleroderma-like fibrotic changes also may be seen in the skin.

Chronic eosinophilic leukemia can occur at any time of life but is most common in adult men between 40 and 50 years of age. The diagnosis can be made with certainty in those with eosinophilia (>1500/mm³) and a *PDGFR* gene rearrangement, which is best detected by fluorescence in situ hybridization. Some patients with an identical clinical picture lack *PDGFR* rearrangements; in these cases (previously termed *idiopathic hypereosinophilic syndrome*), chronic eosinophilic leukemia can be diagnosed only once reactive causes of eosinophilia (eg, helminthic infection, allergy, paraneoplastic syndromes) have been excluded and the marrow proliferation has been proven to be clonal.

Chronic eosinophilic leukemia associated with *PDGFR* rearrangements responds very well to imatinib, which inhibits both the PDGFR-α and -β tyrosine kinases. Imatinib rapidly lowers the eosinophil count and prevents or reverses the related tissue damage. It remains to be seen if this response will be sustained over time.

MYELODYSPLASTIC SYNDROMES

Myelodysplastic syndromes encompass a diverse group of hematopoietic neoplasms caused by acquired mutations that disrupt the normal maturation of myeloid progenitors, leading to cytopenias in the peripheral blood. In myelodysplastic syndrome, hematopoiesis is ineffective, meaning that many marrow progenitors undergo apoptosis before they give rise to formed elements, and those cells that are produced are often malformed (dysplastic). Because most patients present with anemia, myelodysplastic syndrome is often also referred to as *refractory anemia*.

In most instances, myelodysplastic syndrome arises sporadically, but some cases are related to genotoxic exposures. Prior cancer therapy in the form of either radiotherapy or certain types of chemotherapy (particularly DNA alkylating agents) can lead to myelodysplastic syndrome, as can environmental exposure to radiation (eg, the Chernobyl disaster) or certain toxins (eg, benzene).

Myelodysplastic syndrome is caused by acquired mutations, but little is known at present about the causative genes. Activating mutations in tyrosine kinases, the hallmark of myeloproliferative disorders, appear to be absent. The most common chromosomal aberrations are deletions of chromosomes 5q and 7q. One of the genes deleted from chromosome 5 that has been implicated in myelodysplastic syndrome, *RPS14*, encodes a ribosomal protein, which is of interest because several rare inherited diseases associated with bone marrow failure are caused by germline mutations in other ribosomal protein genes.

The classification of myelodysplastic syndrome is complex and beyond the scope of this text. For the student, it is sufficient to understand that the prognosis is related to three variables: the types of cytogenetic aberrations that are present, the number and severity of the cytopenias, and the number of blasts that are present in the marrow. Myelodysplastic syndrome associated with complex cytogenetic aberrations, multiple cytopenias, and increased numbers of blasts has a poor prognosis and survival times of 6 to 18 months, whereas cases on the other end of the continuum, with normal cytogenetics, isolated anemia, and no increase in number of blasts may be associated with survival times of 5 or more years.

Most patients with myelodysplastic syndrome present with vague symptoms related to the slow onset of anemia (fatigue, shortness of breath) or thrombocytopenia (easy bruising, petechiae). The diagnostic hallmark is dysplasia, which can affect all three lineages or only one or two. Characteristic findings include erythroid elements with misshapen nuclei or abnormal iron-laden mitochondria (ringed sideroblasts), neutrophils with only two nuclear lobes (the pseudo-Pelger-Huët anomaly) or abnormal cytoplasmic granulation, and multinucleated or small megakaryocytes with simple nuclei (Fig. 20-8). In addition to dysplasia, the diagnosis is based on the presence of cytopenia(s) and the detection of characteristic cytogenetic aberrations.

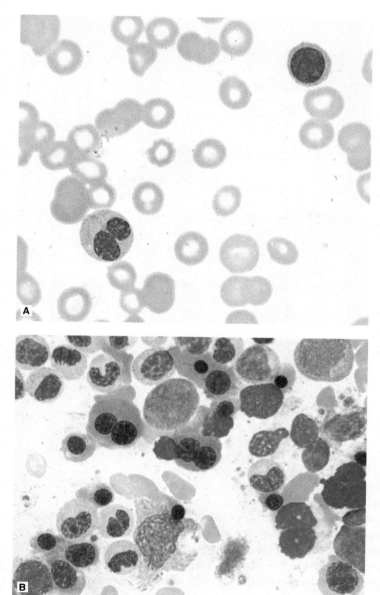

FIGURE 20-8 **Dysplasia in myelodysplastic syndromes.** A) Pseudo-Pelger-Huët cell, a neutrophil with only two nuclear lobes. B) Erythroid dysplasia, in the form of two erythroid precursors near the center of the field with two nuclei. C) Ringed sideroblasts. The blue perinuclear "granules" strung out like a sapphire necklace around the nuclei of the erythroid progenitors are iron-laden mitochondria (Prussian blue stain). D) Megakaryocytic dysplasia. An abnormal megakaryocyte with three separate nuclei is shown.

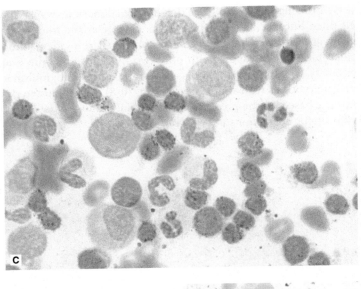

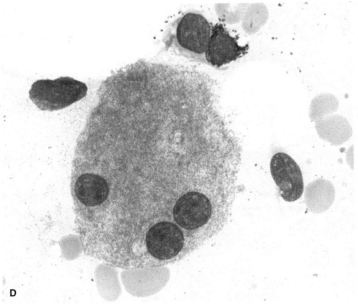

FIGURE 20-8 (*Continued*)   **D**

Myelodysplastic syndrome is primarily a disease of the elderly, with a peak
incidence in individuals >80 years of age. The only definitive therapy is allogeneic stem cell transplantation, which cannot be performed safely in older patients.
Aggressive chemotherapy is usually not effective; although it initially clears the
marrow of tumor cells, the myelodysplastic syndrome progenitors typically grow
back quickly once chemotherapy is stopped, and most patients never achieve a true
remission. This experience has led to the idea that myelodysplastic syndrome often
arises in marrows in which normal hematopoietic stem cells or progenitors are lost

or depleted, allowing mutated, defective myelodysplastic syndrome progenitors to predominate. Most patients receive palliative treatments that seek to improve the peripheral blood counts. Red cell transfusions can alleviate anemia but if the transfusion requirement is high, iron chelation therapy is required. As mentioned in Chapter 5, the ineffective hematopoiesis that is characteristic of myelodysplastic syndrome causes increased iron uptake by suppressing plasma hepcidin levels, which exacerbates the risk of iron overload in transfusion-dependent patients. Patients with anemia and 5q– as a sole cytogenetic abnormality have excellent responses to the thalidomide analog lenalidomide through uncertain mechanisms. A subset of patients responds to 5-azacytidine or decitabine, inhibitors of DNA methylation that are hypothesized to improve marrow function by reactivating unknown genes that are inappropriately silenced in myelodysplastic syndrome.

Despite these diverse therapies, the overall prognosis is poor. Many patients progress to acute myeloid leukemia (defined as >20% blasts in the bone marrow), with those with high-risk disease doing so more rapidly and most frequently. When acute myeloid leukemia supervenes, it usually responds poorly to chemotherapy and is associated with median survival times of only a few months.

SELF-ASSESSMENT STUDY QUESTIONS

1 Which protein is most likely to be mutated in the hematopoietic cells of patients with the myeloproliferative disorder essential thrombocythemia?
   A. JAK2 tyrosine kinase.
   B. PDGF R (platelet-derived growth factor receptor) alpha.
   C. PDGF R (platelet-derived growth factor receptor) beta.
   D. c-MPL (thrombopoietin receptor).
   E. c-Abelson (ABL) tyrosine kinase.

2. A 65-year-old man who has had severe anemia for the last 4 years, with progressive splenomegaly, was admitted with a small bowel infarction. Laboratory results included a hemoglobin of 7 g/dL, hematocrit 22%, reticulocyte count 4%, mean cell volume 90 fL, white cell count 35,000/mm³, with 66% neutrophils, 8% band cells, 8% monocytes, 5% metamyelocytes, 3% myelocytes, 5% eosinophils, and 5% basophils. The blood film showed misshaped red cells, mostly appearing as tear drops, with occasional nucleated red cells. What is the most likely diagnosis?
   A. Acute myeloid leukemia.
   B. Chronic myeloid leukemia.
   C. Myelodysplastic syndrome.
   D. Primary myelofibrosis.
   E. Leukemoid reaction.

3. A 58-year-old man developed a ruddy complexion. His hemoglobin was 20 g/dL. What two laboratory studies would best establish whether the patient has primary polycythemia vera?

   If the physical examination and laboratory test evaluation failed to document polycythemia vera, what further studies would help evaluate the patient's erythrocytosis, and how should they be interpreted?

4. What are the three most important prognostic factors in myelodysplastic syndromes?

21

Acute Leukemias

Jon C. Aster and Daniel J. DeAngelo

LEARNING OBJECTIVES

After studying this chapter you should understand:

- The pathogenic role of mutations in genes encoding transcription factors and signaling molecules in acute leukemia.
- The diagnostic and prognostic role of immunophenotyping, cytogenetics, and molecular genetics in acute leukemia.
- The general approach to treatment of patients with acute leukemia and the associated short-term complications.
- The unique role of "differentiating" agents in the treatment of acute promyelocytic leukemia.

PATHOGENESIS OF ACUTE LEUKEMIA

Acute leukemias and related disorders are aggressive neoplasms caused by acquired somatic mutations in early hematopoietic progenitors. The most obvious pathologic feature in the acute leukemias is the accumulation of undifferentiated blasts in the marrow and other tissues, indicating that, unlike the myeloproliferative disorders, acute leukemias have defects that block or significantly retard differentiation. We now know that specific subtypes of acute leukemia are often associated with mutations that alter the function of transcription factors that are required for normal differentiation of hematopoietic progenitors (Table 21-1). Sometimes these mutations consist of chromosomal rearrangements that create chimeric fusion genes, in which one or both partners encode a transcription factor; in other cases, the pathogenic mutations are more subtle point mutations or deletions. In most instances, the net result of the mutations is to decrease the function of a transcription factor that is required for the differentiation of cells of one or another of the hematopoietic lineages. An exception is mutations in the *NOTCH1* gene, which increase the transcriptional activity of the NOTCH1 protein.

The expression of *NOTCH1* genes bearing gain-of-function mutations in mouse hematopoietic stem cells causes the rapid development of T-cell acute lymphoblastic leukemia/lymphoma (T-ALL), the disease that is specifically associated with *NOTCH1* mutations in man, proving that these mutations are leukemogenic. However, similar experiments performed with other transcription factor genes bearing leukemia-associated mutations that decrease or interfere with a normal transcriptional activity usually fail to produce acute leukemia or do so only after very long periods of time. In fact, when expressed in hematopoietic stem cells, some mutated transcription factors cause bone marrow failure, suggesting that

TABLE 21-1 Examples of Transcription Factor Mutations Associated with Specific Subtypes of Acute Leukemia

Mutations	Effects	Normal Function of Affected Gene(s)	Associated Acute Leukemia
PML-RARα fusion gene [t(15;17)]	Decreased RARα function	RARα: required for granulopoiesis	Acute promyelocytic leukemia
C/EBPA point mutations	Decreased C/EBPα function	Required for granulopoiesis	Acute myeloid leukemia
PAX5, E2A, and *EBF* deletions	Decreased PAX5, E2A, and EBF function	Required for early stages of B-cell development	B-cell acute lymphoblastic leukemia/lymphoblastic lymphoma
NOTCH1 point mutations	Increased NOTCH1 function	Required for early stages of T-cell development	T-cell acute lymphoblastic leukemia/lymphoblastic lymphoma

their primary effect is to block differentiation rather than to cause proliferation. Further evidence that transcription factor mutations are not sufficient to cause acute leukemia has been gleaned from retrospective studies using blood samples (so-called Guthrie cards) that are obtained routinely from newborns. Analyses of these samples by using sensitive polymerase chain reaction (PCR)-based assays have shown that certain transcription factor mutations were present at birth in children who developed acute leukemia as much as 10 to 12 years later. Thus, even acute leukemia may have a long prodrome, during which "pre-leukemic" clones bearing an initial mutation in a transcription factor gene must acquire other somatic mutations for full-blown disease to appear. These insights have provided support for a model in which the development of acute leukemia requires at least two complementary events, a class 1 mutation that drives proliferation and a class 2 mutation in a transcription factor that arrests differentiation (Fig. 21-1).

The class 1 mutations in at least some acute leukemias appear to be gain-of-function mutations in tyrosine kinases, similar to the mutations that are prevalent in the myeloproliferative disorders (Chapter 20). It has long been recognized that a subset of acute lymphoblastic leukemia/lymphoma of B-cell origin (B-ALL) is associated with the presence of the Philadelphia chromosome and a *BCR-ABL* fusion gene. At the cytogenetic level, this is the same lesion found in chronic myelogenous leukemia (CML), a classic myeloproliferative disorder that, if untreated, usually transforms to blast crisis and a picture identical to that of acute leukemia. At a molecular level, it turns out that the form of BCR-ABL protein in B-ALL is usually 190 kDa in size, slightly smaller than the 210 kDa form usually found in CML. However, the 190 kDa form of BCR-ABL activates the same pathways (RAS, JAK/STAT, and PI-3 kinase/AKT) as the 210 kDa form, differing mainly in having a stronger tyrosine kinase activity. When expressed in the hematopoietic stem cells of mice, both the 210 kDa and 190 kDa forms of BCR-ABL produce a myeloproliferative disorder similar to CML.

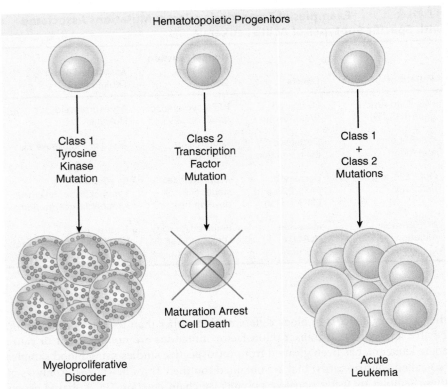

FIGURE 21-1 Types of mutations in hematologic malignancies. Most myeloproliferative disorders (discussed in Chapter 20) have activating class 1 mutations in tyrosine kinases that stimulate growth factor–independent proliferation but leave differentiation relatively intact. Most acute leukemias have mutations that interfere with or alter the activity of one or more transcription factors that are required for normal differentiation. These mutations (class 2), when introduced into the hematopoietic stem cells of mice, cause a maturation arrest but are not sufficient to cause acute leukemia. It is hypothesized that acute leukemias arise from transformed hematopoietic progenitors that acquire both class 1 and class 2 mutations, which collaborate to drive proliferation and block differentiation.

These observations suggested that BCR-ABL–positive ALLs and B-cell blast crises arising in CML might share the same complementary class 2 mutation in some critical transcription factor. Recently, this prediction has been confirmed with the detection of mutations in a gene called *Ikaros* in up to 90% of these two forms of acute leukemia. Ikaros is a transcription factor that regulates early stages of lymphocyte development. The Ikaros mutations result in expression of truncated forms of the protein that interfere with its normal function and thereby prevent the normal differentiation of early lymphoid progenitors. Compellingly, the Ikaros mutations found in the blast crisis stage are absent from the preceding stable phase of CML, linking them directly to the transformation of the myeloproliferative disorder to acute leukemia. It is hypothesized that other transformations, such as the progression of myelodysplastic syndromes to acute myeloid leukemia (AML), are also due to as-yet-unknown acquired class 2 mutations that lead to the loss of some critical transcription factor activity that is required for differentiation.

The mutations that conspire to produce acute leukemia are still being discovered, but it is clear that many different combinations of class 1 and class 2 mutations may be involved, including some that are described later, as well as additional mutations in tumor suppressor genes. The complexity of these molecular details can be daunting, but they are important for two clinically relevant reasons:

- Prognosis. The mutations found in a particular acute leukemia are often predictive of outcome with conventional therapies.
- Targeted therapies. In some instances, the mutated proteins are themselves the therapeutic target.

As targeted therapies become more prevalent, the molecular subtyping of acute leukemia will take on even greater importance. Indeed, it may soon be routine to completely sequence the genomes of acute leukemia cells (as well as other cancers), providing a complete understanding of all of the genetic changes that are responsible for an individual patient's tumor.

ACUTE LYMPHOBLASTIC LEUKEMIA/ LYMPHOBLASTIC LYMPHOMA

Acute lymphoblastic leukemia and lymphoblastic lymphoma encompass different clinical presentations of similar disease entities that are defined by the unbridled proliferation of immature lymphoid cells referred to as lymphoblasts. Acute lymphoblastic leukemia presents in the bone marrow and the peripheral blood, whereas lymphoblastic lymphoma presents as a mass within the bone or soft tissues. These different clinical manifestations relate in part to the origin of the tumor. B-cell tumors almost always arise in the bone marrow (where B cells develop) and present as "leukemias," whereas T-cell tumors often arise in the thymus (where T cells develop) and present as lymphomatous masses. For simplicity we will discuss these two forms of the disease together under the rubric of acute lymphoblastic leukemia/lymphoblastic lymphoma, or ALL.

ALL is the most common cancer of children. There are about 2500 to 3000 new cases of pediatric ALL in the United States per year. The disease also occurs throughout life in adults but makes up a much smaller fraction of the cancer burden in this segment of the population. The factors leading to the pathogenic mutations that drive ALL development are unknown. It most commonly appears sporadically in previously healthy, normal children. There are two major ALL subdivisions, ALL of B-cell origin (B-ALL) and ALL of T-cell origin (T-ALL). These two types of ALL are morphologically identical but differ in terms of their clinical characteristics, immunophenotype, and genetics.

B-CELL ACUTE LYMPHOBLASTIC LEUKEMIA/ LYMPHOBLASTIC LYMPHOMA

B-ALL is the most common type of ALL, comprising roughly 85% of cases. The peak incidence is about age 3 years, which closely coincides with the time of peak bone marrow production of B cells during life. Groups that are at relatively increased risk include children of White or Hispanic origin as well as those with Down syndrome (trisomy 21).

The most common clinical features in B-ALL are related to the replacement of the marrow by lymphoblasts and the resulting pancytopenia. The patient usually presents acutely with several weeks of fatigue or listlessness due to increasing anemia, often accompanied by easy bruising due to thrombocytopenia. Neutropenia may lead to infection, producing fever and sometimes localizing signs. Inspection of the peripheral blood film reveals the presence of lymphoblasts, which may be few or numerous, as well as anemia, thrombocytopenia, and granulocytopenia of variable severity. Unusual patients with lymphomatous presentations may complain of pain in a single long bone or come to attention due to involvement of the skin. B-ALL tends to spread via the meninges to the central nervous system and also may involve other immunologically privileged sites such as the ovary and testis. Splenomegaly, hepatomegaly, and lymphadenopathy may also be present due to tumor infiltration, but these features are usually not prominent.

The diagnosis can be strongly suspected based on morphologic inspection of the blood or the marrow. By definition, the diagnosis in those with leukemic presentations requires that lymphoblasts, cells with fine chromatin, small nucleoli, and scant agranular cytoplasm (Fig. 21-2), comprise at least 25% of the marrow cellularity. However, definitive diagnosis requires immunophenotyping, which is usually carried out by flow cytometry. The tumors cells are positive for terminal deoxynucleotidyl transferase (TdT, an enzyme that is expressed only in immature B and T cells) and certain B-lineage proteins such as CD19, and negative for surface immunoglobulin, which appears only on mature B cells (Fig. 21-3). In unusual lymphomatous presentations, the neoplastic nature of the process is obvious from the effacement of normal tissue by sheets of lymphoblasts, and the diagnosis is

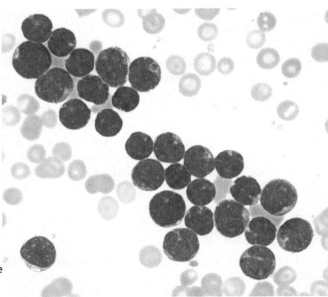

FIGURE 21-2 B-cell acute lymphoblastic leukemia, bone marrow aspirate smear. All of the nucleated cells are lymphoblasts with irregular nuclei, coarse chromatin, and scant amounts of agranular blue cytoplasm.

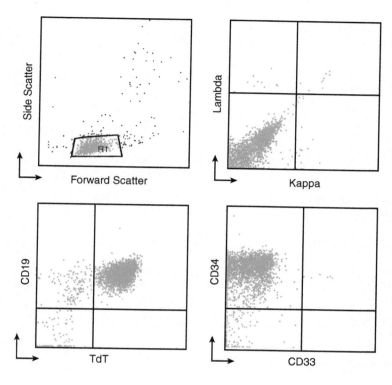

FIGURE 21-3   Flow cytometric findings, B-acute lymphoblastic leukemia (B-ALL). The cells are positive for CD19 (a marker expressed on all B-lineage cells), terminal deoxynucleotidyl transferase (a marker expressed by precursor B and T cells), and CD34 (a hematopoietic stem cell marker present on immature cells) and are negative for kappa and lambda immunoglobulin light chains (which are expressed by mature B cells) and the myeloid marker CD33. This combination of markers is diagnostic of a tumor of precursor B cells.

usually established by performance of immunohistochemistry on tissue sections. The principal diagnostic difficulties arise in children with severe viral infections, in which the immune response may increase the production of normal precursor B cells in the bone marrow while suppressing hematopoiesis, sometimes resulting in modest granulocytopenia. It is usually not difficult to distinguish such processes from B-ALL because reactive populations of lymphoblasts include cells from all stages of early B-cell development and never replace the marrow. In contrast, neoplastic lymphoblasts tend to have a uniform immunophenotype representing one or another stage of early B-cell development.

Subtyping of B-ALL is based on cytogenetics, and particular cytogenetic abnormalities are strongly predictive of clinical outcome; for these reasons, cytogenetic studies should be obtained in all patients with ALL. The most common abnormalities, the involved genes, and their clinical correlates are listed in Table 21-2. Of note, B-ALL associated with *BCR-ABL* fusion genes, rearrangements of the *MLL* gene, or hypodiploidy are associated with poor outcomes with conventional therapies. Outcomes are also worse for patients under 1 or over 10 years. This is partly due to age-dependent differences in the frequency of particular cytogenetic abnormalities (Table 21-2). High white cell counts are also associated with worse outcomes, possibly because they identify patients with unusually high tumor burdens. Overall, B-ALL in children has an excellent prognosis, with complete remissions being obtained in >95% and cures in 75% to 85% of patients. In adults the outcome is more guarded, with cures being obtained in a minority of patients.

TABLE 21-2 Major Cytogenetic Subtypes of B-Cell Acute Lymphoblastic Leukemia/Lymphoblastic Lymphoma

Cytogenetic Abnormality	Involved Genes	Mechanism of Activity	Frequency	Prognosis
t(12;21)	TEL-AML1	Chimeric transcription factor that interferes with AML1 function	25% in children; rare in adults	Excellent
Hyperdiploidy (>50 and <66 chromosomes)	Unknown	Unknown	25% in children; rare in adults	Excellent
Hypodiploidy (<45 chromosomes)	Unknown	Unknown	1%-5%, children and adults	Poor
t(9;22)	BCR-ABL	Constitutively active tyrosine kinase	3% in children, 25% in adults	Poor
t(11q23;v)	MLL and many other genes	Chimeric transcription factor that alters MLL function	Most common subtype in infants; rare in older children	Poor

v, variable other genes.

T-CELL ACUTE LYMPHOBLASTIC LEUKEMIA/ LYMPHOBLASTIC LYMPHOMA

T-ALL makes up roughly 15% of ALL. The peak incidence is at about age 15 years, which coincides roughly with the age at which the thymus reaches its greatest size. For unknown reasons, there is a 2:1 male predominance. About two-thirds of T-ALL present as mediastinal lymphomas associated with large masses centered in the thymus, the organ that gives birth to normal T cells. The enlarging tumor mass often compresses structures such as the major airways and blood vessels, producing cough, shortness of breath, and superior vena cava syndrome, which is characterized by swelling and redness of the face and upper extremities due to blockage of venous return to the heart. The remaining third of cases present with predominantly bone marrow involvement and a leukemic picture identical to that seen with most B-ALL. T-ALL shows a somewhat greater tendency than B-ALL to produce organomegaly and lymphadenopathy, and like B-ALL, often spreads to the central nervous system.

The diagnosis is based on morphologic demonstration of lymphoblasts effacing tissues such as the thymus or bone marrow (Fig. 21-4). As in B-ALL, immunophenotyping is essential to confirm the diagnosis. T-ALL expresses terminal deoxynucleotidyl transferase and variable combinations of T-lineage antigens such as CD1a, CD3, CD4, and CD8 (Fig. 21-5). Unlike in B-ALL, cytogenetics has not proved helpful in predicting patient outcome. In addition to very common activating mutations in NOTCH1, other genetic mechanisms that induce T-ALL include chromosomal rearrangements or other aberrations that lead to increased expression of several other transcription factors, including TAL1, LMO1, and LMO2.

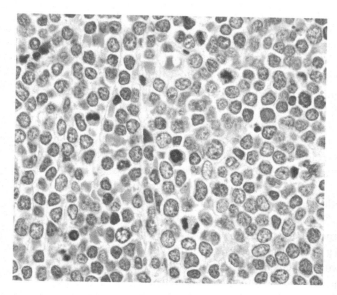

FIGURE 21-4 **T-lymphoblastic lymphoma, thymus.** The tissue is effaced by a population of lymphoblasts with oval nuclei, speckled chromatin, and scant cytoplasm. Mitotic figures are present.

Many of these dysregulated factors appear to interfere with the activity of E2A, a transcription factor that is required for proper B- and T-cell development. Activating mutations in tyrosine kinases are being sought but appear to be uncommon, and the identity of the class 1 mutations in most T-ALLs is uncertain. T-ALL also very commonly has loss-of-function mutations in CDKN2A, a complex locus on chromosome 9q that encodes two tumor suppressors, ARF, which inhibits p53, and p16, which inhibits several kinases that promote cell division.

In the past, T-ALL was considered to have a poorer prognosis than B-ALL, but with newer chemotherapy regimens, this difference no longer holds. Overall, 75% to 80% of T-ALL patients in the pediatric age group are cured, whereas the cure rates in adults are in the 40% to 50% range.

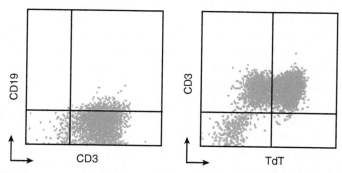

FIGURE 21-5 **Flow cytometric findings, T-cell acute lymphoblastic leukemia/lymphoma (T-ALL) by flow cytometry.** Staining with a panel of antibodies reveals a population of cells that uniformly expresses the T-cell marker CD3 and is partially positive for terminal deoxynucleotidyl transferase, a marker of precursor B and T cells. In contrast, the cells are negative for the pan-B-cell marker CD19. These findings are consistent with a proliferation composed of immature T-cell progenitors.

TREATMENT OF ALL

ALLs, regardless of molecular subtype, are very aggressive tumors with high growth rates and a proclivity to infiltrate many different organs. Unless effective therapy is given, patients succumb to the disease in weeks to a few months, usually due to complications related to bone marrow failure. Currently, childhood B-ALL and T-ALL are treated with an identical regimen that has several phases. The initial goal is to induce remission and clear the central nervous system of any infiltrating lymphoblasts. This is achieved with high doses of intravenous and intrathecal[1] chemotherapy, sometimes with cranial irradiation as well. Several studies have shown that complete clearance of the tumor at the end of induction (4 weeks), as assessed by either very sensitive flow cytometry or PCR-based assays, predicts whether patients will remain in remission, independent of other risk factors. Remission is then consolidated with multiple rounds of high-dose chemotherapy, which is followed with daily low-dose maintenance chemotherapy for up to another 2 to 2.5 years. Young adults also respond well to this very intensive pediatric treatment regimen. It remains to be seen whether use of intensive regimens in selected older adults will also be beneficial.

Along with therapy directed toward the malignant blast cell, supportive measures to prevent complications that are caused or exacerbated by chemotherapy are essential components of treatment. These consist of:

- Transfusions of both red cells and platelets, to reverse cytopenias stemming from leukemia and chemotherapy-induced myelosuppression.

- Careful monitoring for signs and symptoms of infection. In the setting of neutropenia, fever is often the only sign of bacterial or fungal infections, which can be rapidly fatal. Febrile patients require immediate culturing of blood and other body fluids followed by prompt treatment with broad-spectrum antimicrobial agents.

- Meticulous attention to fluid, electrolyte, and acid-base balances. Highly proliferative lymphoblasts are rapidly killed and lysed by chemotherapy, releasing large amounts of metabolites and electrolytes such as uric acid, potassium, and phosphate. These substances must be carefully monitored, and appropriate measures must be taken to prevent toxic buildup during treatment. For example, uric acid released into the blood and filtered by the kidney may precipitate in the renal tubules, leading to acute renal failure. This complication can be prevented by allopurinol, a drug that blocks the conversion of the soluble purines hypoxanthine and xanthine to poorly soluble uric acid.

- Psychological support and encouragement for both the patient and the family. It is essential that caregivers provide clear and unambiguous information, allay fears, and foster hope throughout the arduous and prolonged period from the time of diagnosis through the completion of therapy.

Unconventional therapies are needed for ALL patients with cytogenetic abnormalities that predict a poor prognosis, and for those who either fail to go into remission, or recur during therapy or after therapy is completed. These alternative approaches include intensified chemotherapy and bone marrow transplantation, which is the treatment of choice for patients with B-ALL associated with *BCR-ABL* fusion genes or *MLL* gene rearrangements. Imatinib and dasatinib, tyrosine kinase

[1]Intrathecal therapy: instillation of drugs directly into the cerebral spinal fluid.

inhibitors that are effective in chronic myelogenous leukemia and other myelopro-liferative disorders, also have been used in patients with *BCR-ABL*-positive B-ALL. Most tumors respond well to tyrosine kinase inhibitors initially but recur within a few months. Analysis of recurrent tumors usually shows the presence of *BCR-ABL* mutations that confer resistance to these inhibitors, indicating that the growth of the tumor still depends on signals generated by *BCR-ABL*. Recent studies have shown that administration of tyrosine kinase inhibitors in combination with con-ventional chemotherapy agents produces sustained remissions in most patients with *BCR-ABL*-positive B-ALL, and it appears that at least some of these patients may be cured.

ACUTE MYELOID LEUKEMIA

AML encompasses a group of molecularly distinct entities that share a single mor-phologic feature, the accumulation of undifferentiated blasts of myeloid origin in the bone marrow. Very rarely, tumors identical to AML present as soft tissue masses variously referred to as myeloid sarcoma or granulocytic sarcoma, but such tumors inevitably progress to full-blown AML and are best thought of as unusual presentations of the same disease.

AML is the most common acute leukemia of adults. There are roughly 13,000 cases per year in the United States, with only 10% to 15% of these occurring in children. The incidence of AML begins to rise in middle age and peaks in those over 80 years of age. The risk is increased in those exposed to agents that damage DNA, such as radiotherapy and chemotherapy given for other forms of cancer, as well as patients with rare inherited defects in DNA repair, such as Fanconi anemia (Chapter 4). Certain inherited severe neutropenias, such as that caused by elastase mutations (Chapter 18), are also associated with an increased risk for AML. The incidence is slightly increased in smokers, presumably because of the presence of carcinogens in cigarette smoke, and is increased to a greater degree in individuals exposed to certain toxins, such as benzene. As already noted in Chapter 20, patients with a pre-existing myeloproliferative disorder or a myelodysplastic syndrome are at high risk for progression to AML.

The presentation of AML is similar to ALL, but with some subtle differences. Most signs and symptoms are related to anemia, thrombocytopenia, and neutrope-nia. Splenomegaly and lymphadenopathy are seen less frequently than in ALL, and involvement of the central nervous system is much less common. On the other hand, AML is more likely to infiltrate soft tissues such as the gums, particularly tumors with monocytic differentiation. Myeloid blasts are also larger and stickier than lym-phoblasts. Accordingly, patients with very high blast counts sometimes present with pulmonary or central nervous system symptoms, owing to sludging of blasts in cap-illary beds. Other patients, particularly those with acute promyelocytic leukemia, present with disseminated intravascular coagulation, which ranges from subclini-cal, being detected only by laboratory tests of coagulation, to a severe coagulopathy associated with bleeding complications that may be fatal.

The diagnosis is based on morphologic inspection of the marrow and periph-eral blood coupled with histochemistry, immunophenotyping, and cytogenet-ics. In AML the number of blasts in the peripheral blood varies widely, from 0 to >200,000/mm^3. Thus, the absence of blasts in the peripheral blood (so-called aleukemic leukemia) does not exclude the diagnosis. The marrow is usually markedly hypercellular and contains little or no fat, but the marrow cellularity may also be normal (50% fat) or even decreased, especially in older patients. Regardless of the cellularity, increased numbers of blasts are present. The morphologic findings in AML vary considerably, as illustrated in Fig. 21-6. Individual tumors may be composed predominantly of myeloblasts (granulocytic precursors), monoblasts or early monocytic forms (monocytic precursors), megakaryoblasts, or (rarely) erythroblasts. In many cases, mixtures of blasts with varying degrees of granulocytic and monocytic differentiation are seen. The block in differentiation that is characteristic of AML also varies from nearly complete to partial. In the vast majority of cases, the number of blasts exceeds 20% of the marrow cellularity, which is taken to be diagnostic of AML. Rarely, the number of blasts is <20%, but cytogenetic studies show the presence of an aberration specific for AML (described in the

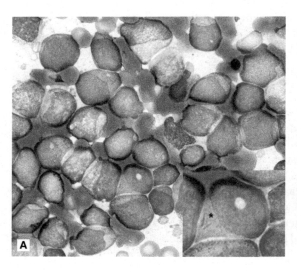
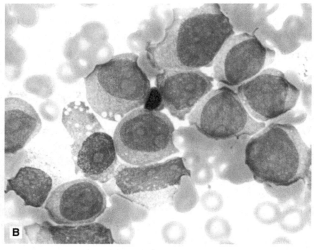
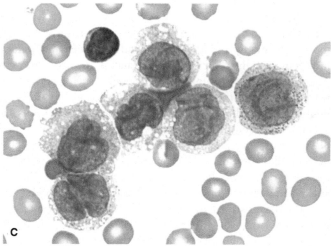

FIGURE 21-6 Acute myeloid leukemia (AML, bone marrow aspirates). A) Myeloblasts. In some AMLs, myeloblasts with coarse chromatin, prominent nucleoli, and moderate amounts of blue cytoplasm predominate. The cytoplasm of several blasts in this field contain fine, needle-like azurophilic Auer rods (inset, asterisk), a finding that is pathognomonic of neoplastic myeloblasts. In other AMLs, the tumor cells exhibit monocytic differentiation. B) Monoblasts with oval nuclei, prominent nucleoli, and abundant basophilic cytoplasm. C) Monocytic tumor cells that show partial differentiation; promonocytes with folded nuclei and gray-blue cytoplasm make up most of the cellularity.

following paragraph), allowing the diagnosis to be made. An additional morphologic finding that is specific for AML is the presence of Auer rods (Fig. 21-6A),
red-purple needle-like inclusions derived from coalescence of abnormal primary
granules that are commonly seen in neoplastic myeloblasts or progranulocytes.
Histochemical stains for myeloperoxidase (a marker of myeloblasts) and nonspecific esterase (a marker of monoblasts) helps to confirm the diagnosis, as does flow
cytometry, which typically reveals the presence of myeloid markers such as CD33,
CD13, and CD117 and/or monocytic markers such as CD14. Many cases are also
positive for CD34, a marker found on hematopoietic stem cells.

Subtyping of AML is based on cytogenetic findings, molecular features, and
clinical context, each of which predicts prognosis and guides therapy. Selected
molecular subtypes that are relatively common or clinically distinct are listed in
Table 21-3. The cytogenetics of AML is complex; over 100 recurrent chromosomal
aberrations have been described. Increasing numbers of other types of recurrent

TABLE 21-3 Selected Molecular Subtypes of Acute Myeloid Leukemia

Tumor	Involved Genes	Oncogenic Mechanism	Comments
AML with t(8;21)	ETO-AML1	Chimeric transcription factor that interferes with AML1 function	5% of AML; frequent blasts with single Auer rods
AML with inv(16)	CBFB-MYH11	Chimeric transcription factor that interferes with CBFB, a binding partner of AML1	5% to 10% of AML; associated with eosinophilia and abnormal violet-purple granules in eosinophilic precursors
AML with t(15;17) acute promyelocytic leukemia	PML-RARA	Chimeric transcription factor that interferes with RARα function	5%-10% of AML; frequent progranulocytes with numerous Auer rods; often associated with "aleukemic" leukemia and disseminated intravascular coagulation
AML with NPM mutations	NPM	Unknown	30% of AML; usually shows monocytic differentiation
AML with C/EBPA mutations	C/EBPA	Decreased C/EBPα function	10%-15% of AML; usually shows evidence of granulocytic differentiation
AML following genotoxic therapy	MLL in subset with 11q23 rearrangements	Altered MLL function in subset with 11q23 rearrangements	MLL rearrangement–associated cases occur 1-5 years following etoposide exposure; cases related to other chemotherapeutic agents or radiation occur 5-10 years after exposure

AML, acute myeloid leukemia; t, translocation; inv, inversion.

mutations also are being described; those that are most common, mutations in the transcription factor C/EBPα and the nuclear transport protein NPM, now define distinct subsets of AML. Finally, AML following genotoxic therapy is genetically and clinically unique and has its own disease category. Of note, gain-of-function mutations in various tyrosine kinases that likely function as pro-growth class 1 mutations have been described in a subset of cases. The most commonly mutated genes are *FLT3* and *c-KIT*, both of which encode receptor tyrosine kinases that are normally expressed in early myeloid progenitors.

AML is generally treated with a standard induction regimen of high-dose chemotherapy followed by consolidation with additional chemotherapy. The drugs and schedules are different from those used to treat ALL, emphasizing the importance of making this diagnostic distinction. The critically important supportive measures used in ALL patients also apply to the management of those with AML.

Overall, patients with AML fare less well than those with ALL. Disease types with particularly poor prognoses, such as AML occurring after genotoxic therapy, may respond better to alternative, more aggressive therapies such as bone marrow transplantation (Chapter 26); however, morbidity and mortality associated with bone marrow transplantation increase sharply with age, excluding many older patients from this option.

Several forms of AML therapy that specifically target mutated oncoproteins are also in current use or under study. Acute promyelocytic leukemia associated with the t(15;17) translocation merits special mention in this regard. This form of AML often presents with leukopenia, few or no circulating blasts, and disseminated intravascular coagulation, the latter caused by procoagulants released from the abnormal azurophilic granules that are present in the neoplastic promyelocytes (Fig. 21-7). At a molecular level, the t(15;17) results in the formation of a chimeric gene encoding a PML-RARα fusion oncoprotein. Normal RARα

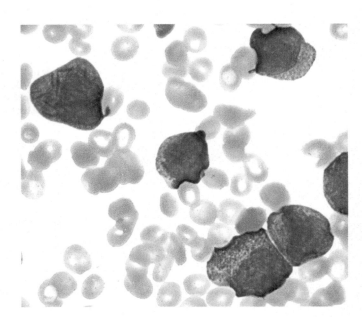

FIGURE 21-7 Acute promyelocytic leukemia (APML), bone marrow aspirate. Scattered hypergranular promyelocytes are present as well as a promyelocyte with multiple Auer rods, a finding that is highly characteristic of this subtype of AML.

(retinoic acid receptor-α) is a transcription factor that associates with a partner protein called RXR and binds to special DNA sequences called *retinoid response elements* (Fig. 21-8). The binding of retinoic acid (vitamin A) to the RARα/RXR complex causes a conformational change that leads to the recruitment of proteins called *coactivators*, which acetylate histones attached to DNA and turn on the transcription of adjacent genes. In myeloid progenitors, the genes regulated by RARα/RXR include some that are required for granulocytic differentiation. PML-RARα retains the ability to bind to RXR and DNA but is much less sensitive to retinoic

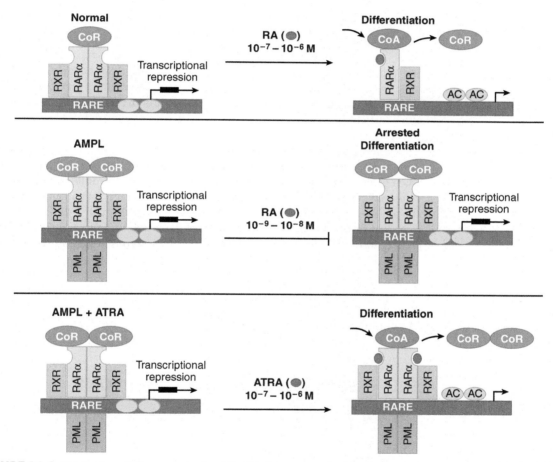

FIGURE 21-8 Mechanism of all-trans retinoic acid action in acute promyelocytic leukemia. In normal myeloid precursors, heterodimers composed of retinoic acid receptor alpha (RARα) and the retinoic X receptor (RXR) bind to specific sequences known as retinoic acid response elements (RAREs) in the promoters of genes that regulate myeloid differentiation. RXR/RARα heterodimers bind to transcriptional co-repressors (CoR) in the absence of retinoic acid (RA), but upon binding, RA releases co-repressors and associates instead with transcriptional co-activators (CoA). This results in the acetylation of histones (AC), leading to the activation of gene expression and granulocytic differentiation. In acute promyelocytic leukemia (APML), a balanced (15;17) chromosomal translocation creates a chimeric gene that drives the expression of a fusion protein consisting of a portion of the promyelocytic leukemia protein (PML) and RARα. The PML-RARα fusion protein retains the capacity to bind to RAREs but has a much higher affinity for co-repressors than RXR-RARα. As a result, physiologic levels of retinoic acid fail to activate gene transcription, resulting in a block in differentiation that contributes to APML. The blockade can be overcome by pharmacologic doses of all-trans retinoic acid (ATRA), which is capable of binding to the PML-RARα fusion protein and displacing co-repressors.

acid. Thus, by occupying retinoid response elements, PML-RARα interferes with gene transcription and blocks differentiation.

Proof of this mechanism comes from treatment of patients with acute promyelocytic leukemia with high doses of all-trans retinoic acid (ATRA), which binds and activates PML-RARα/RXR complexes. Within 1 to 2 days of the start of ATRA treatment, the neutrophil count rises, sometimes reaching levels of 50,000/mm³, and disseminated intravascular coagulation stops. This new cohort of neutrophils harbors the t(15;17), proving that they are the differentiated progeny of the neoplastic promyelocytes. Because neutrophils are short-lived cells with no capacity for cell division, ATRA rapidly clears the bulk of the neoplastic cells. Patients treated with ATRA avoid the cytotoxic complications of conventional chemotherapy but still suffer from other complications. Most notably, shortly after beginning ATRA treatment, some patients develop dyspnea and pulmonary infiltrates due to exudation of fluid from capillaries, a pathologic change that is caused in some way by the differentiating myeloid cells. This complication responds well to temporary cessation of ATRA and treatment with glucocorticoids, which decreases the adhesiveness of neutrophils to endothelium (Chapter 18).

Differentiation therapy with ATRA is sufficient to get most patients with acute promyelocytic leukemia into remission but has not proven to be curative when given alone. To date, it has been used most widely in combination with conventional chemotherapy. More recently, it has been noted that arsenic salts (specifically arsenic trioxide) also target PML-RARα but through a different mechanism that involves increased degradation of the fusion protein. Early trials using a combination of ATRA and arsenic trioxide show response rates of over 90%, and almost all responsive patients have remained in remission, suggesting that this unique combination of targeted therapies will become the treatment of choice in this particular form of AML. Other targeted therapies under evaluation include tyrosine kinase inhibitors, which are being tested on AMLs associated with activating mutations in FLT3, and antibodies specific for myeloid surface proteins (eg, CD33) linked to toxins or radiochemicals.

SELF-ASSESSMENT STUDY QUESTIONS

1. Which of the following provide the most useful prognostic information in patients with acute lymphoblastic or acute myeloid leukemia?
   A. Percent blasts in marrow and cytogenetics.
   B. Patient age and percent blasts in marrow.
   C. Hemoglobin level and cytogenetics.
   D. Patient age and cytogenetics.
   E. Hemoglobin level and platelet count.

2. A 45-year-old librarian presented with fever, weight loss, fatigue, and progressive petechiae and ecchymoses over the last few weeks. Laboratory test results included a hemoglobin of 8 g/dL, hematocrit 25%, reticulocyte count 2%, and white cell count 4,000/mm³ with 10% neutrophils, 5% band cells, 55% promyelocytes, 10% myeloblasts, 5% monocytes, and 15% lymphocytes. The platelet count was 25,000/mm³. What is the most likely cause of the patient's severe purpura?

A. Immune thrombocytopenia.
B. Thrombocytopenia secondary to acute leukemia.
C. Thrombocytopenia due to gram-negative sepsis.
D. Disseminated intravascular coagulation.
E. Infiltration of skin by leukemic cells.

3. What therapy is most likely to benefit this patient?
A. Heparin.
B. Platelet transfusion.
C. Factor VIII concentrate.
D. Imatinib (Gleevec).
E. All-trans retinoic acid.

4. A 14-year-old boy developed shortness of breath, weight loss, and fatigue. A chest radiograph revealed a 12-cm, anterior mediastinal mass. A biopsy of the mass revealed T-cell acute lymphoblastic lymphoma.

What is the most likely molecular pathogenesis?
A. Epstein-Barr virus.
B. Translocation involving the c-*ABL* oncogene.
C. Translocation involving the c-*MYC* oncogene.
D. Translocation involving the *IgH* gene.
E. Activating mutations in the *NOTCH1* gene.

The patient was treated with combination chemotherapy. Over the next 10 days, the tumor mass shrank dramatically, but the patient developed a marked decrease in urine output (oliguria) and a progressive rise in the serum creatinine level from 1.2 mg/dL (upper limit of normal) to 6 mg/dL. The serum calcium level remained normal.

What is the most likely cause of the patient's renal failure?

A. Sepsis and disseminated intravascular coagulation.
B. Obstruction of urine flow from precipitation of uric acid.
C. Obstruction of the ureters by an intra-abdominal lymphoma.
D. Acute pyelonephritis (kidney infection).
E. Hemolytic uremic syndrome.

22 Non-Hodgkin Lymphomas and Chronic Lymphocytic Leukemias

Jon C. Aster and Arnold Freedman

LEARNING OBJECTIVES

After studying this chapter you should understand:

- The major categories of lymphoid neoplasms.
- The role of genomic instability and infectious agents in the pathogenesis of lymphomas.
- The characteristic pathologic and clinical features of chronic lymphocytic leukemia and the major subtypes of non-Hodgkin lymphoma.

INTRODUCTION TO THE LYMPHOID NEOPLASMS

The lymphomas, chronic lymphocytic leukemias, and plasma cell neoplasms are a group of entities that have in common an origin from mature lymphoid cells. However, in other respects, these tumors are remarkably varied in terms of their clinical presentation, behavior, molecular pathogenesis, treatment, and outcome. Historically, these tumors have been grouped according to their typical presentation and their clinical aggressiveness. This remains a useful way to think about these tumors, with the important caveat that even within a particular diagnostic category there is a range of clinical presentations and courses. In recognition of this, the current World Health Organization (WHO) classification of lymphoid neoplasms largely relies on objective pathologic and molecular features to establish specific diagnoses.

Tumors referred to as *lymphomas* most commonly present as a mass within lymph nodes or other secondary lymphoid tissues but also may arise in and affect the function of virtually any organ in the body. Lymphocytic leukemias, by definition, involve the bone marrow and peripheral blood at presentation but also commonly cause lymphadenopathy and splenomegaly. As was discussed in Chapter 19, these distinctions are not absolute; virtually all tumors referred to as *lymphomas* present on occasion with marrow and blood involvement, and leukemias sometimes present as lymphomatous masses. Lymphomas and lymphocytic leukemias also share a propensity to cause immune dysregulation, which gives rise to:

- B symptoms (fever, night sweats, and weight loss).
- Immunosuppression and susceptibility to infection.

- Breakdown of immune tolerance, often leading to production of autoantibodies, particularly against red cells or platelets, and other manifestations of autoimmunity.

Plasma cell tumors have their own distinctive set of signs and symptoms, which are related to destructive bone lesions, kidney failure, and the deleterious effects of complete or partial immunoglobulins secreted by the tumor cells.

The complexity of neoplastic disorders of mature lymphocytes and plasma cells is daunting, rivaling (and reflecting) the complexity of the immune system itself. The most recent WHO classification of lymphoid neoplasms lists over 50 different types, many of which have fascinating biologic and clinical features but are too rare to merit discussion here. Instead, we will focus primarily on the more common tumors (listed in Table 22-1). This handful of neoplasms, which includes several non-Hodgkin lymphomas, chronic lymphocytic leukemia, Hodgkin lymphoma, and plasma cell neoplasms and related disorders, encompasses over 90% of human lymphoid tumors. A few uncommon disorders of exceptional pathogenic interest also will be mentioned.

In this chapter, we present a brief overview of the pathogenesis of lymphoid neoplasms that is relevant to many of the most common subtypes and then discuss the most common forms of non-Hodgkin lymphoma and chronic lymphocytic leukemia in detail. The uncommon T-cell tumors will be mentioned only briefly, and the very rare natural killer (NK) cell tumors (<1% of all lymphoid neoplasms) will not be covered. Hodgkin lymphomas and plasma cell neoplasms are discussed in subsequent chapters.

TABLE 22-1 Common Lymphoid Neoplasms

Neoplasm	Cell of Origin	Implicated Oncogenes	Usual Clinical Behavior
Follicular lymphoma	Germinal center B cell	BCL-2	Indolent
Extranodal marginal zone lymphoma	Post-germinal center B cell	NFκB	Very indolent
Chronic lymphocytic leukemia/ small lymphocytic lymphoma	Germinal center B cell or naïve B cell	BCL-2	Indolent
Diffuse large B-cell lymphoma	Germinal center or post-germinal center B cell	BCL-6, BCL-2	Aggressive
Burkitt lymphoma	Germinal center B cell	c-MYC	Very aggressive
Multiple myeloma	Post-germinal center B cell	Diverse	Variable
Hodgkin lymphoma Classical Nodular lymphocyte predominant	Germinal center or post-germinal center B cell	NFκB	Variable

THE DOUBLE-EDGED SWORD OF GENOMIC INSTABILITY

It is notable that all of the neoplasms listed in Table 22-1, except for a small subset of chronic lymphocytic leukemias, are derived from B lymphocytes that have passed through germinal centers. In contrast, tumors derived from T cells and NK cells are rare, collectively comprising no more than about 10% of lymphoid neoplasms. Thus, relative to T cells or NK cells, germinal center B cells are unusually prone to give rise to lymphoid neoplasms.

The susceptibility of germinal center B cells to transformation is likely related to their inherent genomic instability. Early stages of B- and T-cell development are similar; pre-B cells rearrange their immunoglobulin genes in the bone marrow, emerging as mature naïve B cells expressing immunoglobulin M (IgM), whereas pre-T cells rearrange their T-cell receptor genes in the thymus, emerging as naïve T cells expressing T-cell receptors. Once naïve B and T cells are activated by antigen, however, their paths diverge. Although activated T cells continue to express the same T-cell receptors that they were "born" with, activated B cells migrate into germinal centers and further diversify their immunoglobulin genes through somatic hypermutation and class switching.

Germinal centers are oblong structures found in lymph nodes and the spleen that contain a meshwork of antigen-presenting dendritic cells, small numbers of helper T cells, and scattered phagocytic macrophages (Fig. 22-1). Here, antigen-stimulated B cells begin to divide rapidly and turn on the expression of activation-induced cytosine deaminase, an enzyme that converts cytosine residues in DNA to uracil residues and is required for both somatic hypermutation and class switching (Fig. 22-2). Somatic hypermutation and class switching are essential elements of an effective humoral immune response but are both error prone. Many genes besides the immunoglobulin locus undergo hypermutation in germinal center B cells, although at a lower rate. Similarly, certain chromosomal translocations found in B-cell neoplasms appear to be mistakes that result, in part, from breaks in DNA that are induced during attempted class switching. Some genes, such as *BCL-6*, can be deregulated by either point mutations or chromosomal translocations (Fig. 22-2). Thus, the germinal center reaction is a double-edged sword, permitting effective humoral immunity but also placing germinal center B cells at high risk for mutations that can lead to malignant transformation.

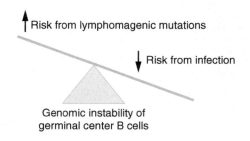

↑ Risk from lymphomagenic mutations

↓ Risk from infection

Genomic instability of germinal center B cells

ROLE OF INFECTIOUS AGENTS IN LYMPHOID NEOPLASMS

Several viruses and a few bacterial infections have been established as cofactors in the development of specific lymphoid malignancies. The clearest associations are with the following agents:

- Epstein-Barr virus (EBV).
- Human herpesvirus-8 (HHV-8, also known as Kaposi sarcoma herpesvirus [KSHV]).

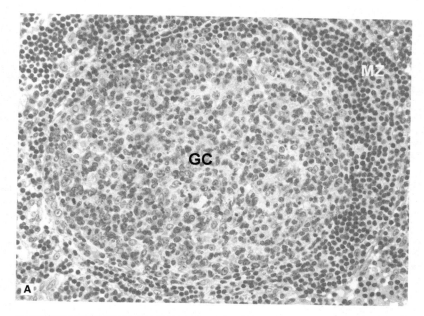

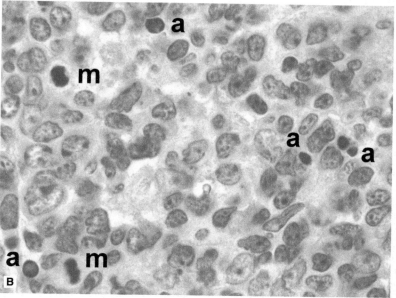

FIGURE 22-1 Reactive germinal center, lymph node. A) A low-power view shows an oblong germinal center (GC) surrounded by a mantle zone (MZ) of small resting B cells that is polarized toward one side of the germinal center. B) A high-power view of the germinal center shows several cells in mitosis (m) and dark-staining nuclear fragments (a) derived from B cells that have undergone apoptotic cell death.

- Human T-cell lymphotropic virus (HTLV-1).
- Human immunodeficiency virus (HIV).
- *Helicobacter pylori.*

EBV is a gamma herpes virus that plays an important etiologic role in several forms of non-Hodgkin lymphoma and Hodgkin lymphoma. Most humans are infected with EBV during their lives, usually in childhood or adolescence. Mature B cells express a receptor for EBV called *CD21* on their cell surfaces that permits the virus

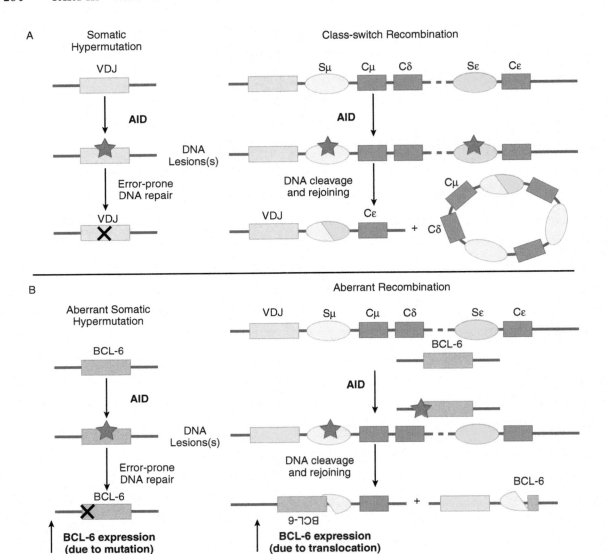

FIGURE 22-2 **Somatic hypermutation, class switching, and lymphomagenic mutations.** A) Normal germinal center B-cell reaction. Antigen-activated germinal center B cells express activation-induced cytosine deaminase (AID), which creates cytosine to uracil mutations within the VDJ segments of the immunoglobulin genes. The resulting uracil:guanine base pair mismatches undergo error-prone DNA repair, leading to mutations. In most cells, these mutations lower the affinity of antibody for antigen; these cells undergo apoptosis (as shown in Fig. 22-1B). However, in a small subset of cells, the AID-induced mutations improve the affinity of antibody for antigen. Signals produced by surface complexes containing these high-affinity antibodies permit cells to survive and subsequently undergo class switching, which also involves AID. Here, AID induces mutations in class-switch regions, non-coding sequences that flank constant region segments. In the example shown, mutations are induced in the mu (Sμ) and epsilon (Sε) switch regions. These lesions are recognized by a complex of proteins and enzymes capable of cutting and rejoining DNA, producing an intragenic recombination event that positions the Cε constant region next to the VDJ segment. As a result, the B cell carrying this IgH chain gene switches from IgM to IgE antibody expression. B) Lymphomagenic AID-mediated mutations. *BCL-6* is an oncogene commonly mutated in human germinal center B-cell lymphomas. In some tumors, point mutations resembling those produced by AID in VDJ segments occur in the promoter region of the *BCL-6* gene. In other instances, the coding region of the *BCL-6* gene is physically translocated into the IgH switch region, an event that likely stems from a mistake during attempted class switching. Both events produce an oncogenic increase in BCL-6 expression.

to enter the cell. Once internalized, EBV produces a number of viral proteins that immortalize B cells and cause them to proliferate in an uncontrolled fashion. In healthy people, T cells mount an immune response to viral antigens displayed on the surface of infected B cells. Cytokines produced by these T cells are responsible for the clinical syndrome known as infectious mononucleosis (Chapter 18). The host T-cell response kills most infected B cells, but a small number of cells turn off the expression of most viral proteins and escape immune destruction, creating a long-lived pool of latently infected B cells. If such cells are activated at some later time by antigen, they may again turn on the expression of EBV proteins that lead to B-cell transformation.

EBV contributes to the development of lymphoid neoplasms in several ways. The best understood is in the context of T-cell immunodeficiency, such as occurs following bone marrow transplantation or in patients treated with high doses of immunosuppressive drugs (eg, organ transplant recipients). If T-cell immunity falls below a certain threshold, lurking EBV-infected B cells may become activated and begin to proliferate in an uncontrolled fashion, giving rise to tumors that may occur in virtually any tissue. These EBV-positive tumors often can be brought under control by lowering the dose of immunosuppressive drugs (although at the risk of organ rejection or graft-versus-host disease, depending on the clinical setting) and by treatment with rituximab, an antibody specific for the B-cell antigen CD20. Other EBV-positive lymphoid tumors include subsets of Burkitt lymphoma, diffuse large B-cell lymphomas (particularly in the elderly), Hodgkin lymphoma, and rare T-cell and NK-cell tumors. The precise role of EBV in these lymphomas is less clear-cut, but molecular analyses have consistently shown that the EBV genomes within the tumor cells are monoclonal, meaning that all of these tumors originate from a single EBV-infected cell, a finding that is taken as strong evidence of a direct pathogenic role for the virus.

HHV-8, another human herpesvirus, is strongly associated with primary effusion lymphoma, a rare, aggressive, B-cell lymphoma that arises within chronic effusions, typically in the pleural or peritoneal spaces. Defective immunity sets the stage for these tumors, which are largely confined to HIV-infected patients and the elderly. Many (but not all) of these tumors are co-infected with EBV, a unique example of two transforming viruses collaborating to cause a human cancer. HHV-8 is also the cause of Kaposi sarcoma, another tumor largely confined to immunosuppressed individuals.

HTLV-1 is the only retrovirus directly associated with a human cancer, a rare tumor called adult T-cell leukemia/lymphoma. HTLV-1 is endemic in southeast Japan, certain parts of the Caribbean, western Africa, and South America. The virus infects and persists in CD4-positive T cells as a provirus integrated in the host cell DNA. After an asymptomatic period that usually spans decades, a small fraction of infected individuals develop adult T-cell leukemia/lymphoma, an aggressive tumor of HTLV-1–infected CD4-positive T cells. The mechanism of T-cell transformation in the unfortunate few who develop tumors is not understood.

Although HIV also infects CD4-positive T cells, it is associated with a greatly heightened risk of B-cell lymphomas. Early in the course of HIV infection, T-cell dysregulation produces a marked hyperplasia of germinal center B cells, resulting in generalized lymphadenopathy. Untreated, late-stage HIV infection with severe T-cell immunodeficiency (AIDS) is associated with a high incidence of aggressive EBV-positive B-cell lymphomas, which usually occur in extranodal sites such as the brain. These late-stage EBV-positive tumors are mostly prevented by antiretro-viral therapy, but even in the era of highly effective therapy, HIV-positive patients have an increased incidence of EBV-negative, B-cell lymphomas. It may be that the germinal center B cells that proliferate extensively in early HIV infection accumulate oncogenic mutations that increase the risk of lymphoma.

Helicobacter pylori is a bacterium that colonizes the mucous layer overlying the pyloric epithelium of the stomach. It induces both an acute and chronic immune response and is an important cause of peptic ulcer. It is also strongly associated with gastric extranodal marginal zone lymphoma, a type of B-cell lymphoma that appears to be caused by chronic inflammation. The process begins as a straight-forward inflammatory reaction that produces a gastritis. With persistence of the process and occurrence of mutations that give certain responding B cells a growth or survival advantage, a clonal B-cell neoplasm arises. Initially, however, this B-cell clone remains dependent on T helper cells that are specific for *Helicobacter* anti-gens. At this point, the tumor cannot grow beyond the stomach and, remarkably, often regresses completely if *H. pylori* is eliminated with antibiotics. Eventually, however, the tumor may acquire additional mutations that relieve the dependency on T-cell help; such tumors are refractory to antibiotic therapy and can spread to extragastric sites. Similar extranodal marginal zone lymphomas occur in tissues involved by chronic autoimmune reactions (such as the thyroid gland in Hashim-oto thyroiditis and the salivary gland in Sjögren syndrome), further supporting the idea that long-standing immune stimulation can lead to certain lymphomas.

Although the infectious agents and unique features of germinal center B cells described earlier are important factors, the causes of lymphoid neoplasms remain incompletely understood. Occasional families have multiple afflicted members, suggesting the existence of genetic factors. Of concern, the incidence of lymphoma is increasing in the United States, particularly in the elderly, presumably due to currently unknown environmental factors.

We will now turn to the common forms of non-Hodgkin lymphomas and lymphocytic leukemia, beginning with the more indolent disorders.

CHRONIC LYMPHOCYTIC LEUKEMIA/SMALL LYMPHOCYTIC LYMPHOMA

Chronic lymphocytic leukemia/small lymphocytic lymphoma (CLL/SLL) is a relatively common tumor that affects about 15,000 people per year in the United States. It is a disease of older adults, with a median age at diagnosis of around 70 years. Most patients present with leukemia (CLL), whereas a small minority present with lymphoma (SLL). In earlier classifications of lymphoid malignancies, CLL and SLL were considered to be separate entities, but they are now accepted to be different clinical manifestations of the same disease.

The molecular causes of CLL/SLL are not well-understood. Unlike other lym-phoid neoplasms (discussed in the following), CLL/SLL is not associated with recurrent chromosomal translocations. Instead, it is characterized by the pres-ence of deletions involving portions of chromosomes 11, 13, 14, and 17 as well as trisomy 12. Of some interest, the deletions involving chromosome 13 appear to remove genes encoding several microRNAs, short, non-coding RNAs that negatively

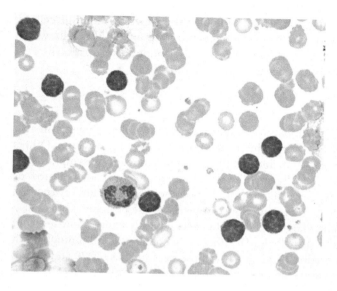

FIGURE 22-3   Chronic lymphocytic leukemia (CLL), peripheral smear. A lymphocytosis of small round lymphocytes with condensed chromatin and scant cytoplasm is evident. A disrupted "smudge" cell (lower left), characteristic of CLL, is also present.

regulate the expression of other genes. The microRNAs on chromosome 13 that are lost from CLL/SLL cells appear to repress the expression of genes that promote cell growth. Deletions on chromosome 17 may contribute to the inactivation of *p53*, a critically important tumor suppressor gene.

In CLL, peripheral blood smears reveal increased numbers of mainly small, round lymphocytes, which are fragile and often disrupted (smudge cells) (Fig. 22-3). In CLL/SLL, the bone marrow usually contains aggregates, clusters, or sheets of similar-appearing tumor cells. Lymph nodes are typically expanded by a diffuse infiltrate of small lymphocytes (Fig. 22-4) and patchy collections of larger, mitotically active cells known as *proliferation centers*, which are characteristic of CLL/SLL.

The microenvironment within lymph nodes and other tissues sustains the growth and survival of the tumor cells. For example, lymph nodes contain reactive

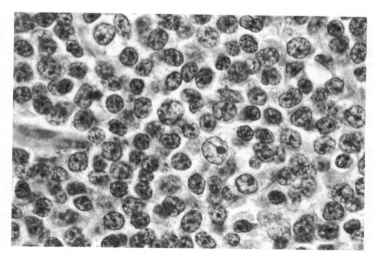

FIGURE 22-4   Chronic lymphocytic leukemia/ small lymphocytic lymphoma (CLL/SLL), lymph node. The lymph node contains an infiltrate consisting of a monotonous collection of small, round lymphocytes mixed with a few larger cells with nucleoli (so-called prolymphocytes, which represent CLL/SLL cells that are actively dividing).

T cells that express CD40 ligand, which stimulates the growth of CLL/SLL cells by activating the CD40 receptor, and also monocyte-derived "nurse-like" cells, which express several factors that activate NF-κB, a transcription factor that turns on a number of genes that enhance the survival of CLL/SLL cells.

DIAGNOSIS

A high proportion of CLL patients are diagnosed while completely asymptomatic, with the disease being discovered due to the presence of lymphocytosis. Others with SLL often come to attention due to diffuse lymphadenopathy. B symptoms are unusual. The diagnosis is usually established by a tissue biopsy of bone marrow or lymph node showing the characteristic morphology coupled with flow cytometry, although if lymphocytosis is present, flow cytometry of the peripheral blood also can be used to make the diagnosis. CLL/SLL cells typically express low levels of surface immunoglobulin (usually IgM); either kappa or lambda immunoglobulin light chain (proving clonality); and pan-B-cell markers such as CD20 and CD23. CD5, a marker mainly expressed on mature T cells, is also expressed by CLL/SLL cells and a few other kinds of B-cell neoplasms.

STAGING

Staging of CLL/SLL is based on the degree of lymphocytosis, other peripheral blood counts, and the presence or absence of lymphadenopathy and organomegaly (Table 22-2). Prognosis is correlated with disease stage. Cytogenetic analysis is also helpful in gauging the prognosis. Specifically, tumors with 13q deletions have the best outcome, whereas those with 11q and 17p deletions have the least favorable prognosis. Additional factors associated with a worse prognosis include the expression of ZAP-70, a signaling protein that is not found in normal B cells. Curiously, tumors with unmutated Ig genes (ie, tumors that have not experienced a germinal center reaction) also have a worse prognosis. Those with SLL are staged by using an approach that is generally applied to all patients with lymphoma (described in the following under *follicular lymphoma*).

TABLE 22-2 Staging of Chronic Lymphocytic Leukemia*

Stage	Findings	Median Survival Time
0	Asymptomatic lymphocytosis	11.5 years
1	Lymphocytosis and lymphadenopathy	11 years
2	Lymphocytosis, lymphadenopathy, and organomegaly**	7.8 years
3	Lymphocytosis and anemia, with or without lymphadenopathy and organomegaly**	about 5 years
4	Lymphocytosis and thrombocytopenia, with or without lymphadenopathy, organomegaly, and anemia	about 5 years

*Based on the Rai classification.
**Organomegaly, enlargement of spleen and/or liver

CLINICAL FEATURES AND TREATMENT

Treatment is usually withheld until patients become symptomatic, which, in those with very early disease, occurs on average 10 or more years after diagnosis; sometimes, no therapy is ever needed. Symptoms are most commonly related to the following:

- Cytopenias caused by replacement of normal marrow progenitors by tumor cells.

- Infections due to poorly understood defects in high-affinity antibody production by normal B cells. Bacterial infections are most common.

- Autoantibodies, which may produce immune thrombocytopenic purpura or immunohemolytic anemia. The autoantibodies are produced by reactive B cells rather than the tumor cells and are another manifestation of the disruption of normal immune function by CLL/SLL.

- Transformation to either an aggressive lymphoma resembling diffuse large B-cell lymphoma (so-called Richter transformation) or an aggressive leukemia resembling B-cell prolymphocytic leukemia. Transformation occurs in about 5% to 10% of patients and represents an ominous development, because such tumors respond poorly to therapy.

CLL/SLL is not currently curable but can be controlled, often for many years, with relatively gentle forms of chemotherapy and/or the anti-B-cell monoclonal antibody rituximab. Patients may eventually succumb due to the development of resistant disease, superimposed infections, or, less commonly, transformation to a more aggressive lymphoma.

FOLLICULAR LYMPHOMA

This is the most common indolent lymphoma. There are about 20,000 new cases per year in the United States. Most patients are asymptomatic at presentation, presenting with only painless lymphadenopathy.

Over 90% of follicular lymphomas are associated with the presence of a (14;18) translocation that juxtaposes the *BCL-2* and IgH genes. The net effect of the translocation is to cause the overexpression of BCL-2, an important inhibitor of apoptosis. Normal germinal center B cells down-regulate BCL-2, which is believed to permit the death of cells that fail to produce high-affinity antibodies during the germinal center reaction, whereas follicular lymphoma cells typically express high levels of BCL-2 protein. Remarkably, germinal center B cells harboring the (14;18) translocation appear to arise from time to time in most normal individuals, very few of whom develop follicular lymphoma. Thus, additional unknown mutations must collaborate with the (14;18) translocation to produce full-blown disease.

DIAGNOSIS

The diagnosis is usually established by lymph node biopsy, which reveals replacement of normal architecture by neoplastic follicles that mimic the appearance of normal germinal centers (Fig. 22-5). Like normal follicles, neoplastic follicles contain a dense meshwork of dendritic cells and scattered T cells, both of which express factors such as CD40 ligand that support the growth and survival of the lymphoma cells. Unlike reactive follicles, in the neoplastic follicles of follicular lymphoma, mitoses are infrequent, single cell necrosis (apoptosis) is usually absent, and BCL-2 protein expression is the rule (Fig. 22-6).

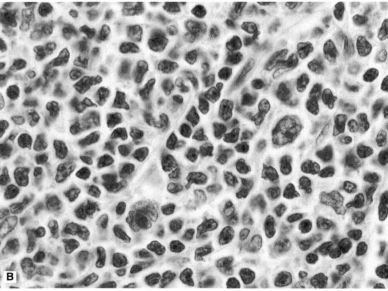

FIGURE 22-5 **Follicular lymphoma, lymph node.** A) At low power, the lymph node is effaced by nodules of neoplastic cells. B) At high power, most of the cells are small, irregular (cleaved) lymphocytes along with a few large lymphoid cells. Note that the mitotic figures and apoptotic cells characteristic of normal germinal centers (Fig. 22-1) are absent.

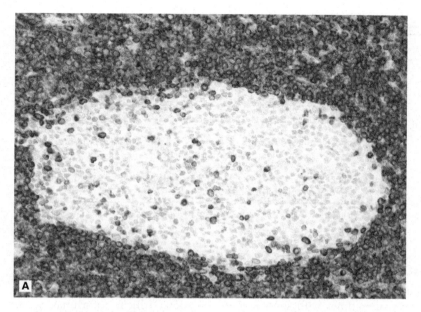

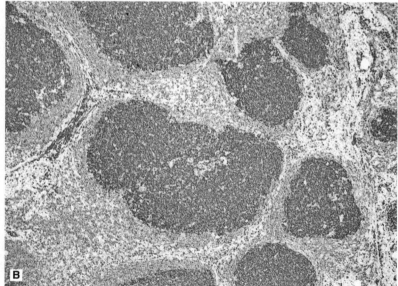

FIGURE 22-6 BCL-2 expression, reactive germinal center versus follicular lymphoma. A) Normal germinal center. The germinal center B cells are negative for BCL-2 protein by immunohistochemistry, whereas the mantle zone B cells and a few germinal center T cells are strongly positive. B) Follicular lymphoma. The neoplastic follicles exhibit strong immunohistochemical staining for BCL-2 protein. Virtually all follicular lymphomas expressing BCL-2 have a (14;18) translocation that fuses the *BCL-2* gene to transcription-promoting elements in the IgH gene.

STAGING

Staging of follicular lymphoma is performed by using a system applicable to all lymphomas that is based on the extent and distribution of disease (Table 22-3). In follicular lymphoma, radiologic imaging typically reveals involvement of multiple lymph node groups on both sides of the diaphragm, and bone marrow biopsy shows overt marrow involvement in over 70% of cases. Thus, most patients have stage IV disease at the time of diagnosis.

TABLE 22-3 Ann Arbor Staging of Lymphoma*

Stage	Distribution of Disease
I	Involvement of a single lymph node group (I) or a single extralymphatic organ or site (IE)
II	Involvement of two or more lymph node groups on the same side of the diaphragm without (II) or with (IIE) localized involvement of an extralymphatic organ or site
III	Involvement of lymph node groups on both sides of the diaphragm without (III) or with (IIIE) localized involvement of an extralymphatic organ or site
IV	Extensive involvement of one or more extralymphatic organs or sites (eg, bone marrow), with or without lymphatic involvement

*Patients are further staged based on the presence (B) or absence (A) of B symptoms.

CLINICAL FEATURES AND TREATMENT

The natural history of follicular lymphoma is one of waxing and waning lymph-adenopathy, sometimes with spontaneous remissions, which, unfortunately, are transient, lasting a median of about 12 months. Patients who are asymptomatic with minimal disease burden require no treatment and are followed expectantly. Treatment is reserved for patients with local symptoms due to progressive or bulky disease with masses of >10 cm, compromised organ function due to disease, B symptoms, symptomatic extranodal disease (eg, pleural effusions), or cytopenias due to bone marrow involvement. Rare patients with early-stage disease can be treated with local radiation, which sometimes produces longstanding remissions and apparent cures in up to 50% of these patients. The majority of patients with advanced-stage disease are treated with chemotherapy and rituximab. Initially this produces excellent responses, but over time, tumors tend to develop resistance to therapy. At present, follicular lymphoma is not usually curable. Of even greater concern, follicular lymphomas can transform to more aggressive tumors resembling diffuse large B-cell lymphoma that often respond poorly to even aggressive chemotherapy. The risk for transformation is about 3% per year.

DIFFUSE LARGE B-CELL LYMPHOMA

Diffuse large B-cell lymphoma (DLBCL) is the most common form of lymphoma in the United States, with about 25,000 newly diagnosed cases per year. It can arise at any age but is most common in older adults; the median age at presentation is 64 years. About two-thirds of DLBCL present within lymph nodes, with the remaining third presenting in extranodal sites, the most common of which is the gastrointestinal tract. However, almost any organ can be involved, either primarily or secondarily.

In DLBCL, the most common molecular lesions are chromosomal transloca-tions and point mutations involving *BCL-6*, a gene encoding a transcription factor required for the development of germinal center B cells. As shown in Figure 22-2, both types of mutations are believed to stem from mistakes that occur during attempted class switching and/or somatic hypermutation in germinal center B cells. These mutations up-regulate the expression of BCL-6, a transcriptional repressor that turns off genes required for the differentiation and/or death of germinal center B cells, thereby promoting their survival and continued proliferation. Molecular analyses and gene expression profiling have revealed that DLBCL is heterogeneous, being composed of at least three major molecular subtypes with differing prognoses.

DIAGNOSIS

Regardless of subtype, DLBCL is an aggressive tumor. Patients usually present with a rapidly enlarging mass or systemic manifestations of lymphoma (B symptoms). In contradistinction to indolent lymphomas and lymphocytic leukemias, the serum lactate dehydrogenase level is elevated in about 50% of patients. The diagnosis is made by tissue biopsy, which, in typical cases, reveals diffuse effacement of tissue architecture by large lymphoid cells (Fig. 22-7), often accompanied by a high mitotic rate and areas of necrosis. Immunophenotyping (either flow cytometry or immunohistochemistry) is essential to establishing the diagnosis. Tumors are typically positive for pan-B-cell markers (eg, CD20), usually express BCL-6, and show variable expression of CD10, BCL-2, and surface immunoglobulin.

STAGING AND PROGNOSIS

Staging is based on physical examination, radiologic studies, and bone marrow examination. Due to the high metabolic rate of the tumor cells, DLBCL is markedly positive by positron emission tomography (PET) scanning (Fig. 22-8), which is increasingly used with conventional radiography and computerized tomography (CT) scanning to stage patients and monitor their responses to therapy. A worse prognosis is associated with patient age >60 years, stage III or IV disease, an elevated serum lactate dehydrogenase level, poor performance status (a high level of disability and debilitation), and more than one extranodal site of involvement.

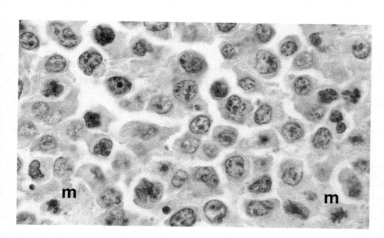

FIGURE 22-7 Diffuse large B-cell lymphoma, lymph node. This high-power field contains a diffuse infiltrate of large lymphoid cells with round to irregular nuclei, open chromatin, several nucleoli, and moderately abundant cytoplasm. Several cells in mitosis (m) are present.

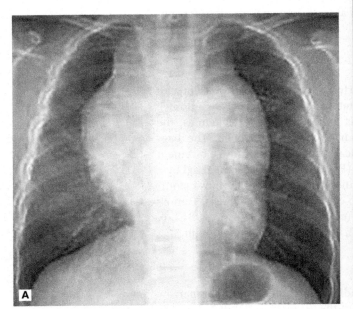
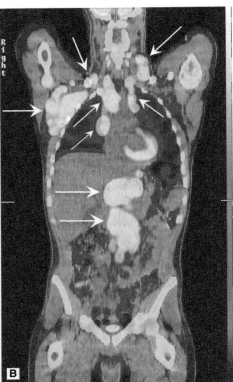

FIGURE 22-8 **Staging of diffuse large B-cell lymphoma (DLBCL) A) Radiologic detection of a large lymphomatous mass involving the mediastinum B) Identification of sites involved by DLBCL by positron emission tomography (PET).** The patient has been injected with ^{18}F deoxyglucose, a radioactive compound that is taken up rapidly by metabolically active tissues and emits positrons upon decay. The image shown represents a three-dimensional reconstruction of the positron emission pattern. The arrows denote abnormal uptake of ^{18}F-deoxyglucose in retroperitoneal, mediastinal, right axillary, and cervical lymph nodes, which is consistent with involvement by lymphoma. (Courtesy of Dr. Ann LaCasce, Dana-Farber Cancer Institute.)

TREATMENT

Patients with DLBCL are treated with combination chemotherapy (CHOP, which consists of cyclophosphamide, doxorubicin, vincristine, and prednisone) plus rituximab. Overall, roughly 50% of patients are cured with this regimen. Patients who fail to respond or relapse generally have a poor prognosis. Only about 25% of relapsed patients treated with aggressive therapies such as stem cell transplantation survive for more than 5 years. A variety of experimental approaches, including targeted therapies, is being explored in this patient group.

BURKITT LYMPHOMA

This highly aggressive lymphoma arises in three distinct clinical settings. It is endemic in subequatorial Africa, where it often occurs in children or young people. In endemic Burkitt lymphoma, the tumor cells are always latently infected with EBV; indeed, Anthony Epstein and Yvonne Barr discovered EBV in 1964 in lymphoma specimens sent to London by Denis Burkitt, who was then working in Kampala, Uganda. Most patients with sporadic Burkitt lymphoma are also infected with malaria, which is believed to be a cofactor in the tumor's development. In the United States, Burkitt lymphoma mainly occurs in sporadic form in children and adolescents, in whom it is also associated with EBV, but only in about 30% of cases. Finally, Burkitt lymphoma may occur in association with immunodeficiency, particularly in those infected with HIV; here too, a minority of cases is associated with EBV.

The molecular hallmark of Burkitt lymphoma is chromosomal translocations involving the *c-MYC* oncogene on chromosome 8q. Usually, *c-MYC* is translocated into the IgH locus on chromosome 14; less commonly, its partners are the kappa or lambda light chain loci on chromosomes 2 and 22, respectively. The net effect of all of these rearrangements is the same: the overexpression of c-MYC protein. c-MYC is a transcription factor that serves as a master regulator of genes that govern cellular metabolism, and its overexpression drives a pattern of gene expression that maximizes cell growth. In line with this, Burkitt lymphoma is one of the fastest growing human tumors.

DIAGNOSIS

Most Burkitt lymphomas arise in extranodal sites, often within the abdomen, such as the gut. The rapidly growing tumor mass produces local symptoms that usually bring the tumor to attention. Biopsy reveals diffuse effacement of tissue by intermediate-sized tumor cells, many of which are either in mitosis or are undergoing apoptosis and being consumed by reactive macrophages (Fig. 22-9). The process creates clear spaces within histologic sections of the tumor, producing a characteristic "starry sky" appearance. By immunohistochemistry, tumors are positive for B-cell (eg, CD20) and germinal center B-cell markers (CD10 and BCL-6) but almost always fail to express BCL-2. Typically, markers of actively growing cells (such as Ki-67) are positive in every cell in the tumor. Cytogenetic analysis (either karyotyping or fluorescence in situ hybridization) is used to detect the characteristic *c-MYC* rearrangements.

CLINICAL FEATURES

Prognosis and treatment are influenced by stage, patient age, and clinical setting. Endemic Burkitt lymphoma is often localized to a single extranodal site and is exquisitely sensitive to chemotherapy, but these features do not hold for sporadic or immunodeficiency-associated disease. In addition, sporadic and HIV-associated Burkitt lymphomas show a strong tendency to spread to the central nervous system, often necessitating prophylactic treatment of this site. Excellent outcomes in sporadic Burkitt lymphoma have been achieved with very intensive chemotherapy regimens of short duration coupled with intrathecal therapy to treat and/or prevent disease in the central nervous system. As in patients with acute leukemia, cytotoxic therapies cause rapid, massive tumor cell death, and special care must be taken to avoid tumor lysis syndrome (Chapter 21). Treatment of HIV-associated disease is more difficult because these patients tend to tolerate high-dose chemotherapy regimens poorly.

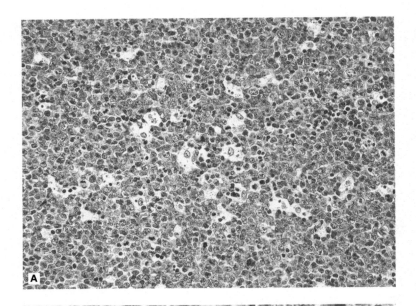

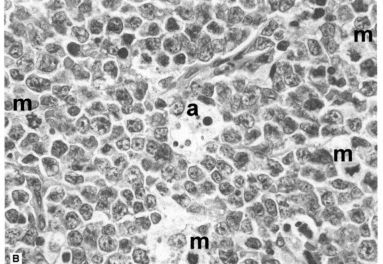

FIGURE 22-9 Burkitt lymphoma, lymph node. A) Intermediate power. The lymph is diffusely effaced by a lymphoid proliferation with interspersed macrophages that produce clear spaces (starry sky appearance). B) High power. The proliferation is composed of lymphoid cells of intermediate size. Note the presence of frequent mitoses (m) and scattered macrophages containing apoptotic cells (a).

T-CELL LYMPHOMAS

T-cell lymphomas are rare but worthy of brief discussion due to their distinctive biological and clinical features. Except for adult T-cell leukemia/lymphoma caused by HTLV-1 infection (already discussed), the causes of these tumors remain mysterious. Some types of T-cell lymphoma preferentially involve particular tissues, a propensity that stems from the expression of homing receptors or *addressins* on their surfaces, which also are used by their normal nontransformed

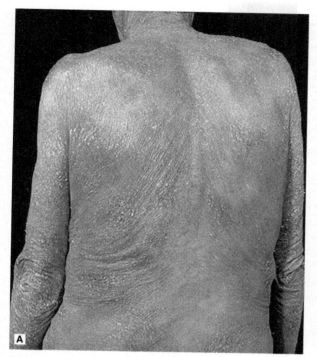
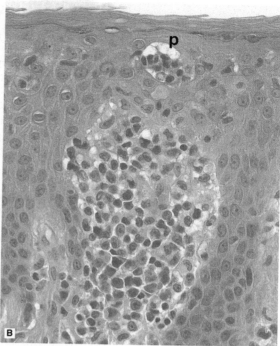

FIGURE 22-10 **Cutaneous T-cell lymphoma.** A) The skin of this patient is heavily involved by lymphoma, which produces diffuse reddening (erythroderma), thickening, and scaling. B) A skin biopsy revealed a dermal infiltrate of irregular lymphoid cells that extends into the epidermis (so-called epidermotropism). A Pautrier abscess (p, an intraepidermal collection of tumor cells) is present, a feature that is commonly seen in cutaneous T-cell lymphoma. (Figure A: Assaf C, Sterry W. Cutaneous lymphoma. In: Wolff K, Goldsmith LA, Katz SI, Gilchrest BA, Paller AS, Leffell DJ, eds. *Fitzpatrick's Dermatology in General Medicine*, 7th edition. New York, United States: McGraw-Hill; 2008: p. 1390.)

counterparts. For example, cutaneous T-cell lymphoma expresses two skin-specific addressins, the adhesion molecule *common leukocyte antigen* and the chemokine receptor *CCR4*, which explain its remarkable tropism for the skin (Fig. 22-10). Other types of T-cell lymphoma home to other tissues, including the small bowel (enteropathy-associated T-cell lymphoma) and even the subcutis (panniculitic T-cell lymphoma). However, like B-cell lymphomas, T-cell lymphomas most commonly present with lymph node involvement. Their diagnosis requires a tissue biopsy and immunophenotyping, often coupled with molecular tests of clonality.

In part due to their rarity and heterogeneity, the molecular pathogenesis of T-cell lymphomas is poorly understood. They often are complicated by B symptoms and immunodysregulation, which may take the form of hypogammaglobulinemia or production of autoantibodies by nontransformed B cells. Cutaneous T-cell lymphoma follows an indolent course but unfortunately is an outlier among T-cell lymphomas, which are generally more aggressive, less responsive to chemotherapy, and much less curable than B-cell lymphomas.

SELF-ASSESSMENT STUDY QUESTIONS

1. A previously healthy, 76-year-old man presented with a 1-month history of fatigue and a 10-pound weight loss over the prior 4 months, in spite of a balanced diet and use of a standard multiple vitamin. He had no fevers or night sweats. The patient did not appear acutely ill. Findings included pallor, slight jaundice, and mild symmetric adenopathy with 1.0-cm lymph nodes palpable in the anterior cervical regions bilaterally, the axillae, and the inguinal region. The liver and spleen were not enlarged, and there was no clubbing, edema, or cyanosis. Neurologic examination results were normal.

   Initial laboratory values:
   Hemoglobin 7.5 g/dL
   Hematocrit 22%
   Mean cell volume 100 fL
   White blood cell count 86,000/mm³
   Differential count 86% lymphocytes, 11% polymorphonuclear cells, 2% monocytes, 1% eosinophils
   Platelet count 151,000/mm³
   Reticulocyte count 11%

   The peripheral blood smear showed predominantly normal-appearing, mature lymphocytes; no blasts were seen. About 30% of the red cells appeared small and lacked central pallor.

   Other laboratory values:
   Lactate dehydrogenase 880 U/L (elevated)
   Total bilirubin 3.6 mg/dL (elevated)
   Direct (conjugated) bilirubin 0.1 mg/dL (normal)
   Iron 80 µg/dL (normal)
   Total iron binding capacity 260 µg/dL (normal)
   Ferritin 400 ng/mL (normal)

   A. What is the bone marrow examination on this patient likely to show?
   B. What is the most likely white cell disorder?
   C. What additional test(s) would confirm the diagnosis?
   D. Why is the patient so anemic?
   E. What additional test(s) would confirm the cause of the anemia?
   F. On the blood film, many of the red cells appear small, and yet the mean cell volume is elevated. Give a plausible explanation for this apparent contradiction.
   G. Why is the nonconjugated bilirubin level elevated?

2. All of the following have been associated with non-Hodgkin lymphoma except:
   A. *Helicobacter pylori* gastritis.
   B. Treatment with immunosuppressive agents.
   C. Patient age greater than 60.
   D. Epstein-Barr virus.
   E. Human herpesvirus-8.
   F. Cytomegalovirus.

3. Match the tumor and the molecular lesion.

   A. Follicular lymphoma
   B. Adult T-cell leukemia
   C. Diffuse large B-cell lymphoma
   D. Burkitt lymphoma
   E. Chronic lymphocytic leukemia

   1. Translocations involving *c-MYC*
   2. Translocations involving *BCL-2*
   3. Mutations involving *BCL-6*
   4. Retroviral infection
   5. Deletions of chromosome 13

Hodgkin Lymphoma

Jon C. Aster and Arnold Freedman

LEARNING OBJECTIVES

After studying this chapter you should understand:

- The origin of the tumor cell of Hodgkin lymphoma, the Reed-Sternberg cell.
- The origin of the reactive infiltrate that surrounds Reed-Sternberg cells.
- The pathologic and clinical distinctions between Hodgkin lymphoma and non-Hodgkin lymphoma.

Hodgkin lymphoma bears the name of Thomas Hodgkin, who described the disease in 1832. It affects about 8500 patients each year in the United States and is distinguished from all other forms of lymphoma (the non-Hodgkin lymphomas) by several unique pathologic and biologic features.

- The presence of Reed-Sternberg cells or variants and peculiar tumor giant cells within an exuberant tissue response consisting of reactive lymphocytes, granulocytes, macrophages, and plasma cells. Unlike virtually all other forms of cancer, in Hodgkin lymphoma the tumor cells make up a small fraction (often <1%) of the overall tumor mass.

- A strong tendency to arise within a single lymph node group and to spread in a predictable, stepwise fashion from one lymph node group to the next. As a result, staging has a greater influence on the treatment of Hodgkin lymphoma than on non-Hodgkin lymphomas.

CLASSIFICATION OF HODGKIN LYMPHOMA

Hodgkin lymphoma is divided into five major pathologic subtypes based on differences in the appearance of the Reed-Sternberg cells and variants as well as the composition of the reactive cellular response:

- Nodular sclerosis. This form is most common in young adults and sometimes occurs in adolescents and even children. It is characterized by two pathologic findings: 1) the presence of a particular type of Reed-Sternberg cell variant, the *lacunar cell* (Fig. 23-1A), and 2) the presence of large bands of collagen that are deposited by reactive fibroblasts. The reactive background consists of a variable mixture of lymphocytes (mainly T cells), granulocytes (particularly eosinophils), macrophages, and plasma cells. The nodular sclerosis subtype is only rarely associated with Epstein-Barr virus (EBV).

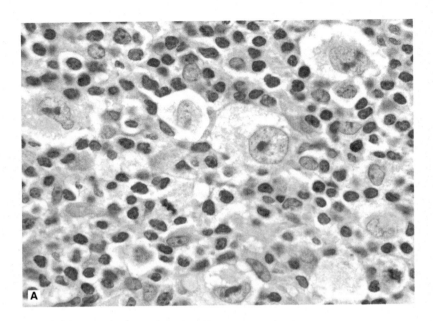

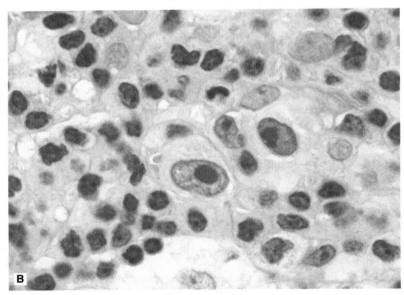

FIGURE 23-1 Reed-Sternberg cells. A) Lacunar variants are seen within spaces created by tearing away of the wispy cytoplasm during tissue sectioning. B) Mononuclear variant. A large mononuclear variant with a single, enormous, eosinophilic nucleolus is present in the middle of the field. C) Diagnostic Reed-Sternberg cell. A classic Reed-Sternberg cell with two nuclei, each with a large nucleolus, and abundant cytoplasm is shown. D) L&H variants. Two typical lymphocytic and histiocytic variants with polypoid, folded nuclei are denoted with asterisks.

- Mixed cellularity. This subtype is most common in older males in the United States but also occurs in young adults and children, particularly in parts of the developing world such as Peru. Lymph nodes are diffusely effaced by a polymorphous infiltrate composed of a mixture of inflammatory cells, scattered classic Reed-Sternberg cells (Fig. 23-1C), and relatively frequent mononuclear Reed-Sternberg variants (Fig. 23-1B). About 70% of cases are associated with EBV (Fig. 23-2).

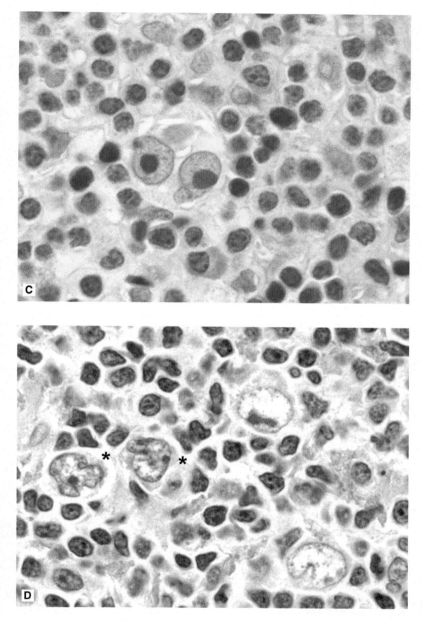

FIGURE 23-1 (*Continued*)

- Lymphocyte rich. This is an uncommon subtype in which the predominant cellular response consists of lymphocytes. About 40% of cases are associated with EBV.

- Lymphocyte depleted. This is a rare subtype except in human immunodeficiency virus (HIV)-positive patients. Frequent Reed-Sternberg cells are seen in involved tissue sections, whereas the host response to these cells is relatively

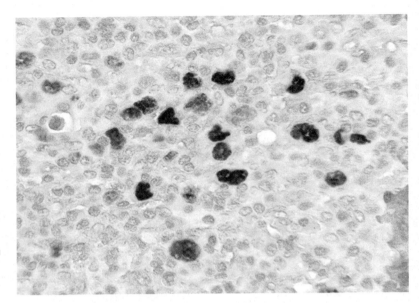

FIGURE 23-2 **Detection of Epstein-Barr virus (EBV) in Reed-Sternberg cells.** EBV small nuclear ribonucleic acids were detected with a chromogenic in situ staining method that produces a brown color. In this field, the nuclei of multiple Reed-Sternberg cells stain positively.

sparse. It is almost always associated with EBV, particularly in those who are HIV positive.

- Nodular lymphocyte predominant. This uncommon subtype (5% of cases) most often arises in young to middle-aged males within axillary or cervical lymph nodes. The tumor cells have nuclei that are lobulated or popcorn kernel–like (Fig. 23-1D); classic Reed-Sternberg cells are rare or absent. For historic reasons, the tumor cells in this subtype are referred to as *lymphocytic and histiocytic* variants, or L&H cells. L&H cells are typically present within nodular aggregates of B lymphocytes, which represent expanded B-cell follicles. This form of Hodgkin lymphoma is not associated with EBV.

Until relatively recently, the nature of the malignant Reed-Sternberg cells in Hodgkin lymphoma was obscure, in part because their paucity in tissues made them very difficult to study. This long-standing mystery was finally solved by elegant studies using individual Reed-Sternberg cells isolated from tissues. These revealed that in all forms of Hodgkin lymphoma the Reed-Sternberg cells have clonal rearranged immunoglobulin heavy chain genes that have undergone somatic hypermutation, proving that these cells are derived from germinal center B cells. Nevertheless, except in the nodular lymphocyte predominant subtype, Reed-Sternberg cells fail to express most B-cell markers and often instead express markers of other cell types, such as granulocytes, macrophages, or even hematopoietic stem cells. This wholesale reprogramming of gene expression contributed mightily to difficulties in determining the origin of Reed-Sternberg cells. The mechanisms underlying this phenomenon are largely unknown.

The characteristic tissue reaction in Hodgkin lymphoma is elicited by a variety of chemokines and cytokines produced by Reed-Sternberg cells, which include chemoattractants and growth factors for T cells, granulocytes, and macrophages

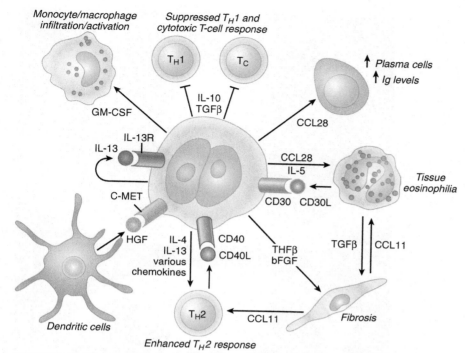

FIGURE 23-3 Cross-talk between Reed-Sternberg cells and inflammatory cells. Some of the more important receptors and factors that contribute to the brisk inflammatory response around Reed-Sternberg cells in tissues are shown. (Diseases of White Blood Cells, Lymph Nodes, Spleen, and Thymus. In: Kumar V, Abbas A, Fausto N, and Aster JC, eds. *Robbins Pathologic Basis of Disease*. 8th ed. Philadelphia, United States: Elsevier; 2010: p.621.)

(Fig. 23-3). Various subtypes elaborate different combinations of factors, some of the most important of which include the following:

- Interleukin (IL)-4, IL-10, and IL-13, which act together to promote humoral immunity and suppress cellular immunity.

- Granulocyte-macrophage colony-stimulating factor (GM-CSF), which can lead to hyperplasia of marrow granulocytic and monocytic progenitors, leukocytosis, and infiltration of lymphomatous tissues by neutrophils and macrophages.

- CCL28 and IL-5, which increase marrow production of eosinophils and provoke peripheral blood and tissue eosinophilia.

- Tumor necrosis factor (TNF)-beta (lymphotoxin) and basic fibroblast growth factor, which activate fibroblasts and stimulate fibrosis, particularly in the nodular sclerosis subtype.

Although the etiology of Hodgkin lymphoma is incompletely understood, some of the molecular events that lead to its development have been discovered. In cases associated with EBV, the tumor cells express latent membrane protein-1, an EBV protein that acts like a constitutively active version of the TNF receptor.

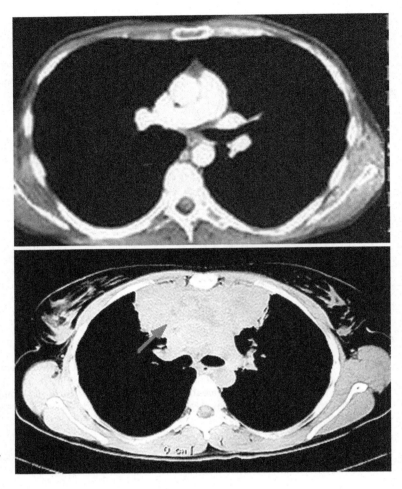

FIGURE 23-4 Mediastinal involvement by Hodgkin lymphoma, nodular sclerosis subtype. The upper image is a normal chest computed tomography (CT) scan. The lower image is the chest CT scan of a patient with a large mediastinal mass that proved on biopsy to be nodular sclerosis Hodgkin lymphoma.

Latent membrane protein-1 turns on nuclear factor-kappa B (NF-κB), a transcription factor that promotes the growth and survival of B cells. It was subsequently determined that EBV-negative cases are often associated with mutations that disrupt the function of IκB and A20, two negative regulators of NF-κB. Thus, activation of NF-κB is believed to be a central event in the pathogenesis of Hodgkin lymphoma.

Regardless of the subtype, most patients with Hodgkin lymphoma present with painless lymphadenopathy, most commonly in the cervical or supraclavicular region.[1] The nodular sclerosis type usually also involves the mediastinum (Fig. 23-4), often inducing chest discomfort, cough, or dyspnea. On occasion, lymphomatous masses in the mediastinum impinge on blood return to the heart and produce superior vena cava syndrome, associated with plethora (redness)

---

[1]An extreme example of lymphadenopathy in Hodgkin disease is shown in the frontispiece that precedes this section on hematologic malignancies (p 199).

and swelling of the face and upper extremities. About one-third of patients have so-called B symptoms such as weight loss and night sweats, and many also complain of pruritus. Laboratory studies often show leukocytosis and eosinophilia, sometimes accompanied by anemia related to the systemic inflammatory state induced by the tumor (anemia of chronic inflammation).

DIAGNOSIS

The diagnosis requires a biopsy of involved tissues, usually a lymph node, and is primarily based on the identification of typical Reed-Sternberg cells and variants within the appropriate cellular background. Cells resembling Reed-Sternberg cells can be found on occasion in non-Hodgkin lymphomas and even in some solid tumors, and immunohistochemical studies are typically carried out to confirm suspected cases of Hodgkin lymphoma. In the nodular sclerosis, mixed cellularity, lymphocyte-rich, and lymphocyte-depleted subtypes (sometimes referred to together as *classical Hodgkin lymphoma*), the tumor cells are usually positive for CD15 (an adhesion molecule often expressed on myeloid cells), always positive for CD30 (a member of the tumor necrosis factor receptor family), and negative for CD45 (leukocyte common antigen). In classical Hodgkin lymphoma, the tumor cells are also positive for PAX-5, a transcription factor that is a master regulator of B-cell development, but the tumor cells of classical Hodgkin lymphoma usually are negative for other B-cell markers (eg, CD20). A significant proportion of classical Hodgkin lymphomas (particularly the mixed cellularity and uncommon lymphocyte-depleted subtypes) is positive for EBV. In contrast, the L&H variants of nodular lymphocyte-predominant Hodgkin lymphoma are uniformly positive for B-cell markers such as CD20 and negative for CD15, CD30, and EBV, further distinguishing this subtype.

PROGNOSIS AND TREATMENT

The overall prognosis for patients with Hodgkin lymphoma is excellent, even in those with advanced disease. As mentioned previously, staging plays a key role in guiding the selection of therapy. Patients with localized, low-stage disease without B symptoms (stages IA and IIA) are currently treated with involved field radiation and limited chemotherapy, whereas those with high-stage disease are treated with combination chemotherapy, sometimes with radiotherapy if bulky masses are present. Responses to both are excellent, and, overall, 60% to 90% of patients are now cured.

The treatment of Hodgkin lymphoma represents a major success in oncology but has come with a price. More patients now die of complications of therapy than from Hodgkin lymphoma itself. These iatrogenic complications take the form of accelerated cardiovascular disease, valvular heart disease, and a wide variety of secondary malignancies (including melanoma, sarcoma, and breast cancer), all of which appear to be related mainly to radiation exposure 15 to 20 years prior to the development of these adverse events. Earlier chemotherapy regimens were also culpable, because they contained alkylating agents that were potent inducers of myelodysplastic syndromes and secondary acute myeloid leukemias. Newer chemotherapy regimens do not appear to be leukemogenic, and clinical research is now being conducted to evaluate treatment with chemotherapy alone, in hope of developing safe, curative treatment regimens that minimize or completely avoid complications associated with radiotherapy.

SELF-ASSESSMENT STUDY QUESTIONS:

1. The best evidence that Reed-Sternberg cells are derived from B cells came from:
    A. DNA sequencing.
    B. Immunophenotyping.
    C. Histology.
    D. Southern blotting.
    E. Viral studies.

2. The inflammatory response to Reed-Sternberg cells in Hodgkin lymphoma is:
    A. Triggered by products released from dying Reed-Sternberg cells.
    B. Generated by EBV antigens expressed by Reed-Sternberg cells.
    C. Rarely accompanied by systemic symptoms.
    D. Not usually associated with detectable laboratory test result abnormalities.
    E. The product of factors expressed by Reed-Sternberg cells.

3. Which of the following statements concerning the treatment of Hodgkin lymphoma is not true?
    A. It is guided by imaging to assess the stage of disease.
    B. It often includes splenectomy.
    C. It is based on a diagnosis rendered on a tissue sample.
    D. It is highly effective, even in advanced disease.
    E. It may include radiation, chemotherapy, or a combination of both modalities.

Multiple Myeloma and Related Disorders

Jon C. Aster

L E A R N I N G   O B J E C T I V E S

After studying this chapter you should understand:

- The causes and consequences of bone disease, renal dysfunction, and immunodeficiency in multiple myeloma.
- The diagnosis and treatment of multiple myeloma.
- The major pathologic and clinical features of the other plasma cell and lymphoplasmacytic neoplasms.

Neoplasms composed of plasma cells have special biological and clinical features related to their capacity to secrete complete or partial immunoglobulin (Ig) proteins. By far the most important of these tumors is multiple myeloma, which is diagnosed in about 15,000 patients per year in the United States. It is a tumor of older adults, with a median age at diagnosis of 69 years. For unknown reasons, it is more common in people of African descent.

MULTIPLE MYELOMA

As the name implies, at diagnosis multiple myeloma typically involves multiple bones of the axial skeleton, particularly the vertebrae, skull, proximal long bones of the extremities, and the ribs. The pathophysiology of the disease is primarily related to four factors:

- Pathogenic antibodies or antibody fragments. Normal antibodies are composed of two heavy chains encoded by the IgH locus and two light chains, which may be encoded by either the Ig kappa or the Ig lambda locus. Multiple myeloma cells most commonly secrete IgG or IgA antibodies. However, in addition to complete antibodies, neoplastic plasma cells usually also secrete free, unpaired Ig light chains; indeed, in about 20% of cases, only light chains are secreted. The small size of the light chains (around 25 kDa) permits them to pass from the blood through the filtration slits of the renal glomeruli and into the renal tubules. Once in the urinary space, Ig light chains are toxic to renal epithelial cells and tend to form precipitates and obstructive casts, both of which contribute to renal dysfunction (Fig. 24-1). Free light chains, particularly lambda light chains, are also prone to form

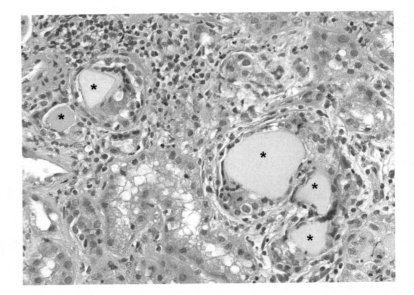

FIGURE 24-1 **Myeloma kidney.**
The asterisks mark renal tubules that are obstructed by light pink casts composed of immunoglobulin light chains mixed with a number of other proteins. The casts have elicited an inflammatory response consisting of macrophages, lymphocytes, and a few eosinophils. (Courtesy of Dr. Helmut Rennke, Department of Pathology, Brigham and Women's Hospital.)

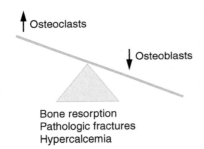

↑ Osteoclasts

↓ Osteoblasts

Bone resorption
Pathologic fractures
Hypercalcemia

amyloid, fibrillar deposits that may be found in the renal glomeruli (Fig. 24-2) and the perivascular spaces of many tissues, including the liver, spleen, and heart. Renal amyloidosis often causes nephrotic syndrome, the spilling of albumin and other plasma proteins into the urine. Alternatively, instead of forming amyloid, free light chains sometimes accumulate in amorphous linear deposits in the kidney and other tissues that produce light chain deposition disease (Fig. 24-3). In more than 85% of cases these light chain deposits are composed of kappa light chains. Light chain deposition disease most commonly presents as renal dysfunction but can also cause clinically significant hepatic or cardiac failure.

- Bone resorption. Bone resorption is caused by tumor-derived factors such as MIP1α and modulators of the Wnt signaling pathway, which act together to suppress osteoblast function and enhance osteoclast function (Fig. 24-4). Tilting this balance leads to marked thinning of bone, setting the stage for pathologic fractures, bone pain, and often hypercalcemia.

- Suppression of humoral immunity. The proliferation of malignant plasma cells somehow inhibits normal B-cell function and the production of normal antibodies, resulting in an increased susceptibility to bacterial infections.

- Renal failure. The deleterious effects of free light chains and light chain deposits on renal function already have been mentioned. These effects are compounded by bacterial infections (pyelonephritis) and hypercalcemia. The kidney is very vulnerable to this panoply of deleterious insults, which lead to overt renal failure in roughly 50% of myeloma patients.

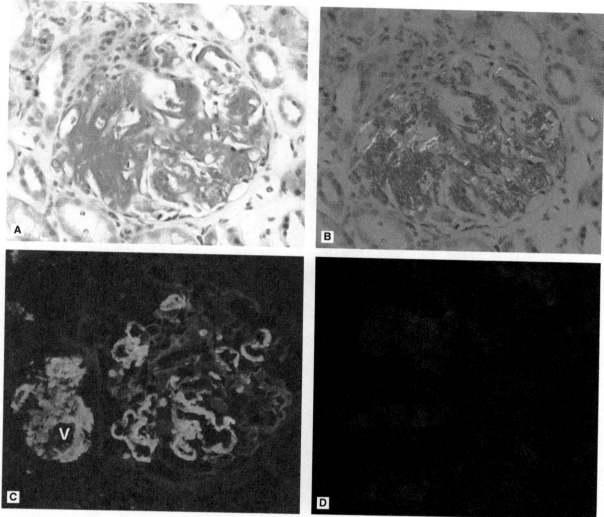

FIGURE 24-2 **Light chain amyloidosis.** A) The capillary walls of this glomerulus contain amorphous deposits that stain positive with the dye Congo red, which selectively binds to amyloid. B) When viewed under polarized light, amyloid stained with Congo red appears green (so-called apple green birefringence), a highly characteristic feature. C, D) Immunofluorescent staining carried out with antibodies specific for lambda (C) and kappa (D) immunoglobulin light chains demonstrates that the amyloid is derived from lambda light chain. Note in *C* that amyloid is deposited both in the capillaries of the glomerulus and in the adjacent wall of the afferent vessel (V), highlighting the tendency of amyloid to deposit in vessel walls throughout the body. (Courtesy of Dr. Helmut Rennke, Department of Pathology, Brigham and Women's Hospital.)

The IgH genes of myeloma cells have undergone class switching and somatic hypermutation, indicating that the tumor is composed of the progeny of an antigen-stimulated germinal center B cell. One IgH gene is typically productively rearranged, permitting the cell to make a monoclonal immunoglobulin, whereas in about 60% to 70% of cases the second IgH gene is involved by one of a diverse set of chromosomal translocations associated with myeloma. The most

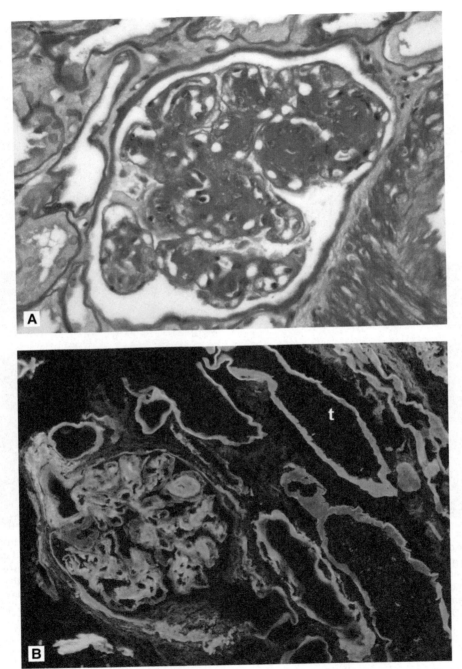

FIGURE 24-3 Light chain deposition disease. A) The glomerulus contains deposits that are positive with the periodic acid-Schiff (PAS) stain. B) Immunofluorescent staining carried out with antibodies specific for kappa and lambda immunoglobulin light chains demonstrates linear deposits of kappa light chain in the glomerulus and in the basement membranes of the renal tubules (t). (Courtesy of Dr. Helmut Rennke, Department of Pathology, Brigham and Women's Hospital.)

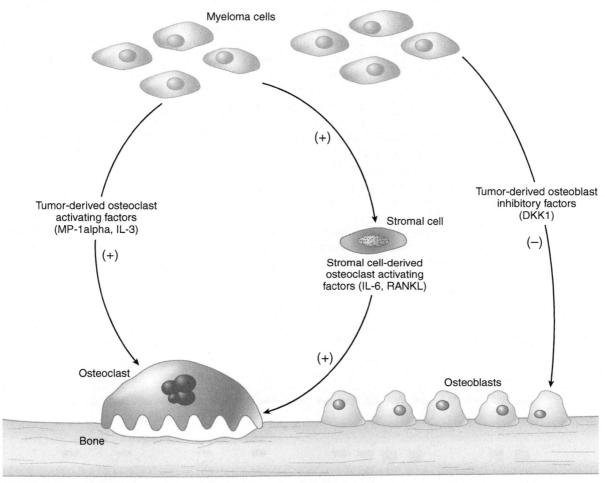

FIGURE 24-4 Mechanisms of bone resorption in multiple myeloma. Myeloma cells stimulate the maturation and function of osteoclasts both directly, via release of factors such as macrophage inhibitory factor-1 alpha and interleukin (IL)-3, and indirectly by stimulating marrow stromal cells to release osteoclastogenic factors such as receptor activator of NF-kappa B ligand (RANKL) and IL-6. At the same time, myeloma cells also release factors such as Dickkopf-1 (DKK-1) that suppress the activity of osteoblasts. The net effect of these alterations is to strongly favor bone resorption. (Modified with permission from Roodman, GD. Pathogenesis of myeloma bone disease. Leukemia 2009:23; 435-441.)

common genes participating along with IgH in these translocations are cyclin D1, an important cell cycle regulator; FGFR3, a receptor tyrosine kinase; and c-MAF, a transcription factor. It appears that most if not all tumors are associated with dysregulation of one of the three human D cyclin genes (cyclin D1, D2, and D3). Many tumors also have deletions of chromosome 13q, the site of the retinoblastoma (Rb) tumor suppressor gene. D cyclin dysregulation and loss of Rb function likely act together to promote the proliferation of the neoplastic plasma cells. Myeloma cells also rely on interactions with stromal cells in the bone marrow microenvironment for signals that enhance their growth and survival. The molecular details of this dependency are still being defined, but certain therapies appear to act, at least in part, by disrupting the interaction of myeloma cells with stromal cells in the marrow.

Myeloma usually presents insidiously with symptoms related to anemia, renal failure, bone resorption, or hypercalcemia. Occasional patients experience the sudden onset of pain due to a pathologic fracture in a long bone, a rib, or a vertebra. Other patients become ill due to bacterial infections brought on by the acquired hypogammaglobulinemia. The diagnosis is based on a combination of laboratory, radiologic, and pathologic findings. Greater than 80% of tumors secrete excessive amounts of a complete monoclonal antibody (an M protein), which can be detected and quantified by serum protein electrophoresis (Fig. 24-5A). Once an M protein is identified, the specific type of antibody (eg, IgA, IgG, kappa or lambda light chain) is determined by immunofixation (Fig. 24-5B), which typically also confirms a decrease in normal polyclonal antibodies. Free light chains in the urine

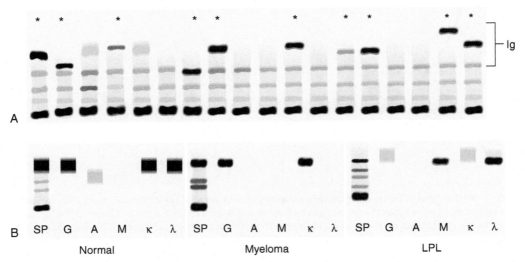

FIGURE 24-5 M protein detection and characterization. A) Serum protein electrophoresis. In this test, serum proteins are separated based on size and charge by electrophoresis in an agarose gel, which is then stained with a protein dye. Lanes marked with an asterisk contain a sharply focused band within the region of the gel to which immunoglobulin (Ig) migrates, an appearance that is indicative of the presence of a monoclonal immunoglobulin (an M protein). Note that each M protein migrates differently, reflecting the fact that each has its own unique amino acid sequence. The amount of M protein is quantified based on its staining intensity. B) Once an M protein is detected, it is further characterized by immunofixation. In this assay, the same sample is loaded in multiple lanes and separated by electrophoresis as in A. One lane is stained for total protein (SP), whereas the other individual lanes are incubated with antibodies specific for various immunoglobulin heavy chains (G, A, or M) and light chains (κ, *kappa* or λ, *lambda*) and then washed extensively. Any antibody-antibody complexes that form in the gel are resistant to removal during washing; these "immunofixed" proteins are detected with a protein stain. Immunoglobulins in normal serum (*left panel*) are of many different types and therefore appear as a broad smear. In contrast, in multiple myeloma, a single major sharp immunoglobulin band is seen in the lanes stained for IgG heavy chain and kappa light chain, indicating the presence of an IgG-kappa M protein. Note also that normal immunoglobulins are suppressed in this sample, a hallmark of myeloma. The right hand panel contains serum from a patient with lymphoplasmacytic lymphoma (LPL) that is associated with production of an IgM-lambda M protein. Unlike the myeloma sample, this serum has relatively preserved levels of polyclonal immunoglobulin.

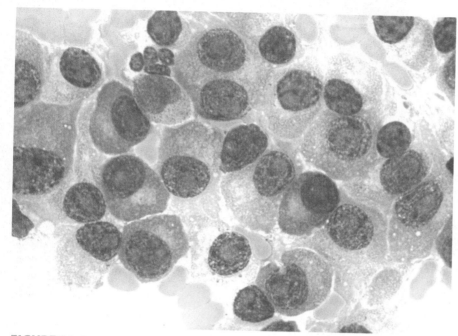

FIGURE 24-6 **Multiple myeloma, bone marrow aspirate.** Most of the cellularity consists of abnormally large plasma cells with enormous nucleoli, a feature that is often seen in multiple myeloma.

(Bence Jones proteins) can be detected and quantified by using the same methods and also can be measured in the serum by using recently developed, highly sensitive free light chain tests. Of note, standard urine dipstick tests detect only negatively charged proteins, such as albumin, and do not detect free light chains, which typically bear a net positive charge.

The other key diagnostic tests include bone marrow examination (biopsy and aspirate), radiologic surveys, and additional laboratory studies. In most patients with full-blown disease, more than 30% of the marrow cellularity consists of plasma cells, which often exhibit unusual morphologic features, including prominent nucleoli (Fig. 24-6), multinucleation, or intracellular inclusions composed of immunoglobulin that may take the form of globular droplets or even crystals. However, in some symptomatic patients, the marrow sample contains only a low percentage of plasma cells; in these instances, other criteria must be used to establish the diagnosis. These include the radiologic identification of characteristic "punched out" lytic skeletal lesions (Fig. 24-7), which are produced by expanding masses of plasma cells (plasmacytomas), and the laboratory documentation of hypercalcemia, renal failure, and anemia.

The course in multiple myeloma is highly variable. Some patients with minimal symptoms have an indolent or smoldering form of the disease that is compatible with survival for a decade or more. Most patients, however, have progressive disease with all of its systemic complications. High concentrations of M-protein

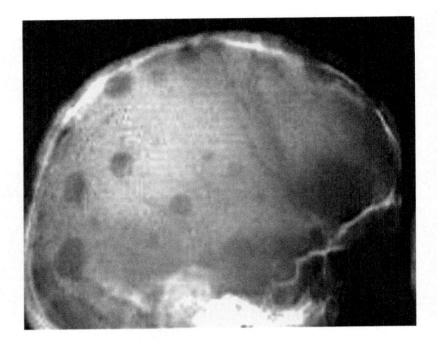

FIGURE 24-7 Lytic bone lesions, multiple myeloma. This radiograph of the skull shows multiple radiolucencies, each corresponding to a plasmacytoma associated with bone resorption. (Courtesy of Dr. Paul Richardson, Dana-Farber Cancer Institute.)

in the serum or light chains in the urine, multiple lytic bone lesions, moderately severe anemia (hemoglobin <8.5 g/dL), or marked hypercalcemia (calcium >12 mg/dL) are all associated with a worse prognosis.

Until recently, most patients were treated with standard chemotherapy, which usually produced transient responses and was associated with an average survival of 3 to 5 years. The picture has brightened considerably with the addition of proteasome inhibitors, thalidomide analogs such as lenalidomide, and bisphosphonates to the therapeutic armamentarium. Plasma cells are very sensitive to proteasome inhibitors, possibly because these drugs prevent the degradation of misfolded proteins (such as unpaired light chains), inducing a stress response that leads to apoptosis. Thalidomide analogs may act by interfering with interactions between myeloma cells and the marrow stroma. Bisphosphonates, drugs that inhibit osteoclast activity, are used to minimize bone resorption and thereby lessen hypercalcemia and pathologic fractures. Bone marrow transplantation is being tested experimentally. To date, no treatment has been proven to be curative in myeloma, but these new treatments have roughly doubled the median survival, providing reason for optimism.

OTHER PLASMA CELL NEOPLASMS

In addition to multiple myeloma, a number of other closely related plasma cell tumors have been described:

- Solitary osseous plasmacytoma. As the name implies, this is an isolated destructive lesion of bone. Over the course of 10 years, about 70% of these tumors evolve to multiple myeloma.

- Extraosseous plasmacytoma. These clonal plasma cell proliferations arise in soft tissues, most commonly in the oropharynx and gastrointestinal tract. They are usually localized and, unlike solitary osseous plasmacytoma, only rarely progress to systemic disease. Many are seemingly cured by simple excision.

- Monoclonal gammopathy of uncertain significance (MGUS). Roughly 3% of people over age 50 and 5% of people over age 70 have low levels of a M-protein in their sera. People with MGUS are by definition asymptomatic. The clonal plasma cells in MGUS harbor many of the same genetic aberrations found in full-blown myeloma, such as chromosomal translocations involving the IgH gene, indicating that MGUS is a precursor lesion. Indeed, MGUS transforms to myeloma at a rate of about 1% per year.

- Monoclonal immunoglobulin deposition diseases. Sometimes patients develop symptomatic amyloidosis or light chain deposition disease before sufficient tumor burden develops to meet the diagnostic criteria for myeloma.

The prognosis in this group of disorders is generally excellent, the principle risk being progression to full-blown myeloma with all of its attendant clinical problems. The exception is in monoclonal immunoglobulin deposition diseases, particularly amyloidosis, which has a poor prognosis even in the absence of progression to myeloma. Most affected patients eventually succumb to the accumulation of amyloid in the kidney, liver, and heart, which leads to renal failure, liver failure, and restrictive cardiomyopathy, sometimes complicated by cardiac conduction defects.

LYMPHOPLASMACYTIC LYMPHOMA

This rare B-cell lymphoma is mentioned briefly because its clinical features, like those of myeloma, often stem from the overproduction of a monoclonal antibody. Lymphoplasmacytic lymphoma is an indolent tumor of older adults (median age, mid-60s) that typically involves the marrow, lymph nodes, and spleen at diagnosis. The tumor is usually composed of a mixture of small lymphocytes, plasma cells, and intermediate cells sometimes referred to as plasmacytoid lymphocytes (Fig. 24-8). The plasma cell component of the tumor secretes a monoclonal immunoglobulin, most commonly IgM.

Patients generally present with one or more of the following:

- Anemia due to replacement of the bone marrow by tumor, increased plasma volume, and hemolysis, which is seen in 15% to 20% of patients and usually is caused by a "cold" autoantibody.

- Neurologic symptoms, most often peripheral neuropathy of uncertain etiology.

- Symptoms related to hyperviscosity, which leads to mucosal bleeding, disturbances of vision and hearing, congestive heart failure, and changes in sensorium. It is restricted to patients with IgM-producing tumors (sometimes referred to as Waldenström macroglobulinemia). IgM circulates in the blood as a 900 kDa pentamer composed of five IgM moieties linked covalently through an attachment called a J chain. The effect of a given molecule

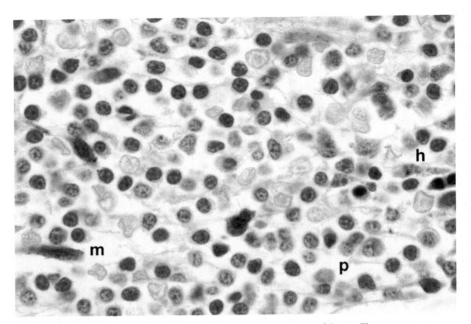

FIGURE 24-8 **Lymphoplasmacytic lymphoma, bone marrow biopsy.** The marrow cellularity consists of small lymphoid cells showing varying degrees of plasmacytic differentiation. Several cells resembling small plasma cells are present (p) as well as strap-like mast cells (m), which are often present as a reactive component of the marrow infiltrates in this disease. Macrophages laden with greenish-brown hemosiderin are also present (h), a reflection of concomitant immunohemolytic anemia in this particular patient.

on the viscosity of a solution increases exponentially with its size; hence, increases in IgM produce hyperviscosity much more readily than other types of antibodies, which have smaller molecular diameters. Symptoms are related in part to pooling of blood in the venous side of the circulation. This effect produces dilation and tortuosity of the retinal veins, which can be appreciated by funduscopic examination.

Unlike myeloma, lymphoplasmacytic lymphoma does not produce excessive free light chains or cause bone resorption and so is not associated with renal failure or pathologic fractures. Amyloidosis can occur but only rarely. B-cell function tends to be preserved, and infections are not as common as in myeloma.

Lymphoplasmacytic lymphoma is not curable, but tumors respond well to combinations of gentle chemotherapy and rituximab, which targets the CD20-positive small lymphocytic component of the tumors. Because most IgM in the body is intravascular, symptoms related to hyperviscosity can be controlled with plasmapheresis. Like other indolent lymphomas, lymphoplasmacytic lymphoma tends to become more refractory to therapy over time. Uncommonly, it transforms to aggressive tumors resembling diffuse large B-cell lymphoma. Overall survival is about 5 years.

SELF-ASSESSMENT STUDY QUESTIONS

1. Match the disorder with the best answer.
   A. Multiple myeloma
   B. Monoclonal gammopathy of uncertain significance
   C. Primary amyloidosis
   D. Lymphoplasmacytic lymphoma
   E. Kappa light chain disease

   1. Nephrotic syndrome
   2. Linear deposits of Ig
   3. Tinnitus and blurred vision
   4. Bacterial pneumonia
   5. Precursor to myeloma

2. Which of the following does not contribute to renal failure in multiple myeloma?
   A. Bacterial infection.
   B. Hypercalcemia.
   C. Free light chains.
   D. Intact immunoglobulin.
   E. Amyloidosis.

A 67-year-old woman noted progressive fatigue beginning 9 months ago. Her husband has observed that she looks increasingly pale. For the past 4 months she has had severe pain in her lower back. Two months ago she was hospitalized with pneumococcal lobar pneumonia. Her hemoglobin at that time was 8 g/dL, and she was transfused with two units of packed red cells. During the last month she has developed anorexia and hiccoughs. On physical examination, she has a resting pulse of 90 beats/minute and a normal BP and respiratory rate. The patient is very pale. She has no icterus and no palpable lymphadenopathy. There is marked tenderness over the third lumbar vertebral body. The remainder of the examination is unremarkable.

   Laboratory values:
   Hemoglobin 5.0 g/dL, hematocrit 15%, normal mean cell volume, reticulocyte count 1.1%
   Normal white blood cell count and differential counts and normal platelet count
   Serum: Blood urea nitrogen 100 mg/dL, creatinine 5.8 mg/dL, calcium 12 mg/dL
   Anterior/posterior and lateral radiographs of the lower spine show marked osteoporosis and a lytic lesion in the third lumbar vertebra

3. Which of the following is the most likely diagnosis?
   A. Burkitt lymphoma.
   B. Myeloid metaplasia and myelofibrosis.
   C. Hemolytic uremic syndrome.
   D. Multiple myeloma.
   E. Renal cell carcinoma metastatic to the bone marrow.

4. What is the most likely pathophysiologic explanation for the patient's development of pneumococcal lobar pneumonia?
   A. Impaired granulocyte function.
   B. Obstruction of a bronchus from lung metastasis.
   C. Acquired hypogammaglobulinemia.
   D. Impaired T-cell immunity secondary to lymphoma.
   E. Splinting and hypoventilation from back pain leading to atelectasis.

Additional Review Questions: Chapters 18 through 24

1. Heme malignancy pathogenesis. Fill in the blank with A, B, C, or D. Choose the *best* answer, and use each choice only once.

   ____ 1. Acute leukemia
   ____ 2. Chronic myeloproliferative disorders
   ____ 3. Myelodysplastic syndromes
   ____ 4. Mature B-cell lymphomas

   A. Chromosomal gains and losses
   B. Activating tyrosine kinase mutations
   C. Translocations involving hematopoietic differentiation genes
   D. Translocations involving immunoglobulin loci

2. Leukemia/myeloproliferative disorders clinical presentation. Fill in the blank with A–I. Choose the *best* answer, and use each choice only once.

   Diagnosis
   ____ 1. Acute myeloid leukemia
   ____ 2. T-cell acute lymphoblastic leukemia
   ____ 3. Myelodysplastic syndrome
   ____ 4. Precursor B-cell acute lymphoblastic leukemia
   ____ 5. Chronic lymphocytic leukemia
   ____ 6. Chronic myeloid leukemia
   ____ 7. Essential thrombocytosis
   ____ 8. Polycythemia vera
   ____ 9. Idiopathic myelofibrosis

   Clinical presentation
   A. An older adult with hepatosplenomegaly, abnormally dense bones on radiographs, and mild pancytopenia and teardrop RBCs
   B. A 60-year-old woman, 7 years after adjuvant chemotherapy for breast cancer with pancytopenia
   C. A teenage boy with a white blood cell count of 120,000/mm³ and a mediastinal mass
   D. A 4-year-old child with petechiae and pancytopenia
   E. An incidental finding in an otherwise well 67-year-old man
   F. A 45-year-old woman with splenomegaly, neutrophilic leukocytosis, peripheral basophilia, and thrombocytosis
   G. An 80-year-old man with a plethoric complexion, hematocrit of 65%, and platelet count of 1,400,000/mm³
   H. A 50-year-old woman with headaches and a platelet count of 1,200,000/mm³
   I. A 32-year-old man presenting to his dentist with fleshy bleeding gums and easy bruising

3. Heme malignancy treatment and prognosis. Fill in the blank with A–F. Choose the *best* answer, and use each choice only once.

   ____ 1. Acute myeloid leukemia
   ____ 2. Pediatric acute lymphoblastic leukemia
   ____ 3. Adult acute lymphoblastic leukemia
   ____ 4. Chronic myeloproliferative disorders
   ____ 5. Indolent lymphomas
   ____ 6. Aggressive lymphomas

   A. "Chronic" diseases, not thought of as curable by chemotherapy or hematopoietic stem cell transplantation (HSCT)
   B. Curable only by HSCT only
   C. More than 85% curable with conventional chemotherapy
   D. About 30% to 40% curable with conventional chemotherapy
   E. About 40% to 60% curable with conventional chemotherapy
   F. Grave prognosis if evolving in an older patient with a prior history of myelodysplastic syndrome

4. Cytogenetics triplet matching. Match the cytogenetic abnormality with the genes involved and the specific diagnosis. Choose the *best* answer, and use each choice only once. Answers should be in the form 1/A/I, 2/B/II, etc.

1. t(15;17)	A. (IgH;BCL2)	I. B-lymphoblastic leukemia or chronic myeloid leukemia
2. t(14;18)	B. (PML;RARa)	
3. t(8;14)	C. (c-myc;IgH)	II. Follicular lymphoma
4. t(9;22)	D. (BCR;ABL)	III. Acute promyelocytic leukemia
		IV. Burkitt lymphoma

25

Blood Transfusion

H. Franklin Bunn and Richard Kaufman

LEARNING OBJECTIVES

After studying this chapter you should be able to:

■ Describe the structures of the ABO and Rh blood group antigens.

■ Understand how blood is typed and cross-matched.

■ Name the clinical and laboratory features of acute and delayed transfusion reactions.

■ Identify and prioritize the different risks associated with blood transfusion.

In 1492, as Pope Innocent VIII lapsed into a coma, the blood of three boys was infused—into his mouth! Considerable progress has been made since then, particularly following Karl Landsteiner's discovery of the ABO blood group antigens in 1901. Blood transfusions have had a larger impact on medicine and surgery than any other therapeutic advance in hematology. In the United States, approximately 15 million units of blood are transfused each year.

This chapter begins with the fractionation of donor blood into cellular and plasma components that are used in transfusion. An overview of the important blood group antigens is followed by a consideration of methods used for typing and cross-matching units of blood. After reviewing the indications for transfusing red cells, platelets, and plasma, we discuss the hemolytic, immunologic, inflammatory, and infectious risks posed by transfusion therapy. The chapter ends with a perspective on current and future developments in transfusion medicine.

DONOR BLOOD COMPONENTS

The standard blood donation involves phlebotomy through a large-bore needle inserted into an arm vein. Approximately 450 mL are transferred into a sterile plastic bag containing citrate phosphate dextrose (CPD)-adenine. Citrate (C) prevents coagulation by chelating calcium ions. The phosphate (P) buffer maintains the pH at physiologic levels. Dextrose (D) provides a source of energy during blood storage. Adenine enhances the viability of the stored red cells.

As noted in Chapter 1, when a tube of anticoagulated blood sediments in a gravitational field, the relatively dense red cells go to the bottom, and the less dense white cells and platelets form a "buffy coat" layer on the upper surface of the red cells, whereas cell-free plasma is least dense and collects at the top of the tube. In the blood bank, the bag of freshly collected donor blood is first centrifuged at relatively low speed, allowing separation into packed red cells and platelet-rich plasma (Fig. 25-1). The platelet-rich plasma is then spun at a higher speed, enabling separation into cell-free plasma and a platelet concentrate (Fig. 25-1).

Packed red cells are stored at 4°C for up to 42 days. In most medical centers, the white blood cells are removed by a filter, a maneuver that lowers the incidence of febrile reactions and human leukocyte antigen (HLA) alloimmunization and reduces the risk of infection with cytomegalovirus. Patients undergoing hematopoietic stem cell transplantation receive red cell units that have been irradiated in order to reduce the risk of graft-versus-host disease. The fresh plasma is frozen and stored at −18°C or colder for up to 1 year. The platelet concentrate is stored at 20°C for a maximum of 5 days. Typically, to prepare a transfusable dose of platelets, concentrates from six donors are pooled. An alternative way to collect platelets in numbers sufficient for transfusion involves circulating venous blood from a donor through an apheresis machine, which continuously removes platelets and returns red cells and plasma to the donor. Platelet units are also irradiated prior to administration to transplant patients.

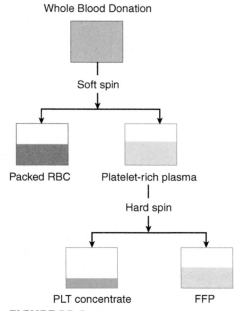

FIGURE 25-1 **The separation of a 450-mL (one pint) unit of donor blood into packed red cells (RBC), platelet concentrate (PLT), and plasma FFP, fresh frozen plasma.**

BLOOD GROUP ANTIGENS

As explained in Chapter 10, red cell stability, pliability, and ion transport depend on specific membrane proteins. In fact, there are over 100 red cell surface membrane proteins. Many of these are polymorphic and have come to attention because they induce clinically significant immune responses when transfused into mismatched recipients. In the past, the blood antigens responsible for these immune responses have been identified by immunologic methods, but in recent years the genes that encode these proteins have been cloned and sequenced, allowing their structure and sometimes function to be established. Figure 25-2 depicts the membrane topology of a number of the well-defined red cell antigens.

A blood group system consists of carbohydrate or protein red cell antigens produced by alleles of a single genetic locus or by closely linked alleles. Most blood group antigens stem from single nucleotide polymorphisms. For example, the S and s alleles of the glycophorin B gene differ by a single nucleotide polymorphism in codon 29, with the S allele encoding a methionine residue (ATG) and the s allele encoding a threonine residue (ACG). Most red cell antigens are proteins expressed on the cell surface, but some, most notably those of the ABO system, stem from differences in carbohydrates linked to surface proteins or glycolipids.

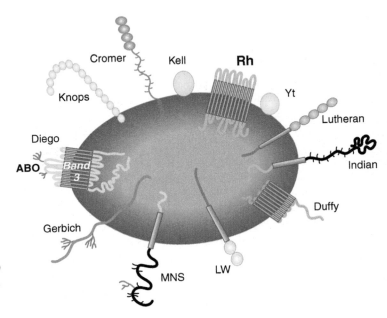

FIGURE 25-2 The topology of red cell membrane proteins that are well-characterized antigens. Also shown is the ABO system, in which the antigens are carbohydrate. (Modified with permission from Dr. Elizabeth Sjöberg-Wester.)

THE ABO SYSTEM

The A and B antigens are defined by the terminal sugar that is attached to glycoproteins and glycosphingolipids by specific transferases. As shown in Figure 25-3, the precursor for these terminal sugars is the H antigen, which has the sequence R-acetylglucosamine-galactose-fucose, where R is a core carbohydrate moiety. The A antigen is formed by a glycosyltransferase that catalyzes the addition of an N-acetylgalactosamine to the subterminal galactose, whereas the B antigen is formed by an allelic variant that catalyzes the addition of another galactose residue to the core galactose. Most populations also contain a common allele lacking enzymatic activity that is designated O. Because OO homozygotes lack A and B terminal transferases, they express only the unmodified H antigen on their red cell surfaces. These individuals have the O blood type. Those who have type A or type B red cells are either homozygotes (AA or BB) or heterozygotes (AO or BO) (Table 25-1). Those with type AB red cells inherit one A allele and one B allele from their two parents.

From fetal development throughout life, individuals are exposed to A and B antigens from a variety of sources and, as a result, develop antigen-specific "natural" IgG and IgM immunoglobulins even in the absence of blood transfusion. The IgM antibodies fix

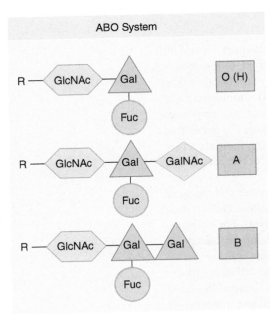

FIGURE 25-3 The terminal polysaccharide structures of H substance as well as A and B antigens.

complement and, as explained in more detail, later in this chapter, cause intravascular hemolysis. As shown in Table 25-1, individuals with type A red cells have anti-B antibodies in their plasma, whereas those with type B red cells have anti-A. Individuals with type O red cells have both anti-A and anti-B antibodies in their plasma. They are sometimes called *universal donors* and, indeed, during the Vietnam War, group O blood was sometimes administered on the battlefield to recipients, irrespective of blood type. Conversely, group AB individuals lack both anti-A and anti-B in their plasma and are sometimes called *universal recipients*.

TABLE 25-1 ABO System

Genotype	RBC Antigens	Serum Antibody
AA or AO	A	Anti-B
BB or BO	B	Anti-A
AB	AB	None
OO	O	Anti-A, anti-B

THE Rh SYSTEM

The proteins that comprise the Rh system are encoded by two homologous genes on chromosome 1. Both proteins are complex transmembrane proteins that span the plasma membrane of the red cell 12 times. As depicted in Figure 25-4, one protein contains the D antigen and another the C, c, E, and e antigens. The Rh system also contains 45 other less immunogenic and less well-characterized antigens. D is extraordinarily immunogenic and therefore the most important protein antigen in transfusion practice. *Rh positive* and *Rh negative* refer to the presence or absence of D antigen on the surface of the red cell. About 15% of White North-American individuals are Rh (D) negative. They do not form alloantibodies to D unless exposed to red cells from either a fetus or transfusions. Much less commonly, alloantibodies can form against C, c, E, and e antigens that, as shown in Figure 25-4, are created by amino acid replacements in protein domains located on the external surface of the red cell. Alloantibodies against Rh antigens are IgG immunoglobulins that are opsonins but do not fix complement. Macrophages recognize and phagocytose the IgG-coated red cells, leading to extravascular hemolysis. Of note, most cases of autoimmune hemolysis due to warm IgG antibodies (Chapter 11) are caused by autoantibodies against the Rh antigens.

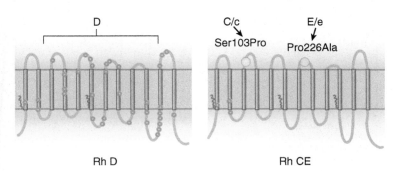

Rh proteins

Rh D

Rh CE

C/c Ser103Pro

E/e Pro226Ala

FIGURE 25-4 The topology of Rh proteins containing the D antigen (left) and the C, c, E, and e antigens (right).

As discussed later in this chapter, the D antigen is also responsible for the development of hemolytic disease of the fetus and newborn, and the Rh system is a major contributor to incompatibility of transfused blood. In addition, a number of red cell antigens outside the Rh system can engender alloantibodies. The most commonly encountered alloantibodies are detected by routine screening, as described in the following section.

PRETRANSFUSION TESTING

When a unit of donor blood is collected, it is typed for the presence of A and B antigens as well as D antigen on the red cells. The addition of serum containing a high titer of anti-A antibody will result in prompt clumping (agglutination) of type A or AB red cells, whereas type O red cells remain in a uniform suspension. In a like manner, this simple agglutination test is also used to determine whether red cells express B and D antigens.

Pretransfusion testing
ABO/Rh typing
Antibody screen
Cross-match

The blood of a patient who is to receive red cell transfusions undergoes the same ABO and D typing as described earlier for donor units. In addition, the patient's serum is tested for the presence of alloantibodies other than anti-A and anti-B. Figure 25-5 shows an example of the use of red cells from two individuals carefully selected to differ not only in the Rh C, c, E, and e antigens but also in other antigen systems (Kell and Duffy). If the patient's serum fails to agglutinate cells from either of these donors, it lacks alloantibodies to these antigens. Note, however, that the patient's serum in fact agglutinates the red cells of donor 2. This result indicates that the patient has alloantibodies to E, c, or Fy^b, or possibly a combination thereof, but no alloantibodies to D, C, e, K, k, or Fy^a. The blood bank then uses additional panels of red cells to identify the patient's specific alloantibody or alloantibodies. This information allows the blood bank to select units that not only have the same ABO and D type as the patient but also lack the antigens to which the patient is immune. As a further safeguard, each selected donor unit is then tested against serum from the patient by means of the indirect antiglobulin test (indirect Coombs test, Fig. 11-3) to ensure that the unit is fully compatible.

Donor	Rh					Kell		Duffy		Serum reaction
	D	C	E	c	e	K	k	Fy^a	Fy^b	
1	+	+	O	O	+	+	+	+	O	O
2	+	O	+	+	O	O	+	O	+	3+

FIGURE 25-5 Use of two panels of antigenically characterized red cells to test a patient's serum for the presence of alloantibodies. The interpretation of the results shown is explained in the text.

+ Antigen present
O Antigen absent
3+ Agglutination = unexpected antibody present, ID required

INDICATIONS FOR TRANSFUSION

RED CELLS

The sole purpose of transfusing red cells is to enhance the oxygen carrying capacity of the blood. The most clear-cut indication is acute blood loss, usually from surgery, trauma, or severe gastrointestinal hemorrhage. Among physical signs, postural hypotension is particularly informative, because it usually indicates hypovolemia and therefore the need for restoration of both red cell mass and plasma volume. For more information on anemia due to blood loss, see Chapter 3. The decision as to whether or when to transfuse a patient with subacute or chronic anemia is more nuanced. Many independent factors must be considered, including the etiology of the anemia, the coexistence of underlying disorders, and the patient's age, symptoms, and signs. In patients with the anemia of renal failure, erythropoietin therapy is nearly always sufficient to restore the red cell mass. Transfusions also may be avoided if the anemic patient is known to have an uncomplicated deficiency of iron, cobalamin, or folate, because such patients respond rapidly to appropriate replacement therapy. Patients with long-standing anemia, particularly younger and sedentary individuals, are able to tolerate severe anemia remarkably well, owing to compensatory mechanisms discussed in Chapter 3. In contrast, if the anemia is of recent onset, it is often less well-tolerated, particularly if the patient is physically active. In patients with symptoms of angina pectoris or episodes of transient cerebral ischemia, the threshold for transfusion is relatively low because of concern that continued hypoxia may lead to damage of a vital organ. For all these reasons, it is difficult and indeed inadvisable to assign a target hemoglobin or hematocrit level below which a patient should be transfused. During the last decade evidence has accumulated indicating that red cell transfusions are used too liberally among both medical and surgical patients. In fact, some studies have shown that the more restrictive use of blood transfusions in patients with moderate anemia significantly lowers the mortality rate.

PLATELETS

As discussed earlier, a platelet unit is prepared either as a pool from six individual blood units or from a single donor by apheresis. As mentioned in Chapter 14, the normal life span of platelets in the circulation is 7 to 9 days. However, platelets have a significantly shorter life span when transfused to thrombocytopenic patients. Moreover, after receiving platelets, some recipients develop an immune response, most commonly to mismatched major histocompatibility antigens (HLA antigens), which further accelerates the clearance of donor platelets. For these reasons, platelet transfusions should be administered sparingly. Platelet transfusions are much more effective in thrombocytopenias due to underproduction than in those caused by enhanced platelet destruction. The primary indication for platelet transfusion is bleeding owing either to thrombocytopenia or much less often to defective platelet function. In addition, platelets are commonly transfused to patients who are not bleeding but whose platelet counts are so low that there is high risk of significant hemorrhage. As with red cell transfusions, in recent years the indications for prophylactic platelet transfusion have become more restrictive. As shown in Figure 25-6, patients with normally functioning platelets do not develop significant gastrointestinal blood loss unless the platelet count falls below

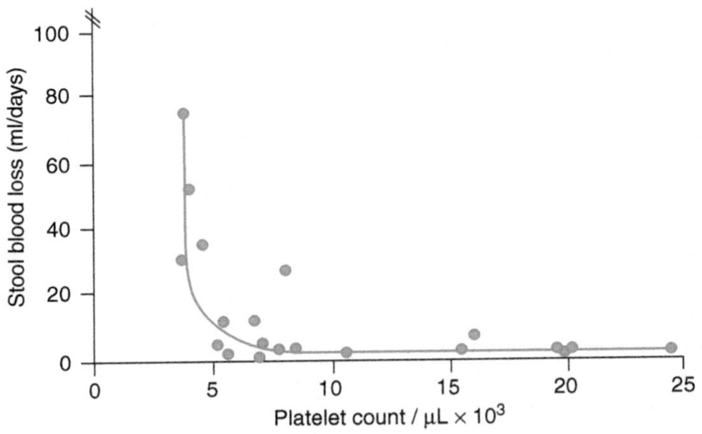

FIGURE 25-6 Blood loss detected in the stool in patients with different degrees of thrombocytopenia. (Modified with permission from Slichter SJ, Harker L. Thrombocytopenia: mechanisms and management of defects in platelet production. *Clin Haematol* 1978;7:523-39.)

$5000/mm^3$. A prospective study has shown that there is no significant difference in the risk of major hemorrhage in a group of patients transfused with platelet counts of $<10,000/mm^3$ compared with a group with a transfusion threshold of $<20,000/mm^3$.

PLASMA

The primary indication for transfusion of fresh frozen plasma is correction of deficiencies of multiple clotting factors, as may occur in liver disease, overdosing of warfarin, and disseminated intravascular coagulation (all described in detail in Chapter 16). In contrast, patients who have inherited single clotting factor deficiencies are treated with specific replacement therapy (described in Chapter 15). Patients with acute massive hemorrhage benefit from infusion of fresh frozen plasma for two reasons. Because they are hypovolemic, they respond favorably to the administration of a colloid load that is retained within the intravascular space. Moreover, many of these patients have low levels of clotting factors either because of disseminated intravascular coagulation or dilution from loss of plasma and high-volume fluid replacement. Blood banks maintain a supply of cryoprecipitate, which is prepared by collecting the protein precipitate that forms when plasma is cooled to 4°C. Cryoprecipitate contains factor VIII, von Willebrand factor, factor XIII, fibronectin, and fibrinogen, all of which except fibrinogen can replaced by administration of either recombinant protein products or highly purified concentrates. Thus, cryoprecipitate is primarily used for treatment of hypofibrinogenemia.

RISKS OF TRANSFUSION

HEMOLYTIC REACTIONS

As summarized in Table 25-2, hemolysis due to the administration of antigenically incompatible red cells can be either immediate or delayed. Immediate hemolytic reactions are nearly always due to ABO incompatibility. For example, if an individual with type B blood receives a unit of type A blood by mistake, the recipient's preexisting IgM anti-A antibodies will cause complement fixation and intravascular lysis of the

TABLE 25-2 Hemolytic Transfusion Reactions

	Acute	Delayed
Timing	Immediate	3-10 days after transfusion
Mechanism	Preformed antibody	Anamnestic antibody response
Antibody	IgM or complement-fixing IgG (eg, anti-A or anti-B)	IgG, no complement fixation (eg, anti-Rh)
Site of hemolysis	Usually intravascular	Usually extravascular
Clinical sequelae	Severe cases: shock, disseminated intravascular coagulation, acute renal failure	Usually none

transfused red cells. The patient's clinical presentation depends on how much blood was infused before the error was suspected and the transfusion stopped. Patients generally develop fever and chills, often accompanied by dyspnea, tachycardia, hemoglobinuria, and severe pain, usually in the lower back. Transfusion of a large volume of ABO-incompatible blood often produces hypotensive shock, oliguria, and disseminated intravascular coagulation. Note that all of these findings except for hypotension are likely to be missed if the patient is in the operating room under general anesthesia. At the first signal that incompatible blood may have been administered, the infusion must be stopped and serologic testing repeated on the donor and recipient blood. During this time it is critical to maintain intravenous access and careful monitoring of blood pressure and urine output. Fortunately, contemporary blood banking has a series of safeguards in place that make this complication very rare. In New York State, 9,000,000 units of blood were transfused over the decade 1990 through 1999. A total of 462 patients (about 1 per 20,000 units given) suffered adverse consequences from administration of ABO-incompatible blood.

Delayed hemolytic transfusion reactions are more commonly encountered and seldom caused by error. As mentioned earlier, patients develop alloantibodies to protein antigens only after pregnancy or transfusions. The Rh D antigen is highly immunogenic and will trigger detectable levels of anti-D after a single exposure. In contrast, antigens such as Rh C, c, E, and e as well as Kell and Duffy (Fig. 25-5) and others, shown in Figure 25-2, are less immunogenic, but in some cases nevertheless trigger a primary immune response in an antigen-negative recipient. This primary response may not cause the development of a sufficiently high antibody titer to be detectable by the screening procedure described in Figure 25-5. However, if at a later point in time the recipient is transfused with a second unit containing this antigen, within 3 to 10 days an anamnestic immunologic response will raise the titer of antibody to sufficient levels to cause clinically significant hemolysis. As mentioned at the beginning of this chapter, anti-Rh antibody is an IgG and does not fix complement. Accordingly, the hemolysis is extravascular and not nearly as severe as that encountered in immediate hemolytic reactions due to ABO incompatibility. Figure 25-7 depicts a typical delayed transfusion reaction. This complication should be suspected in any patient who develops an unexplained drop in hemoglobin or hematocrit within a week of receiving transfused red cells. Often the patient has no

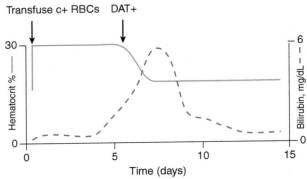

FIGURE 25-7 **Time course of a typical delayed hemolytic transfusion reaction due to the anamnestic induction of anti-c antibodies.** On day 0, the patient was transfused with Rh c+ red cells, resulting in the desired increment in hematocrit level. By day 5, a rise in the serum bilirubin level suggested the possibility of hemolysis. At this time, the direct antiglobulin test result was positive. As the antibody-coated donor red cells were rapidly cleared from the circulation, the serum bilirubin level rose further, and the hematocrit level fell rapidly. DAT, direct antiglobulin test.

symptoms or signs but occasionally may develop fever, chills, and jaundice, and rarely hemoglobinuria. The diagnosis is established either by documenting the presence of antibody-coated red cells in the patient's blood by the direct antiglobulin test (Chapter 11, Fig. 11-3A) or by the indirect antiglobulin test (Chapter 11, Fig. 11-3B), in which the patient's serum is tested against a panel of red cells with characterized antigens as well as against the donor red cells that were recently infused. Often the direct antiglobulin test is negative because the antibody-coated red cells have been rapidly cleared by resident macrophages. Delayed hemolytic transfusion reactions usually do not require therapy. However, the patient's hemoglobin and hematocrit levels should be closely monitored, and care must be given to ensure that future red cell transfusions are antigen negative.

Hemolytic disease of the fetus and newborn (HDFN) involves an immunologic response following the "transfusion" of red cells from the fetus into the maternal circulation. By far the most common cause of HDFN is maternal Rh D alloimmunization. The pathogenesis is similar to that of a delayed hemolytic transfusion reaction; a typical scenario is as follows. An Rh-negative mother is carrying a fetus that has inherited the D antigen from its father. During the first pregnancy, leakage of fetal red cells across the placenta results in the mother becoming immunized against the D antigen. However the amount of anti-D antibody that crosses the placenta into the fetal circulation is too low to cause hemolysis. With subsequent pregnancies, the mother mounts an anamnestic immunologic response to D+ fetal red cells, putting the fetus and newborn at high risk of developing alloimmune hemolysis. The baby develops severe anemia and generalized edema (hydrops) owing to tissue hypoxia. In addition, the high levels of nonconjugated bilirubin in fetal and neonatal plasma can cross the blood-brain barrier and accumulate in the brain, particularly in the basal ganglia, causing irreversible neurologic damage (kernicterus). If signs of fetal distress during the third trimester trigger a hematologic investigation leading to the diagnosis of HDFN, intrauterine transfusion will prevent the development of hydrops and kernicterus. Fortunately, HDFN is rarely encountered today thanks to the discovery 50 years ago that the administration of anti-D immunoglobulin (RhoGAM, Ortho Clinical Diagnostics, Rochester, NY) to Rh-negative mothers after their first delivery safely and effectively suppresses sensitization to Rh D and prevents the development of HDFN in subsequent pregnancies.

TRANSFUSION-RELATED LUNG INJURY

Approximately one in 3000 patients develops acute interstitial pneumonitis within 6 hours of transfusion, accompanied by dyspnea, tachycardia, hypoxemia, fever, and hypotension. Figure 25-8 shows the rapid development of bilateral pulmonary infiltrates in a patient whose lungs were normal prior to transfusion. This

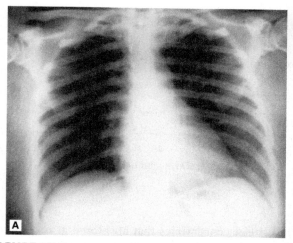
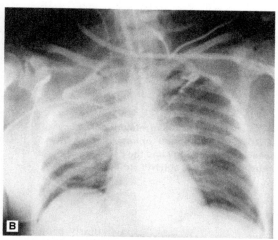

FIGURE 25-8 Development of transfusion-related acute lung injury (TRALI) following blood transfusion. A. Pre transfusion; B. Post-transfusion showing rapid emergence of bilateral pulmonary infiltrates. (Modified with permission from Bux J. Transfusion-related acute lung injury (TRALI): a serious adverse event of blood transfusion. *Vox Sang* 2005;89:1-10.)

acute process is often difficult to distinguish from pulmonary edema, pulmonary embolus, bacterial pneumonia, pulmonary hemorrhage, or acute respiratory distress syndrome. It is likely that transfusion-related acute lung injury (TRALI) is a form of acute respiratory distress syndrome caused by donor antibodies that bind to and activate either recipient neutrophils or pulmonary endothelial cells. In many cases, the causative antibodies appear to be against HLA antigens. Other cases are associated with pathogenic antibodies against a polymorphic antigen expressed on neutrophils, called choline transporter-like protein 2 (CLT2); these antibodies are particularly prone to cause severe and often fatal TRALI. TRALI is the most commonly encountered serious complication of transfusion therapy. The treatment of TRALI is primarily supportive. All patients require oxygen and most need ventilator assistance. These episodes usually resolve over 48 to 96 hours, but the mortality is 5% to 25%. The risk of TRALI can be reduced by the use of plasma from male donors, because women may become HLA-alloimmunized during pregnancy. Cases of suspected TRALI are investigated by the blood bank. Donors of blood products believed to have caused TRALI are permanently banned from donating blood.

TRANSMISSION OF INFECTIOUS PATHOGENS

A variety of bacterial, viral, and parasitic infections can be transmitted by transfusion of blood or blood products. Current transfusion practice mandates routine screening for the pathogens listed in Table 25-3. Bacterial contamination is

TABLE 25-3 Infectious Disease Screening

Human immunodeficiency viruses 1 and 2 (HIV1 and HIV2)
Hepatitis B virus
Hepatitis C virus
Human T-cell lymphotropic viruses 1 and 2 (HTLV1 and HTLV2)
West Nile virus
Syphilis
Trypanosomiasis (Chagas disease)
Bacteria (platelets)

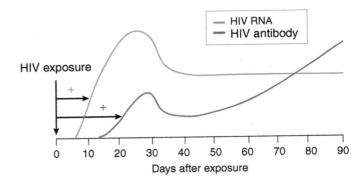

FIGURE 25-9 **The human immunodeficiency virus (HIV) "window period" or time intervals between exposure to HIV and the detection of HIV ribonucleic acid (RNA) and HIV antibody.**

particularly problematic in platelet concentrates that are stored at room temperature. Occasional cases of malaria in the United States have arisen through transfusion of blood from a donor who has recently returned from a tropical area. The viral pathogens of most concern are human immunodeficiency virus (HIV), hepatitis C, and hepatitis B. However, thanks to highly sensitive and specific immunologic and genetic methods for detection, the risk of transmission of these viruses via blood products has fallen several orders of magnitude over the last 25 years. As Figure 25-9 shows, there is only a short (10 day) window of time between exposure to HIV infection and its detection by testing for HIV RNA in the blood. Despite these advances, the lay public continues to harbor fears that HIV and hepatitis are the most likely serious complications of transfusion therapy. In fact, as Table 25-4 shows, TRALI and administration of incompatible blood pose much higher risks than viral pathogens.

TABLE 25-4 Risks of Blood Transfusion

	Per-Unit Risk
Transfusion-related acute lung injury	1/3000
Incompatible blood	1/14,000
Pathogen	
Bacteria (platelets)	1/75,000
Hepatitis B virus	1/200,000
Hepatitis C virus	1/2,000,000
Human immunodeficiency virus	1/2,000,000

SELF-ASSESSMENT STUDY QUESTIONS

1. You are running a large military blood bank in Afghanistan. During the height of the "troop surge," you anticipate a much higher number of severe military and civilian casualties. You need to issue blood to battalion field stations scattered around the country for emergency administration in settings where no typing or cross-matching is possible. The number of potential blood donors among military personnel far exceeds the number of units you can draw, refrigerate, and transport to the field stations. Therefore you give highest priority to donors with which of the following blood types?
   A. Group O, Rh negative.
   B. Group O, Rh positive.
   C. Group AB, Rh negative.
   D. Group AB, Rh positive.
   E. Group A, Rh negative.

2. A 32-year-old woman with acute myeloid leukemia had induction chemotherapy with a combination of strongly myelosuppressive agents. Ten days after initiation of therapy, she has shaking chills, dysphagia, and dyspnea. Physical examination revealed a temperature of 103°F, oral and pharyngeal mucositis, rales in her right lower lungs, and small petechiae on her lower legs.

   Laboratory values:
   Hemoglobin 5.9 g/dL, hematocrit 17.8%, mean cell volume 90 fL, reticulocyte count 0.3%
   White blood cell count 980/mm³ with 12% neutrophils, 2% monocytes, 3% myeloblasts, and 83% lymphocytes
   Platelet count 22,000/mm³
   Radiography results:
   Chest radiograph shows a small, faint, right lower lobe infiltrate

   The blood bank should administer which of the following products?
   A. Neutrophils, platelets, and packed red cells.
   B. Platelets and packed red cells.
   C. Packed red cells.
   D. Neutrophils and packed red cells.
   E. Whole blood.

3. Which of the following is currently the most commonly encountered serious complication of blood transfusion therapy?
   A. Sepsis from bacteria that have contaminated the blood.
   B. Transmission of HIV.
   C. Transmission of hepatitis C.
   D. Acute hemolytic reaction from an ABO mismatch.
   E. Transfusion-related acute lung injury.

26 Hematopoietic Stem Cell Transplantation

Jon C. Aster and Joseph H. Antin

LEARNING OBJECTIVES

After studying this chapter you should understand:

- The clinical applications and complications of hematopoietic stem cell transplantation.
- The major types of hematopoietic stem cell transplantation.
- The genetics of allogeneic hematopoietic stem cell transplantation.
- The causes of graft rejection and graft failure.
- The pathogenesis of graft-versus-host disease and the graft-versus-tumor effect.

The era of hematopoietic stem cell transplantation (HSCT) began in the 1950s, when pioneering studies by E. Donnall Thomas, James Till, and Ernest McCulloch demonstrated the ability of unfractionated bone marrow cells to "rescue" animals from hematopoietic failure induced by otherwise lethal doses of radiation. Such studies had profound implications and consequences for basic research, because they proved the existence of multipotent hematopoietic stem cells and provided a powerful new experimental tool for studying the immune system.

From very early days, it was evident that HSCT also had enormous therapeutic potential but was prone to cause serious and all too frequently fatal complications. HSCT remains as close to a high-wire act as exists in medicine, one in which patients receive potentially lethal doses of chemotherapy and/or radiation. However, as we will discuss, advances in stem cell biology, immunology, and pharmacology have allowed the development of more effective, less toxic HSCT strategies. As a result, HSCT is now being used to treat an increasing number of disorders and a broader spectrum of patients than ever before. This chapter serves as an overview of some of the salient features of this fascinating, rapidly evolving area of hematology.

CLINICAL APPLICATIONS OF HSCT

HSCT has proven to be effective in the following clinical settings:

- Correction of genetic and acquired defects in hematopoietic stem cells (HSC). Until the dream of gene therapy for germline defects is realized,

HSCT is often the only hope for those suffering from severe genetic disorders that affect the function of the HSC or its progeny. Replacing the defective HSCs of the patient with HSCs obtained from a normal donor can cure such diseases. HSCT has been used to treat many genetic diseases, including those affecting lymphocytes (eg, severe combined immunodeficiency, X-linked agammaglobulinemia), red cells (eg, severe thalassemia, sickle cell disease), and monocytes/macrophages (eg, Gaucher disease).

- Support for high-dose cancer treatment. The dose-limiting toxicity of radiotherapy and many conventional chemotherapy agents is bone marrow failure due to ablation of HSCs. HSCT overcomes this limitation by providing the patient with healthy HSCs, which can completely reconstitute hematopoiesis and the immune system over a period of weeks to months.

- Generation of graft-versus-tumor effect. When a recipient receives HSCs from another individual who is not an identical twin, the transplanted HSCs give rise to a "new" immune system that may recognize the patient's tumor as non-self and mount an immune response against it. It is now clear that this graft-versus-tumor effect is a very important benefit of HSCT in certain types of cancer, particularly myeloid leukemias.

- Generation of organ graft tolerance. HSCT has sometimes been used to alleviate solid-organ rejection. These types of procedures typically involve the transplantation of HSCs along with a solid organ, such as a kidney or a single lobe of the liver.

- Salvage from genotoxic chemicals or radiation. To date, this indication has applied mainly to rare individuals exposed to nuclear power plant accidents (eg, Chernobyl). It is sobering to consider, however, that the United States government is currently expending large amounts of time and money planning for the consequences of a terrorist attack involving a so-called dirty bomb containing radioisotopes. Such an attack has the potential to cause severe bone marrow damage to hundreds or thousands of people, many of whom may need to undergo HSCT if they are to survive.

There are three types of HSCT. *Autologous* transplants are performed with the patient's own HSCs. These have the advantage of avoiding immunologic complications but fail to generate the graft-versus-tumor effect and thus produce higher rates of relapse in those being treated for myeloid leukemias. *Syngeneic* transplants use HSCs from identical twins and have the same advantages and disadvantages as autologous transplants. *Allogeneic* transplants are done with stem cells obtained from a genetically distinct donor.

The most important determinants of the immunologic consequences of allogeneic HSCT are the class 1 and class 2 major histocompatibility complex (MHC) antigens, also known as human leukocyte antigens (HLA). You will recall that class 1 and class 2 MHC molecules present short peptides derived from intracellular and extracellular antigens, respectively. Although many genes in the MHC locus influence immunity, experience has shown that, for patients undergoing allogeneic HSCT, the most important are the HLA-A, HLA-B, and HLA-C class 1 antigens and the HLA-DR class 2 antigens. The roles of the class 2 antigens HLA-DQ and HLA-DP are less clear. The genes encoding these HLA antigens are closely linked on chromosome 6 and thus are inherited en bloc in what is referred to as a *haplotype*. An allogeneic HSCT in which the haplotypes of the donor and the recipient are identical is called a matched transplant. HSCT can be performed with one or two mismatched antigens, but the risks of the procedure are substantially higher than with an HLA-identical donor.

Another important variable in allogeneic transplantation is whether the HSCs are from a related family member or an unrelated donor. In addition to the MHC loci, poorly characterized "minor" histocompatibility complex loci have lesser but still significant immunologic effects. Allogeneic transplants from related donors are generally performed between siblings, who have a greater degree of identity at these minor loci than do unrelated donors. As shown in Figure 26-1, there is a 25% chance that any sibling will be fully matched at the MHC loci. In contrast, it is rare for a patient to have a full HLA match with a parent or a child. Of note, one or more of the minor histocompatibility complex antigens is located on the Y chromosome. As a result, the transplantation of HSCs from female donors into male recipients produces more graft-versus-tumor effect but also is more prone to result in significant graft-versus-host disease (GVHD) (described later).

HSCs from several different sources are used clinically. Most allogeneic transplants from related donors are performed with whole, unfractionated bone marrow or with HSCs harvested from peripheral blood. The latter are typically obtained a few days after administration of a hematopoietic cytokine such as G-CSF (granulocyte colony stimulating factor (Chapter 2)). Allogeneic transplants from unrelated donors may be performed with bone marrow, HSCs harvested from the peripheral blood, or blood obtained from the placenta at birth (so-called umbilical cord blood). Cord blood has the advantage of being available as a byproduct of every child's birth. There is a national initiative to establish public cord blood banks, with an eye toward future use in unrelated allogeneic HSCTs. The principle disadvantage of cord blood is that the number of HSCs in any sample is relatively small, a limitation that can be overcome by pooling of cord blood from two or more donors.

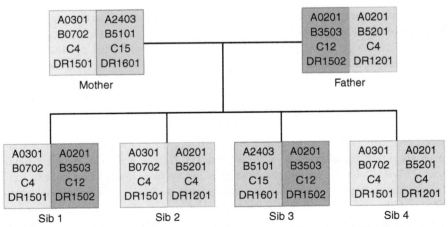

FIGURE 26-1 Inheritance of HLA haplotypes. Note how different HLA-A, HLA-B, HLA-C, and HLA-DR alleles segregate together in this pedigree due to their close linkage on chromosome 6. Two of the children (sibs 2 and 4) are HLA identical, having inherited the same pair of haplotypes from their parents.

Autologous transplantation is generally performed on cancer patients with peripheral blood HSCs obtained at 7-10 days after a dose of chemotherapy with GCSF stimulation. Recovery from the chemotherapy stimulates HSC proliferation and mobilization.

CONVENTIONAL HSCT: CONDITIONING AND ENGRAFTMENT

All forms of HSCT require some conditioning of the recipient with myelotoxic therapies. Conditioning is required to kill or mobilize sufficient numbers of host HSCs to open up the stem cell niche in the marrow (Chapter 2), creating space for the HSCs in the graft. Conditioning also may serve to eradicate a host immune system that has run amok (eg, aplastic anemia, Chapter 4) or to destroy tumor cells that may be resistant to standard doses of chemotherapy and radiation (eg, the transformed HSCs that cause chronic myelogenous leukemia, Chapter 20). The precise conditioning regimen used is tailored to the disorder being treated. For nonneoplastic disorders, common regimens consist of chemotherapy with or without anti-thymocyte globulin, an antibody that recognizes and leads to the killing of T cells. For neoplastic disorders, conditioning is usually done with high-dose chemotherapy regimens, sometimes in combination with total body irradiation.

Several days after conditioning, donor HSCs are transfused into the peripheral blood of the recipient. If all goes well, the marrow and the peripheral blood are reconstituted by donor-derived hematopoietic cells and their progeny (Fig. 26-2). The earliest formed elements that appear in the recipient are derived from late myeloid progenitors, followed by a second cohort of cells derived from early myeloid progenitors. However, sustained reconstitution requires engraftment of HSCs, the only marrow cells that possess the key properties of multipotency and self-renewing capacity.

On average, it takes about 3 weeks for the marrow to engraft and begin to produce mature myeloid cells (platelets, red cells, and neutrophils). However, the pace and timing of reconstitution in the recipient varies depending on several factors including the source of the HSCs. In general, unfractionated bone marrow has greater numbers of early progenitors and HSCs than does cord blood, and, as a result, patients receiving

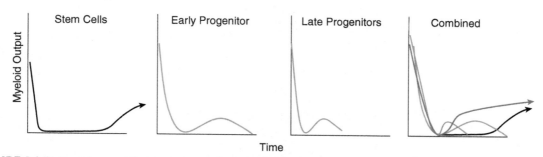

FIGURE 26-2 Engraftment following hematopoietic stem cell transplantation. At early times posttransplant, formed myeloid elements are derived from committed myeloid progenitors. Sustained reconstitution of hematopoiesis occurs later and depends on the engraftment of hematopoietic stem cells.

unfractionated bone marrow tend to engraft more rapidly. During the critical pre-engraftment period, these patients are profoundly immunosuppressed and are completely dependent on transfusion of red cells to maintain oxygen delivery to tissues and transfusion of platelets to prevent bleeding. Because of agranulocytosis there is a very high risk of severe and potentially fatal bacterial and fungal infections during the first 2 or 3 weeks, prior to the production of adequate numbers of neutrophils from the allograft. Measures aimed at reducing the morbidity and mortality associated with infections in the immediate posttransplant period include housing of patients in special positive-pressure rooms supplied with filtered air to limit exposure to pathogens and aggressive treatment with broad-spectrum antibiotics at the earliest sign of infection.

Other complications in the early posttransplant period are directly related to cellular injuries induced by conditioning. Nearly all patients have mucositis, particularly of the soft palate and esophagus, causing swallowing to be painful and difficult. These mucosal lesions are potential sites of entry of pathogenic bacteria. An even more serious complication is veno-occlusive disease, which appears to be caused by damage to endothelial cells lining the venous sinusoids of the liver. Although the precise pathogenesis is unknown, the injury induces fibrin deposition and obstruction of hepatic sinusoids (leading some to suggest that this entity would be better entitled *sinusoidal obstruction syndrome*). The blockage of blood flow causes liver engorgement and tender hepatomegaly and can lead to hypoxic centrilobular hepatic necrosis and liver failure in severe cases.

Graft failure and graft rejection are other serious early complications of HSCT. The incidence of graft rejection is proportional to the degree of immunologic dissimilarity between the donor and the recipient and thus is relatively high in unrelated allogeneic HSCTs. Graft rejection also is increased by prior immunization of the recipient by transfusions of red cells or platelets. Graft failure may stem from an insufficiency of HSCs in the stem cell preparation, damage to the marrow microenvironment caused by the conditioning regimen, or infection. Patients who fail to engraft must undergo another transplant, typically with HSCs from an unrelated donor, if they are to recover. Understandably, second transplants are associated with a high rate of graft failure and morbidity and mortality related to a second round of conditioning.

Once neutrophils appear, the recipient's risk of bacterial and fungal infections declines dramatically. However, as described in the following section, in allogeneic transplant recipients reconstitution of the lymphoid arm of the immune system is a much more complicated process, one involving a delicate balance between immunosuppression and GVHD, an assault on the host mediated by lymphocytes derived from the graft. Under the best of circumstances, recovery of adaptive immunity in allogeneic HSCT recipients requires many months, and, as a result, these patients are at high risk for viral infections and Epstein-Barr virus (EBV)–driven B-cell tumors for an extended period of time after transplantation.

GRAFT VERSUS HOST DISEASE

HSC preparations used in allogeneic transplants contain varying numbers of mature T cells. These cells as well as newly produced lymphocytes derived from donor HSCs have the capacity to "see" host cells as foreign. Curiously, the tissues most prone to GVHD are the skin, the gastrointestinal mucosa, and the bile ducts.

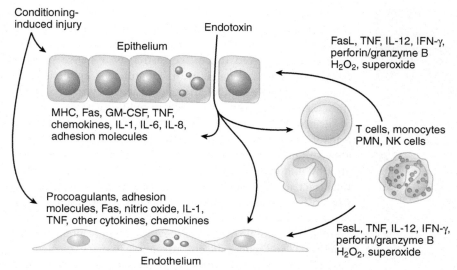

FIGURE 26-3 Pathogenesis of graft-versus-host disease. Cells and soluble factors proposed to be involved are shown (see text for details). (Adapted from Antin JH, Approaches to graft versus host disease. Pediatr Transplant 2005, Suppl 7:71-5.)

The common feature of these tissues is that they line parts of the body that are constantly exposed to bacteria and other pathogens.

The pathogenesis of GVHD is still incompletely understood, but a plausible scenario involves the following series of events (Fig. 26-3). The initiating trigger is believed to be epithelial cell injury caused by a number of factors, including the conditioning regimen, proinflammatory stimuli such as endotoxin, and cytomegalovirus infection. Injured epithelial cells secrete a number of soluble proinflammatory factors that activate resident dendritic cells, tissue macrophages, and endothelial cells, which also may be activated directly by molecules derived from bacteria such as endotoxin. Once a proinflammatory state is established, graft-derived T cells specific for recipient histocompatibility antigens are recruited. CD8-positive cytotoxic T cells selectively target the epithelial cells, inducing their death by apoptosis and in the process amplifying the initial stimulus—epithelial cell injury.

Early in the posttransplant period (generally within the first 100, days), GVHD is caused by mature T cells present in the preparation of donor cells. This form of the disease (acute GVHD) can appear quickly and have dramatic clinical manifestations. The incidence of acute GVHD can be reduced by treating the graft with anti-T-cell antibodies prior to infusion into the recipient, but this proves to be a trade-off, because T-cell depletion increases the risk of recurrence of the original tumor as well as the development of new EBV-positive B-cell tumors. Beyond 100 days, GVHD appears to be mainly mediated by both new T cells and B cells that are produced from HSCs or other early progenitors in the graft. This phase of the disease tends to follow a more indolent course (hence the name *chronic GVHD*) but nevertheless can have devastating consequences.

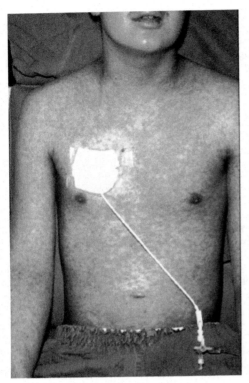

FIGURE 26-4 **Acute graft-versus-host disease.** A patient with the characteristic rash is shown. For unknown reasons, the rash often appears first on the hands and feet.

Acute GVHD presents with rash, diarrhea, and elevated liver function tests. The rash is often diffuse and can be quite striking (Fig. 26-4). The microscopic features are similar in each of the involved tissues, consisting of a sparse infiltrate of lymphocytes associated with apoptosis of epithelial cells (Fig. 26-5). The extent of the epithelial injury varies widely, from a few scattered necrotic cells in mild disease to denuding of surfaces in the most severe cases. Severe acute GVHD often leads to sepsis and a fatal outcome. Chronic GVHD is associated with more subtle forms of tissue injury that lead to fibrosis, atrophy, and loss of function (Fig. 26-6). The skin, gastrointestinal tract, and liver are prominently involved, but other tissues, particularly the lung, also may be affected. Atrophy and fibrosis of the skin may lead to scleroderma-like changes and loss of hair. Fibrosis of mucosal surfaces of the gut may prevent absorption of nutrients and render the gut susceptible to mechanical injury. Fibrosis also may seriously impact pulmonary and hepatic function. In those patients who received total body irradiation as part of the conditioning regimen, fibrosis related to late-stage radiation toxicity also may contribute to organ failure.

The clinical challenge is to control GVHD while allowing sufficient immune activity to generate a graft-versus-tumor effect (in those being treated for cancer) and foster immune reconstitution. This balance is achieved by careful titration of immunosuppressive agents that inhibit T-cell activation (cyclosporine, tacrolimus, sirolimus), interfere with T-cell proliferation (methotrexate, mycophenolate), or kill T cells (anti-thymocyte globulin, prednisone).

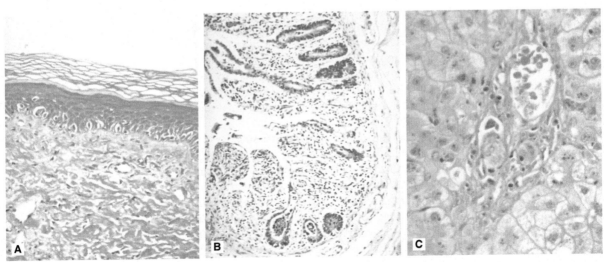

FIGURE 26-5 **Acute graft-versus-host disease.** A) The skin shows a scant lymphocytic infiltrate that "tags" the dermal-epidermal junction. B) Severe acute graft-versus-host disease has partially denuded the colonic epithelium. C) A hepatic portal region is shown that contains a sparse lymphocytic infiltrate and lacks recognizable bile ducts, due to the immune attack on these cells.

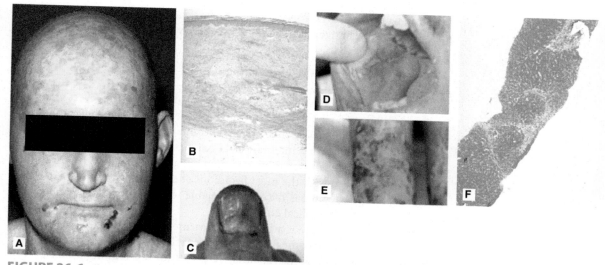

FIGURE 26-6 **Chronic graft-versus-host disease (GVHD).** A) Gross appearance of severe chronic GVHD. Note the loss of hair, atrophy, and fragility of the skin and jaundice due to underlying liver dysfunction. B) A biopsy of skin shows atrophic epidermis and dense dermal fibrosis. C) The nails may become pitted and dysmorphic, also due to a derangement of collagen production. Fibrosis and atrophy may lead to chronic ulceration of the oral mucosa (D) and the skin (E). F) The liver also may develop fibrosis centered on the hepatic triads.

GRAFT-VERSUS-TUMOR EFFECT

Many clinical studies have now established the therapeutic importance in allogeneic transplants of the so-called graft-versus-tumor effect. This activity stems from recognition and killing of host tumor cells by immune cells in the graft. Because the tumors in which this beneficial effect is most clearly demonstrated are chronic myelogenous leukemia, acute myeloid leukemia, and acute lymphoblastic leukemia, it is often referred to as graft-versus-leukemia effect, or GVL.

GVL and GVHD go hand in hand, because the incidence of leukemia relapse is directly related to the immunologic similarity of the donor and recipient. Thus, relapse in leukemia occurs most frequently in syngeneic transplant recipients and least frequently when donors suffer from some degree of acute and/or chronic GVHD (Fig. 26-7). In diseases like chronic myelogenous leukemia that are particularly sensitive to GVL, the effect may be augmented by infusion of donor leukocytes (as described in Chapter 20). A major question for the field is whether GVL can be

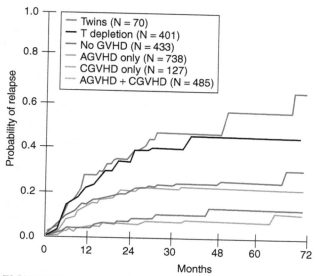

FIGURE 26-7 **Relationship of graft-versus-host disease (GVHD) and leukemia relapse.** Pooled results are shown for patients treated for acute lymphoblastic leukemia, chronic myelogenous leukemia, and acute myeloid leukemia. *AGVHD,* acute GVHD; *CGVHD,* chronic GVHD; *T depletion,* T-cell–depleted allograft. (Adapted from Horowitz M, Gale R, Sondel P. Graft-versus-leukemia reactions after bone marrow transplantation. Blood. 1990;75:555-562.)

teased apart from GVHD. This may be possible if cancer-specific minor histocompatibility complex antigens can generate an effective GVL response.

THE FUTURE OF HSCT

Historically, the use of allogeneic HSCT has been curtailed by the severe complications caused by myeloablative conditioning regimens and the inability to identify suitable donors for many patients. The latter limitation has been solved in part by the creation of national and international bone marrow registries containing lists of haplotyped donors, a resource that is now being supplemented by cord blood banks. However, even with the most fastidious attention to clinical care, conventional conditioning regimens have unacceptable toxicities for older patients and those with underlying medical conditions.

Based on the insight that much of the treatment benefit of allogeneic HSCT in those with leukemia comes from the GVL effect, recent work has focused on the development of nonmyeloablative conditioning regimens that permit at least partial engraftment of donor cells. In principle, such regimens could greatly expand the number of patients who are eligible for HSCT, including those who are older, who require second transplants, or who have organ dysfunction that precludes conventional conditioning regimens. Recent studies have shown that nonmyeloablative conditioning with chemotherapy is indeed much less toxic, often requiring minimal hospitalization, and can be tolerated by children and adults of all ages as well as those with chronic diseases. Radiation is not required, which may lessen the risk of some late complications of HSCT.

An example of the promise of nonmyeloablative HSCT can be seen in the treatment of an adult woman with sickle cell disease (Fig. 26-8). This less toxic strategy is particularly amenable to treatment of sickle cell patients because, unlike those with leukemia, they can tolerate a minor degree of hematopoietic chimerism. This patient received an allogeneic transplant from a brother with sickle cell trait 2 weeks after an exchange transfusion to lower the burden of SS red cells. The conditioning regimen consisted of nonmyeloablative doses of chemotherapy (fludarabine and busulfan). A second exchange transfusion was done after transplantation to tide the patient over until engraftment was complete. As of 6 months post-HSCT, the levels of Hb A and Hb S in the peripheral blood were about 60% Hb A and about 40% Hb S, the levels expected for an individual with sickle cell trait. With establishment of the graft, the peripheral smear normalized, and hemolysis ceased, lowering the erythropoietic drive and decreasing the marrow cellularity to normal. With appropriate prophylaxis, GVHD was held in abeyance.

With additional experience and a more comprehensive understanding of the immunologic facets of HSCT, it should be possible to use nonmyeloablative HSCT in patients with a wide spectrum of neoplastic and nonneoplastic hematologic conditions. Such studies are currently underway in older adult patients with acute myeloid leukemia and other hematologic conditions that have a poor prognosis with conventional therapies.

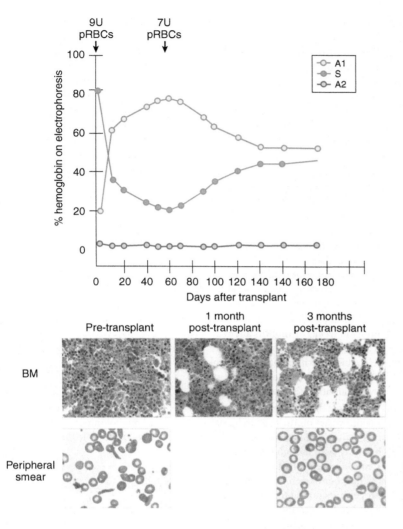

FIGURE 26-8 **Treatment of sickle cell disease with nonmyeloablative hematopoietic stem cell transplantation.** Exchange transfusions were given immediately prior to and 58 days following transplant. See text for details.

SELF-ASSESSMENT STUDY QUESTIONS

1. Current indications for infusion of hematopoietic stem cells include:
   A. Salvage from genotoxic exposures.
   B. Inherited disorders of immunity.
   C. Aggressive forms of leukemia.
   D. Aplastic anemia.
   E. All of the above.

2. Common findings in acute graft-versus-host disease include all of the following except:
   A. Rising transaminase levels.
   B. Bloody diarrhea.
   C. Scaly rash and generalized erythroderma.
   D. Pulmonary fibrosis.
   E. Sepsis.

3. Matching. Fill in the blank with A through I. Choose the *best* answer, and use each choice only once.

____ 1. Transplantation for these disorders requires full myeloablative therapy.

____ 2. No graft-versus-host disease prophylaxis is required in this setting.

____ 3. ABO mismatches in bone marrow transplantation require washing donor red cells out of the hematopoietic stem cell preparation.

____ 4. Success of hematopoietic stem cell transplantation in this setting is evidence that gene therapy delivered in the form of genetically modified autologous stem cells also can work, as tiny amounts of the missing protein are curative.

____ 5. The efficacy of donor lymphocyte infusion weeks or months after transplantation demonstrates that leukemia cell killing by an initial blast of chemotherapy is not all there is to transplantation for malignancies.

____ 6. The source of transplanted cells has a major impact on the time to hematologic reconstitution in transplant recipients because, even though hematopoietic stem cells are present in all sources, the number of stem cells and early progenitors poised to become mature blood cells is variable.

____ 7. Although transplantation is curative, with excellent long-term disease-free survival, gene therapy has not been effective for humans because of the need for high-level tissue-specific expression.

____ 8. Stem cells obtained from marrow, cord blood, or peripheral blood find their way to their proper niche within days.

____ 9. Source of "rescue" hematopoietic stem cells for patients with non-hematopoietic cancers undergoing high-dose myelotoxic chemotherapy.

A. Blood type A-negative donor into blood type O-positive recipient with a high titer of isohemagglutinins

B. Cord blood vs peripheral blood mobilized stem cells vs bone marrow

C. Sickle cell disease

D. Homing

E. Autologous transplantation

F. Paroxysmal nocturnal hemoglobinuria or chronic myelogenous leukemia.

G. Identical twin transplantation for aplastic anemia in one twin.

H. Graft vs leukemia effect

I. Severe combined immunodeficiency due to adenosine deaminase deficiency

Answers to Questions

Chapter 1
1. D   2. B   3. D

Chapter 2
1. A   2. B   3. D

Chapter 3
1. D   2. C   3. B   4. iron deficiency, thalassemia
5. cobalamin deficiency, folate deficiency, hemolysis, aplasia, myelodysplasia, alcohol abuse

Chapter 4
1. E   2. B   3. E

Chapter 5
1. B   2. C   3. A

Chapter 6
1. D   2. A   3. A

Chapter 7
1. D   2. B   3. A

Chapter 8
1. B   2. E   3. B

Chapter 9
1. A   2. E   3. D

Chapter 10
1. B   2. E   3. D

Chapter 11
1. B   2. E   3. A

Chapter 12
1. A   2. C

Chapter 13
1. E   2. B   3. E   4. B

Chapter 14
1. C   2. D   3. D   4. A   5. C

Chapter 15
1. B   2. B

Chapter 16
1. D   2. D

Chapter 17
1. C   2. A   3. A: V, B: AV, C: AV, D: V, E: A, F: AV, G: V, H: V

Chapter 18
1. F   2. D   3. B   4. D

Chapter 19
1. F   2. D   3. Ac, Ba, Cb, Df, Ee, Fd

Chapter 20
1. A   2. D   3. A. Plasma Epo level, JAK2 mutation analysis; B. arterial pO_2, imaging to search for neoplasm; 4. % marrow blasts, cytogenetic findings, platelet count

Chapter 21

1. D   2. D   3. E   4A. E   4B. B

Chapter 22

1A. sheets of mature lymphocytes; 1B. chronic lymphocytic leukemia; 1C. flow cytometry; 1D. Immune hemolysis; 1E. direct antiglobulin (Coombs) test; 1F. spherocytes appear small but they are not – a sphere is larger than a disc of the same diameter; MCV is elevated because of reticulocytosis. 1G. hemolysis results in increased catabolism of heme into bilirubin.   2. F   3. A2, B4, C3, D1, E5

Chapter 23

1. A   2. E   3. B

Chapter 24

1. A.4., B.5., C.1., D.3., E.2.   2. D,   3. D   4. C

Chapter 25

1. A   2. C   3. E

Chapter 26

1. E   2. D   3: 1F, 2G, 3A, 4I, 5H, 6B, 7C, 8D, 9E.

Additional Review Questions – Chapters 18-24

1. 1C, 2B, 3A, 4D
2. 1I, 2C, 3B, 4D, 5E, 6F, 7H, 8G, 9A
3. 1F, 2C, 3D, 4B, 5A, 6E
4. 1 B III, 2 A II, 3 C IV, 4 D I

Index

CPSIA information can be obtained
at www.ICGtesting.com
Printed in the USA

9 780071 713788